TEACHING SOCIAL and EMOTIONAL LEARNING

in Health Education

Applications in School and Community Settings

Mary Connolly, BS, MEd, CAGS, CHES

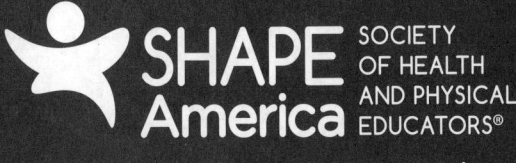

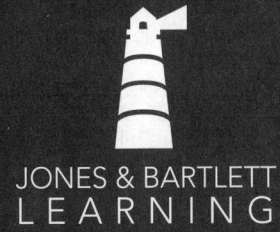

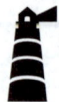

World Headquarters
Jones & Bartlett Learning
25 Mall Road, 6th Floor
Burlington, MA 01803
978-443-5000
info@jblearning.com
www.jblearning.com

Jones & Bartlett Learning books and products are available through most bookstores and online booksellers. To contact Jones & Bartlett Learning directly, call 800-832-0034, fax 978-443-8000, or visit our website, www.jblearning.com.

23238-7

Production Credits
Director of Product Management: Cathy Esperti
Product Manager: Whitney Fekete
Content Strategist: Carol Brewer Guerrero
Content Coordinator: Andrew Labelle
Project Manager: Jessica DeMartin
Project Specialist: Erin Bosco
Senior Digital Project Specialist: Angela Dooley
Director of Marketing: Andrea DeFronzo
VP, Manufacturing and Inventory Control: Therese Connell

Composition: Exela Technologies
Project Management: Exela Technologies
Cover Design: Briana Yates
Senior Media Development Editor: Troy Liston
Rights & Permissions Manager: John Rusk
Rights Specialist: Benjamin Roy
Cover Image (Title Page, Chapter Opener):
  © Omelchenko/Shutterstock, Image ID: 268664435
Printing and Binding: McNaughton & Gunn

Library of Congress Cataloging-in-Publication Data
Names: Connolly, Mary (Health education consultant), author.
Title: Teaching social and emotional learning in health education :
    applications in school and community settings / Mary Connolly.
Description: First edition. | Burlington, MA : Jones & Bartlett Learning,
    2022. | Includes bibliographical references and index.
Identifiers: LCCN 2020052696 | ISBN 9781284206586 (paperback)
Subjects: LCSH: Health education–Study and teaching–United States.
Classification: LCC RA440.3.U5 C68 2022 | DDC 613.071–dc23
LC record available at https://lccn.loc.gov/2020052696

6048

Printed in the United States of America
25 24 23 22 21   10 9 8 7 6 5 4 3 2 1

About SHAPE America

SHAPE America – Society of Health and Physical Educators serves as the voice for 200,000+ health and physical education professionals across the United States. The organization's extensive community includes a diverse membership of health and physical educators, as well as advocates, supporters, and 50+ state affiliate organizations.

© Klaus Vedfelt/DigitalVision/Getty Images

Since its founding in 1885, the organization has defined excellence in physical education. For decades, SHAPE America's National Standards for K-12 Physical Education have served as the foundation for well-designed physical education programs across the country. Additionally, the organization helped develop and owns the National Health Education Standards.

SHAPE America provides programs, resources and advocacy to support health and physical educators at every grade level as they prepare all students to lead a healthy, physically active life. The organization's newest program — health. moves. minds.® — helps teachers and schools incorporate social and emotional learning so students can thrive physically *and* emotionally.

Our Vision

A nation where all children are prepared to lead healthy, physically active lives.

Our Mission

To advance professional practice and promote research related to health and physical education, physical activity, dance and sport.

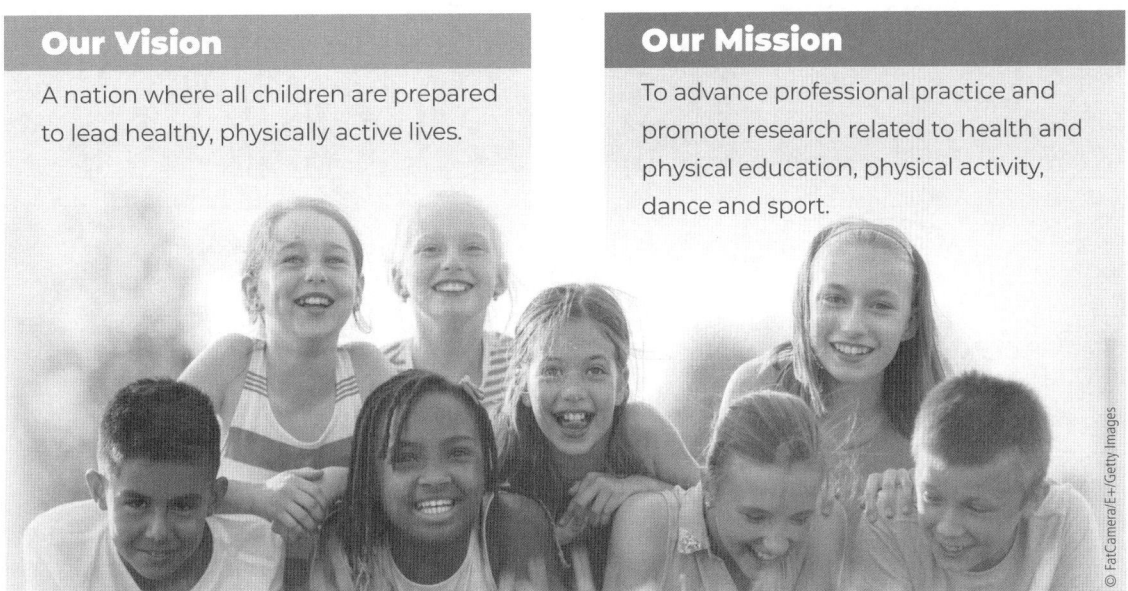

© FatCamera/E+/Getty Images

To learn more, visit
www.shapeamerica.org

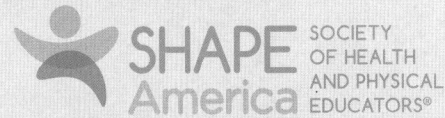

SHAPE America SOCIETY OF HEALTH AND PHYSICAL EDUCATORS®

Brief Contents

Preface   xiii
Walkthrough   xv
About the Author   xxi
Acknowledgments   xxiii

CHAPTER 1   **Introduction to Social Emotional Learning** 1

CHAPTER 2   **Pedagogical Practices** 17

CHAPTER 3   **Teaching Self-Awareness** 35

CHAPTER 4   **Teaching Self-Management** 109

CHAPTER 5   **Teaching Social Awareness** 163

CHAPTER 6   **Teaching Relationship Skills** 203

CHAPTER 7   **Teaching Responsible Decision Making** 253

Glossary   287
Index   289

Contents

Preface xiii

Walkthrough xv

About the Author xxi

Acknowledgments xxiii

CHAPTER 1 Introduction to Social Emotional Learning 1

Social Emotional Learning and The Every
    Student Succeeds Act. 1

SEL and Academic Performance 2

SEL Curriculum 2

National Health Education Standards 2

CASEL Social Emotional Learning
    Competencies 2

The Evolution of Social Emotional Learning . . . 9

    Collaborative for Academic and Social
        Emotional Learning 9

    The Wallace Foundation 10

        Cognitive Regulation *11*

        Emotional Processes *11*

        Social and Interpersonal Skills *12*

        Character *13*

        Mindset *13*

    The Yale Center for Emotional Intelligence—
        RULER Model 13

Whole School, Whole Community, Whole
    Child Connection to Social Emotional
    Learning 13

    Collaboration 13

Chapter Review Questions 15

References 15

CHAPTER 2 Pedagogical Practices 17

Developmental Considerations. 17

Understanding by Design Meets
    Neuroscience and Skills-based Health/
    Social Emotional Learning. 19

Assessment 21

    Formative Assessment 22

        Formative Assessment Tools *23*

    Summative Assessment 23

        Performance Task *26*

Using the Backwards Design to Plan
    Assessment and Instruction 27

    The Steps of Backwards Design 27

        Step 1: Data Analysis. *27*

        Step 2: Standards/SEL Selection *28*

        Step 3: Assessment *28*

        Step 4: Instruction *28*

    Backwards Design Example 29

        Step 1: Data Analysis. *29*

        Step 2: Standards Selection *29*

        Steps 3 and 4: Assessment and Instruction
            for Standard 1 . . . . *30*

        Steps 3 and 4: Assessment and Instruction
            for Standard 7 . . . . *30*

Delivery of Skills-Based Health/SEL 30

    Effective SBH/SEL Teaching Strategies 31

        Skill Practice *31*

        Role Play *31*

        Discussion *31*

        Book/Story *31*

        Teaching Skills *31*

        Vocabulary. *32*

        SBH/SEL Tools and Handouts *32*

        Writing *32*

        Drawing. *32*

        Art/Creative Project. *32*

        Visual Display *32*

        Video *32*

        Song. *32*

        Game. *33*

References 33

CHAPTER 3 Teaching Self-Awareness 35

Social and Emotional Learning (SEL)
    Competencies 35

Introduction 35

Preview 38

   Unit Plan 38

   Skills-Based Lesson Plan 39

   Skills-Based Lesson Infrastructure 39

   Organization 39

Section 1. Recognizing Emotions,
Thoughts, and Values and How They
Influence Behavior 39

   Recognizing/Identifying Emotions 39

      PreK–2: Self-Awareness: Identifying Emotions 40

      Step 3 – Instruction 40

      Grades 3–5: Self-Awareness: Identifying Emotions 41

      Step 3 – Instruction 43

      Grades 6–8: Self-Awareness: Identifying Emotions 45

      Step 3 – Instruction 46

      Grades 9–12: Self-Awareness: Identifying Emotions 48

      Step 3 – Instruction 50

Section 2. Accurately Assessing One's
Interests, Strengths and Limitations,
and Possessing a Well-grounded Sense
of Self-efficacy and Optimism and a
"Growth Mindset." 55

   Accurate Self-Perception/Recognizing Strengths . . . 55

      *PreK–2: Self-Awareness: Accurate Self-perception/
      Recognizing Strengths* 55

      Step 3 – Instruction 56

      *Grades 3–5: Self-Awareness: Accurate Self-Perception/
      Recognizing Strengths* 58

      Step 3 – Instruction 58

      *Grades 6–8: Self-awareness: Accurate self-perception/
      recognizing strengths* 60

      Step 3 – Instruction 61

      *Grades 9–12: Self-Awareness: Accurate Self-Perception/
      Recognizing Strengths* 62

      Step 3 – Instruction 63

   Self-Confidence/Recognizing Strengths 65

      *PreK–2 Lesson: Self-Awareness: Self-Confidence/
      Recognizing Strengths* 65

      Step 3 – Instruction 66

      *Grades 3–5: Self-Awareness: Self-Confidence/
      Recognizing Strengths* 69

      Step 3 – Instruction 69

      *Grades 6–8: Self-Awareness: Self-confidence/
      Recognizing Strengths* 71

      Step 3 – Instruction 71

      *Grades 9–12: Self-Awareness: Self-confidence/
      Recognizing Strengths* 72

      Step 3 – Instruction 74

   Self-Efficacy 76

      PreK–2: Self-Awareness: Self-Efficacy 77

      Step 3 – Instruction 77

      Grades 3–5: Self-Awareness: Self-Efficacy 78

      Step 3 – Instruction 79

      Grades 6–8: Self-Awareness: Self-Efficacy 80

      Step 3 – Instruction 82

      Grades 9–12: Self-Awareness: Self-Efficacy 84

      Step 3 – Instruction 85

Growth Mindset 86

   Importance of Feedback in Helping Students
   Develop a Growth Mindset 87

      *What Is the Relationship between Self-Confidence,
      Self-Efficacy, and Growth Mindset?* 88

      PreK–2: Self-Awareness: Growth Mindset 89

      Step 3 – Instruction 89

      Grades 3–5: Self-Awareness: Growth Mindset 91

      Step 3 – Instruction 92

      Grades 6–8: Self-Awareness: Growth Mindset 93

      Step 3 – Instruction 95

      Grades 9–12: Self-Awareness: Growth Mindset 97

      Step 3 – Instruction 97

Sample Lesson Plan for Analyzing
Influences/Self-Awareness 101

References 104

Chapter 3—Appendix A 106

   Self-Awareness: Scope, Sequence, Content,
   SEL–Competency/Subcompetencies 106

**CHAPTER 4 Teaching
Self-Management 109**

Social and Emotional Learning (SEL)
Competencies 109

Introduction 109

Preview 112

   Skills-Based Unit 112

   Skills-Based Lessons 112

   Organization 113

Section 1. Regulating One's Emotions,
Cognitions, and Behaviors 113

   Impulse Control, Self-Discipline,
   Self-Motivation 113

      *PreK–2: Self-Management: Impulse Control,
      Self-Discipline, Self-Motivation* 113

      Step 3 – Instruction 114

      *Grades 3–5: Self-Management: Impulse Control,
      Self-Discipline, and Self-Motivation* 117

      Step 3 – Instruction 118

      *Grades 6-8: Self-Management: Impulse Control,
      Self-Discipline, Self-Motivation* 119

      Step 3 – Instruction 121

      *Grades 9–12: Self-Management: Impulse Control,
      Self-Discipline, Self-Motivation* 123

      Step 3 – Instruction 124

   Self-Management: Stress Management 125

      PreK-2 125

      Step 3 – Instruction 127

      Grades 3–5: Self-Management: Stress Management 129

Step 3 – Instruction *130*

Grades 6–8: Self-Management: Stress Management *133*

Step 3 – Instruction *134*

Grades 9–12: Self-Management: Stress Management *137*

Step 3 – Instruction *138*

Section 2. Setting and Achieving Personal and Educational Goals/Organizational Skills **141**

PreK–2 Self-Management: Goal Setting 142

Lesson Overview: Goal Setting to Eat Healthy and Increase Physical Activity *142*

Step 3 – Instruction *143*

Grades 3–5: Self-Management: Goal Setting 145

Lesson Overview: Goal Setting to Use MyPlate to Eat Healthy *145*

Step 3 – Instruction *146*

Grades 6–8: Self-Management: Goal Setting 148

Lesson Overview: Goal Setting to Eat Breakfast *148*

Step 3 – Instruction *149*

Grades 9–12: Self-Management: Goal Setting . . . 152

Lesson Overview: Goal Setting to Be with Friends and Not Drink *152*

Step 3 – Instruction *152*

Sample Lesson Plan for Self-Management: Using Yoga and Belly Breathing to Reduce Stress **154**

References **158**

Chapter 4—Appendix A **160**

Self-Management: Scope, Sequence, Content, SEL–Competency/Subcompetencies 160

CHAPTER 5 Teaching Social Awareness 163

Social and Emotional Learning (SEL) Competencies 163

Introduction 163

Preview 165

Unit Plan 165

Skills-Based Lesson Plan 165

Skills-Based Lesson Infrastructure 166

Organization 166

Section 1. Taking the Perspective of and Empathizing with Others, Respecting Others and, Recognizing Community Resources 166

Taking Perspective of and Empathizing with Others, Respecting Others, and Recognizing Community Resources 167

PreK–2: Social-Awareness: Perspective Taking, Empathy, and Community Resources 167

Lesson Overview: Empathy for a Friend and Accessing Community Resources *167*

Step 3 – Instruction *168*

Grades 3–5: Social-Awareness: Perspective-Taking, Empathy, and Community Resources 169

Lesson Overview: Coping with Bullying by Taking Perspective, Being Empathetic, and Accessing Community Resources *169*

Step 3 – Instruction *171*

Grades 6–8: Social-Awareness: Perspective-Taking, Empathy, and Community Resources 173

Lesson Overview: Taking Perspective, Empathizing with, and Recognizing Community Resources for LGBTQ (Lesbian, Gay, Bisexual, Transsexual, and Queer/Questioning) Middle School Students *173*

Step 3 – Instruction *174*

Grades 9–12: Social-Awareness: Perspective Taking, Empathy, and Community Resources 176

Lesson Overview: Physical Activity *176*

Step 3 – Instruction *177*

Section 2. Appreciating Diversity/Respecting Others/Persevering in Addressing Challenges 180

Grades PreK–2: Social-Awareness: Appreciating Diversity/Respecting Others/Persevering in Addressing Challenges 180

Lesson Overview: Respecting Differences *180*

Step 3 – Instruction *180*

Grades 3–5: Social-Awareness: Appreciating Diversity/Respecting Others/Persevering in Addressing Challenges 183

Lesson Overview: Accepting Differences *183*

Step 3 – Instruction *184*

Grades 6–8: Social-Awareness: Appreciating Diversity/Respecting Others/Persevering in Addressing Challenges 187

Lesson Overview: Accepting Differences *187*

Step 3 – Instruction *187*

Grades 9–12: Social-awareness: Appreciating Diversity/Respecting Others/Persevering in Addressing Challenges 191

Lesson Overview: Appreciating Diversity *191*

Step 3 – Instruction *192*

Sample Lesson Plan for Social Awareness . . . 196

References 199

Chapter 5—Appendix A 201

Social Awareness: Scope, Sequence, Content, SEL Competency/Subcompetencies 201

CHAPTER 6 Teaching Relationship Skills 203

Social and Emotional Learning (SEL) Competencies 203

Introduction 203

Preview 204

    Unit Plan 204

    Skills-based Lesson Plan 204

    Skills-based Lesson Infrastructure 205

    Organization 206

Section 1. Establishing and Maintaining
Healthy and Rewarding Relationships/
Communicating Clearly 206

    PreK–2: Relationship Skills: Establishing and
    Maintaining Healthy and Rewarding
    Relationships/Communicating Clearly 207

      Lesson Overview: Expressing Appreciation
      and Respect—Friendship 207

      Step 3 – Instruction 208

    Grades 3–5: Relationship Skills: Establishing
    and Maintaining Healthy and Rewarding
    Relationships/Communication 209

      Lesson Overview: Coping with Grief 209

      Step 3 – Instruction 211

    Grades 6–8: Relationship Skills: Establishing
    and Maintaining Healthy and Rewarding
    Relationships/Communication 212

      Lesson Overview: Conversation Skills—Choosing
      Friends 213

      Step 3 – Instruction 214

    Grades 9–12: Relationship skills: Establishing
    and Maintaining Healthy and Rewarding
    Relationships/Communication–Advocacy 216

      Lesson Overview: Value of Face-to-Face Conversation
      with a Friend Rather than Texting 217

      Step 3 – Instruction 217

Section 2. Negotiating Conflict
Constructively/Seeking and Offering
Help When Needed 219

    Grades PreK–2: Relationship Skills: Negotiating
    Conflict Constructively/Seeking and
    Offering Help When Needed 220

      Lesson Overview: Resolving Conflict—Friendships . . 220

      Step 3 – Instruction 220

    Grades 3–5: Relationship Skills: Negotiating
    Conflict Constructively/Seeking and
    Offering Help When Needed 222

      Lesson Overview: Resolving Conflict—Friendships . . 222

      Step 3 – Instruction 223

    Grades 6–8: Relationship Skills: Negotiating
    Conflict Constructively/Seeking and
    Offering Help When Needed 225

      Lesson Overview: Resolving Conflict: Friendships . . 225

      Step 3 – Instruction 226

    Grades 9–12: Relationship skills: Negotiating
    Conflict Constructively/Seeking and
    Offering Help When Needed 228

      Lesson Overview: Resolving Conflict in a Dating
      Relationship 228

      Step 3 – Instruction 229

Section 3. Resisting Inappropriate Social
Pressure/Seeking and Offering Help
When Needed 231

    Grades PreK–2: Relationship Skills: Resisting
    Inappropriate Social Pressure/Seeking and
    Offering Help When Needed 231

      Lesson Overview: Preventing Injuries on the
      Playground 232

      Step 3 – Instruction 232

    Grades 3–5: Relationship Skills: Resisting
    Inappropriate Social Pressure/Seeking
    and Offering Help When Needed 235

      Lesson Overview: Using Refusal Skills to Reject
      Being Pressured to Be a Bully 235

      Step 3 – Instruction 235

    Grades 6–8: Relationship Skills: Resisting
    Inappropriate Social Pressure/Seeking
    and Offering Help When Needed 237

      Lesson Overview: Using Refusal Skills to Avoid the
      Risks of Being Pressured to Smoke Marijuana . . . 238

      Step 3 – Instruction 238

    Grades 9–12: Relationship Skills: Resisting
    Inappropriate Social Pressure/Seeking
    and Offering Help When Needed 240

      Lesson Overview: Using Refusal Skills
      to Avoid the Risks of Driving with a Newly
      Licensed Driver 240

      Step 3 – Instruction 241

Sample Lesson Plan for Relationship
Skills 243

References 247

Chapter 6—Appendix A 249

    Relationship Skills: Scope, Sequence, Content,
    SEL Competency/Subcompetencies 249

CHAPTER 7 Teaching Responsible Decision Making . . . 253

Social and Emotional Learning (SEL)
Competencies 253

Introduction 253

Preview 258

    Unit Plan 258

    Skills-Based Lesson Plan 258

    Skills-Based Lesson Infrastructure 258

    Organization 258

Making Constructive Choices 259

    PreK–2 Making Constructive Choices 259

      Lesson Overview: Taking Medicine Safely 259

      Step 3 – Instruction 260

    Grades 3–5: Responsible Decision Making 262

      Lesson Overview: Making Responsible Decisions
      about Getting Together with Friends 263

      Step 3 – Instruction 263

Grades 6–8: Responsible Decision Making 267
    Lesson Overview: Alcohol. 267
    Step 3 – Instruction 268
Grades 9–12: Responsible Decision Making 271
    Lesson Overview: Distracted Driving 271
    Step 3 – Instruction 272
Sample Lesson Plan for Responsible
Decision Making 275

References 281
Chapter 7—Appendix A 283
    Responsible Decision Making: Scope, Sequence,
    Content, SEL Competency/Subcompetencies . . . 283

Glossary. **287**
Index **289**

Preface

Social emotional learning (SEL) has become a national movement in our schools. The Collaborative for Academic, Social, and Emotional Learning (CASEL); Transforming Education; The Wallace Foundation; Yale Center for Emotional Intelligence; ASCD; and the Centers for Disease Control and Prevention (CDC) are some of the many leaders in the field.

Often, the implementation plan includes integration into all subject areas. This plan effectively institutionalizes SEL into PreK–12 education but there is an additional strategy that utilizes the expertise of trained, licensed, skills-based health/SEL educators.

Skills-based health education, predicated on the National Health Education Standards, is aligned with the CASEL competencies and consequently, a PreK–12 skills-based health educator is already teaching SEL!

National Health Education Standards	CASEL Competencies
Standard 1—Content	All competencies
Standard 2—Analyzing Influences	Self-Awareness
Standard 3—Accessing Valid Information, Products, Services	Social-Awareness
Standard 4—Interpersonal Communication	Relationship Skills
Standard 5—Decision Making	Responsible Decision Making
Standard 6—Goal Setting	Self-Management
Standard 7—Practicing Healthy Behaviors	Self-Management
Standard 8—Advocacy	Relationship Skills

This text provides health educators with the foundational and pedagogical expertise to specifically teach SEL in their skills-based classroom. Grade span examples provide data rationale for inclusion, the infused performance indicators to reduce the risk factor, and the backwards design of planning assessment and instruction.

Each chapter is organized around the CASEL competency description and is therefore divided into sections. Each contains PreK–2, Grades 3–5, Grades 6–8, and Grades 9–12 infrastructure for a skills-based health/SEL lesson or foundation for a unit.

Each grade span explains and demonstrates how to teach the infused performance indicator. Often, the SEL competency is taught within the content and skill portion of the sample. Student practice is facilitated with interactive worksheets available digitally.

Skillful teachers use the chapter information as a foundation for teaching or to spawn a different idea that works better for their students.

The "secret sauce" is the practice prompt. Here, the grade span example weaves together a story that includes the Standard 1 content, skill, and SEL competency followed by questions that help the students clarify and reinforce information and practice the skill.

For the experienced skills-based health educator, this text will help teach SEL *deliberately* as part of a well-coordinated PreK–12 approved curriculum. Use the resources from CASEL and other organizations to supplement your program. Display the CASEL competencies and make sure students, administrators, and parents know you are teaching SEL as part of your comprehensive program.

Involve the Wellness Team in your Skills-Based health/SEL efforts. SEL is a component of the CDC/ASCD model along with health education and it provides an infrastructure to address whole child issues comprehensively.

It is not easy to change the paradigm, but you are already teaching SEL if you are teaching skills-based health education. Take a leadership role and use your advocacy skills to inform stakeholders of your pedagogical practice.

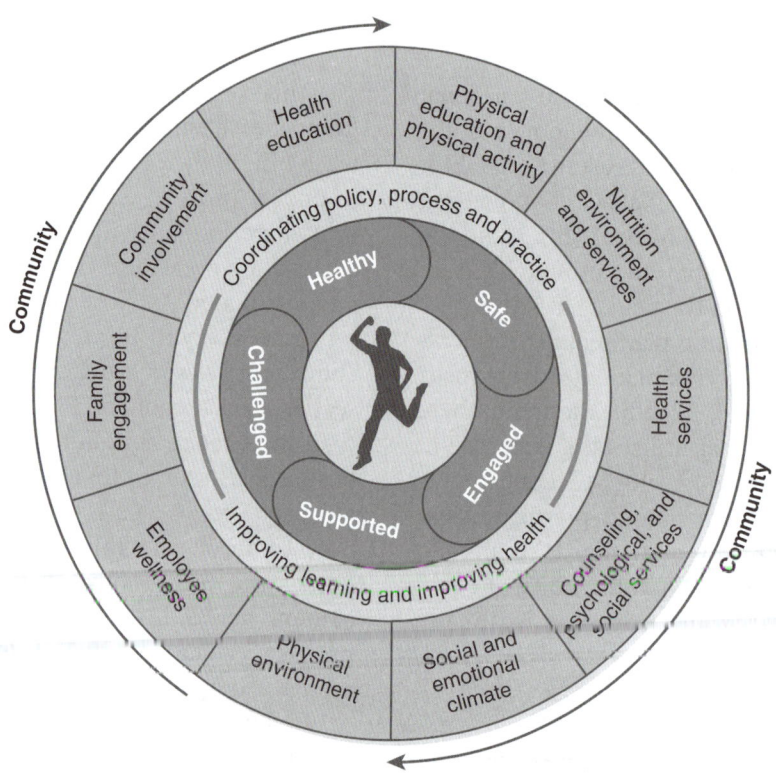

Centers for Disease Control and Prevention, CDC Healthy Schools. (2020, February 27). Whole School, Whole Community, Whole Child (WSCC). Retrieved from Centers for Disease Control and Prevention, CDC Healthy Schools: https:// www.cdc.gov/healthyschools/wscc /index.htm

Walkthrough

Teaching Social and Emotional Learning in Health Education: Applications in School and Community Settings provides the tools that instructors need to successfully incorporate social and emotional learning into the classroom.

The text aligns social and emotional learning to standards-based health education, heavily referencing the National Health Education Standards and the Collaborative for Academic and Social and Emotional Learning (CASEL) competencies.

Chapter Overview

Each CASEL competency has a chapter dedicated to it, and is divided into sections according to grade level groupings: PreK–2, Grades 3–5, Grades 6–8, and Grades 9–12. For each grade span, the infrastructure for a skills-based health/SEL lesson or foundation for a unit is provided.

Grades 6–8: Relationship Skills: Negotiating Conflict Constructively/Seeking and Offering Help When Needed

Between 38.6% and 47.2% of middle school teens report ever being in a physical fight. (Centers for Disease Control and Prevention, 2020)

Middle school teens need to understand that conflict is a natural and important part of our social life. In order to resolve conflict, teens must learn and practice the skill of conflict resolution. Once learned, practiced, and integral to how teens relate to one another, a teen may gain self-confidence and experience improved relationships.

Lesson Overview: Resolving Conflict: Friendships

Students examine the benefits of and barriers to maintaining a healthy relationship and demonstrate their conflict resolutions skills.

Resources:

- Michigan Model for Health

Materials needed:

- Sticky notes
- **Worksheet 6.10 Benefits of and Barriers to Maintaining a Healthy Relationship**
- **Worksheet 6.11 Resolving Conflict**

Table 6.15 provides an overview of the lesson objectives, assessment, and instruction for this lesson.

Table 6.15 Lesson Objectives, Assessment, and Instruction

Step 1 – Lesson Objectives	Step 2 – Assessment
The verb of the *infused* performance indicator and the SEL competency generate the assessment and instruction.	Design the assessment based on the objectives. Ask yourself the question, "What can my students do to show me they have met the standard?"
1.8.7 <u>Describe</u> the benefits of and barriers to practicing healthy behaviors *such as maintaining a healthy relationship.* (Joint Committee on National Health Education Standards, 2007, p. 24)	1.8.7 Student <u>describes</u> the three benefits of and three barriers to practicing healthy behaviors *such as maintaining a healthy relationship.*
4.8.3 <u>Demonstrate</u> effective conflict management or resolution strategies *with peers.* (Joint Committee on National Health Education Standards, 2007, p. 30)	4.8.3 Student <u>demonstrates</u> how to resolve conflict with a peer.
SEL–Relationship skills: Communication, social engagement, relationship building, teamwork	Students <u>demonstrate</u> how to negotiate conflict constructively and seek or offer help when needed.
Step 3 – Instruction	
Design the instruction so that students learn the content, skill, and competency to be successful on the assessment. Ask yourself the question, "What do I need to teach so that the students will be successful when assessed?"	

© Dmelchenko/Shutterstock

Detailed instruction outlines are provided for each grade span, explaining how to teach the infused performance indicator.

Step 3 – Instruction

1. Define
   a. Describe: To use words that help others envision the physical attributes of a person, place, or thing.
   b. Demonstrate: To show how something is accomplished.
   c. Healthy relationship: A relationship that includes honesty, good listening skills, able to trust one another, and mutual respect. (Office on Women's Health, Office of the Assistant Secretary for Health, Human Services, 2015)
2. 1.8.7 Describe the benefits of and barriers to practicing healthy behaviors *such as maintaining a healthy relationship*
   a. Ask the students to define "healthy relationship." Agree on the definition. Use the definition above as a guide.
   b. Ask the students to write down on a sticky note or on the board, the characteristics (benefits of) of a healthy relationship. Students place their comments on the board. As they are posted, place similar responses together to determine which characteristics are the most common.
   c. Once the benefits of a healthy relationship are established and discussed, distribute **Worksheet 6.10 Benefits of and Barriers to Maintaining a Healthy Relationship** to explore the barriers to establishing or maintaining a healthy relationship.
   d. Benefits of maintaining a healthy relationship
      1) **Talk Honestly:** Able to talk honestly; share thoughts, feelings, and experiences. Each respects the privacy of the other. Able to talk through conflicts.
      2) **Good Listener:** Able to express care for what the other person is saying. Look at the other person and minimize distractions. If you don't agree, acknowledge you see the other person's point of view. (perspective taking)
      3) **Trust and Respect:** Each feels valued for who they are, not because of superficial things like clothes, phones, computers, other belongings.
3. 4.8.3 Demonstrate effective conflict management or resolution strategies *with peers*.
   a. Brainstorm common conflicts experienced between peers and place them on the board.
   b. Use **Worksheet 6.11 Resolving Conflict** to review the steps of conflict resolution and model one of the student conflict examples. Provide time for the students to select another example and resolve on their own. Ask for volunteers to role play the scenario, demonstrating how the conflict was resolved.
   c. Conflict resolution skills
      1) Take some time to calm down. Try belly breaths.
      2) Put yourself in the other person's shoes to better understand why they are upset.

Student practice is facilitated with interactive worksheets available digitally in the eBook, and to instructors.

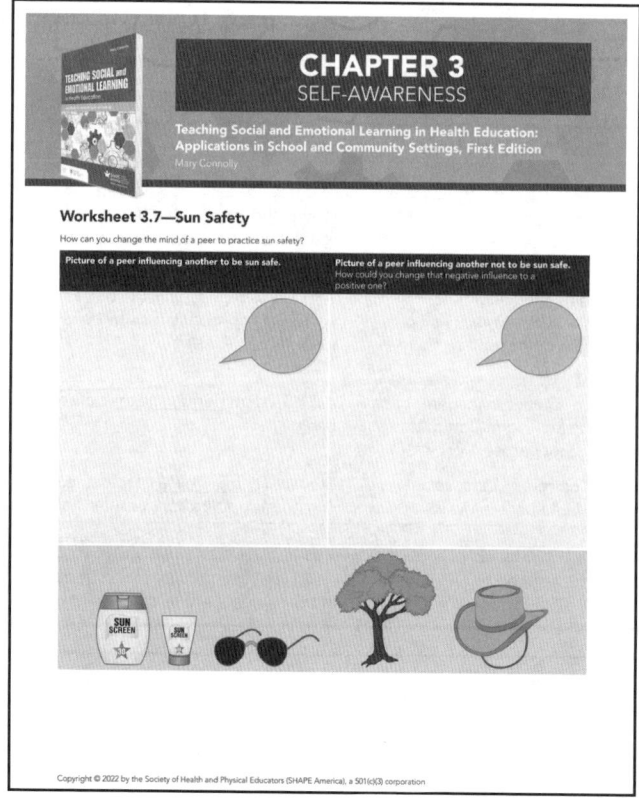

Practice Prompts present scenarios that cover the Standard content, skill, and SEL competency, and present questions to clarify and reinforce information and practice the skill.

4. Read the practice prompt. Students answer the reflection questions and discuss.

Practice Prompt: Jackson

Jackson and Philip have been friends for a long time. Jackson loves skateboarding and has given Philip his old skateboard and helmet so they could go to the park together. Jackson taught Philip how to navigate the ramps at the skatepark and he is getting pretty good.

Now that they are in middle school, Philip is interested in playing for the school soccer team. He tried out and made it! Lately, he is spending more time with his soccer teammates than with Jackson and Jackson is not happy. He thought they would always be friends.

One day, Jackson said, "Hey, since we are not hanging out anymore, I want my old skateboard and helmet back." "Why? asked Philip. "We can still go to the park."

"When you spend all your time with your new soccer teammates, I feel that we are not friends anymore" said Jackson. Philip looked at Jackson while he was talking and listened carefully. He couldn't believe what he was hearing. To calm down, he took a couple of deep breaths before he spoke.

"Wait a minute, Jackson," Philip said. "I am just excited I made the team. I don't want to disappoint anyone so I practice a lot with the team. It doesn't mean I don't want to be your friend or skateboard with you anymore! I love going to the park and working out with you!" Philip said.

"Well, OK, you can keep the skateboard. Let's figure out how to make sure you have the time you need for soccer and still find the time to go boarding," said Jackson.

"I have an idea," Philip said, "Let's set time aside each week to go to the park." "That is a good idea, but the weekends don't always work for me. How about we wait to go boarding until the soccer season is over?" "Or, the days I don't have soccer practice, we go to the park?" said Philip. "I like that idea," said Jackson.

"I like working with the team, but I also like solo sports. The team is very competitive and with Boarding, I compete against myself" said Philip. "That's not entirely true," said Jackson. "You are pretty competitive with me, but you will need more practice to keep up!"

The boys laughed and walked to the bus together. Both felt great that they resolved the problem. They value their friendship and are glad they got through that problem.

Table 6.16 Identifying How Resolving Conflict Affects Personal Health

Question	Answer
What were three benefits of and three barriers to practicing healthy behaviors *such as maintaining a healthy relationship when there is a conflict?* (1.8.7)	Benefits of maintaining a healthy relationship when there is a conflict. ■ **Talk Honestly:** The boys talked honestly share thoughts, feelings, and experiences. They talked through conflicts. ■ **Good Listener:** Each boy expressed care for what the other one was saying. Look at the other person and minimize distractions. ■ **Trust and Respect:** Each boy felt valued for who they were, not for superficial reasons. Barriers to maintaining a healthy relationship when there is a conflict. ■ It was difficult for Jackson to confront Philip because he was angry and hurt. ■ It was difficult, at first, for Philip to understand why Jackson did not want to be his friend anymore. ■ It was challenging for the boys to find a way to spend time boarding because Philip made a commitment to the soccer team and that took a lot of his time.

How did Jackson and Philip resolve their conflict? (4.8.3)	1. Calm down
	  • Philip took some deep breaths before he spoke to calm down.
	2. Put yourself in the other person's shoes to better understand why they are upset.
	  • Philip told Jackson that just because he made the soccer team, it didn't mean he didn't want to be his friend.
	3. Explain how you feel using "I" messages.
	  • Jackson: "When you spend all your time with your new soccer teammates, I feel that we are not friends anymore."
	  • Philip: "I am just excited I made the team. I don't want to disappoint anyone so I practice a lot with the team. It doesn't mean I don't want to be your friend or skateboard with you anymore!"

Resources

- **eBook**
- **Slides in PowerPoint format**
- **Worksheets**
  - Presented in the eBook
  - Also provided digitally for instructor use
- **Sample Lesson Plans**
  - Presented at the end of each chapter
  - Also provided digitally for instructor use
- **Scope and Sequence documents**
  - Presented as chapter appendices
  - Also provided digitally for instructor use

Sample Lesson Plan for Relationship Skills

Unit: *State the unit of the lesson.*	Interpersonal Communication
Topic: *State the topic of the lesson.*	Relationship skills: Negotiating conflict constructively/seeking and offering help when needed
Grade level: *State the grade level of the lesson.*	Grades 3–5
Time allotment: *State the time allotted for the lesson.*	40 minutes
Lesson summary: *Provide a summary of the lesson.*	Students learn to resolve conflict and consequently improve friendships and personal social-emotional health.
Risk behavior data: *Provide time rationale for this lesson by accessing the risk behavior the lesson reduces.*	N/A
Standards and SEL Competency to reduce the risk factor(s): *List the Standard 1 and skills standards and the SEL competency/ subcompetency.*	1.5.1 <u>Describe</u> the relationship between healthy behaviors and personal health. 4.5.3 <u>Demonstrate</u> nonviolent strategies to manage or resolve conflict. SEL–Relationship skills: Communication, social engagement, relationship building, teamwork
Objectives: *The objectives are the infused performance indicators and SEL competency.*	1.5.1 <u>Describe</u> the relationship between healthy behaviors *such as using a skill to resolve conflict* and personal health. 4.5.3 <u>Demonstrate</u> nonviolent strategies to manage or resolve conflict *with a peer.* SEL–Relationship skills: Communication, social engagement, relationship building, teamwork
Lesson assessment: *Design an assessment for each infused performance indicator and SEL competency.*	1.5.1 Student <u>describes</u> *three* relationships between having the skill to resolve conflict and personal health. 4.5.3 Student <u>demonstrates</u> how to resolve conflict with a peer. SEL–Relationship skills: Communication, social engagement, relationship building, teamwork Student <u>demonstrates</u> how to negotiate conflict with a peer.
Lesson instruction: *Provide a detailed description of how content, skill, and SEL competency are taught, "bell to bell."*	Review/Preview Ask the students how they observe their peers resolving conflict. Is the strategy a healthy or unhealthy strategy? Why? What are some nonviolent ways to resolve conflict? Is that strategy healthy or unhealthy? Why? Lesson Objectives Students describe the relationship between using skills to resolve a conflict and personal health and how to use nonviolent strategies to resolve conflict. Define lesson vocabulary, if necessary.

	Lesson
	
	 1. 1.5.1 <u>Describe</u> the relationship between healthy behaviors *such as using a skill to resolve conflict* and personal health.
	   a. Place the following statements around the room and cover them. Read the prompt. Uncover and discuss how the boys in the story accomplished each of the criteria below by resolving their conflict.
	     1) Children improve their ability to get along with others. (social health)
	     2) Children are happier knowing they have the skill to resolve conflict. (emotional health)
	     3) Children have better friendships (social health)
	     4) Children learn better. (intellectual health) (KidsMatter, Learning to Resolve Conflict, 2011)
	   b. **Prompt**: Jay was using the computer but had to be excused to go to the bathroom. When he returned, Jondo was using his computer. "Hey, get up! I was using that computer," said Jay. "I didn't know you were using it, there was no one sitting here a few minutes ago," said Jondo. "That's because I had to go to the bathroom. Get up! I am working on my science assignment and I need to finish," said Jay. Mrs. Solveitall heard the boys arguing and asked, "What is the matter?" Jay explained that he was using the computer but had to get up to go to the bathroom and when he returned, Jondo was using his computer. "I didn't know Jondo was using the computer, Mrs. Solveitall, the screen was off, and the seat was empty, so I sat down and began my work," said Jondo

Chapter 6—Appendix A
Relationship Skills: Scope, Sequence, Content, SEL Competency/Subcompetencies

Note: This page is organized by grade span, Standard 1, skill standards, the HECAT content areas, and SEL Competency/subcompetencies.

The HECAT content areas include: AOD – Alcohol and Other Drugs; HE – Healthy Eating; MEH – Mental/Emotional Health; PHW – Personal Health and Wellness; PA – Physical Activity; S – Safety; SH – Sexual Health; T – Tobacco; V – Violence Prevention

Establishing and Maintaining Healthy and Rewarding Relationships/Communicating Clearly

Grade Span	Standard 1	Skill	HECAT Content Areas and Specific Content	SEL Competency and Subcompetencies
PreK–2	1.2.1 Identify that healthy behaviors, *such as expressing appreciation and demonstrating respect,* affect personal health.	4.2.1 Demonstrate one healthy way to express needs, wants, and feelings by using "i" messages.	Mental/Emotional health- expressing appreciation and respect — Friendship	Relationship skills: Communication
3-5	1.5.2 Identify examples of emotional, intellectual, physical, and social health *that occur when experiencing a loss.*	4.5.1 Demonstrate effective verbal and nonverbal communication skills to enhance *the* health *of a friend experiencing a loss.*	Mental/Emotional health — Coping with grief.	Relationship skills: Communication, social engagement, relationship building, teamwork
6-8	1.8.2. Describe the interrelationships of emotional, intellectual, physical, and social health in adolescence *when communicating about whether or not to make a friend.*	4.8.1. Apply effective verbal and nonverbal communication skills to enhance health *when discussing positive and negative friendships.*	Mental/Emotional health: Conversation skills-choosing friends	Relationship skills: Communication, social engagement, relationship building, teamwork
9–12	1.12.7 Compare and contrast the benefits of and barriers to practicing a variety of healthy behaviors *such as talking face to face rather than by texting.*	8.12.4. Adapt health messages and communication techniques *about the value of person-to-person communication rather than texting* to a specific target audience.	Mental/Emotional health: value of face-to-face conversation with a friend rather than texting.	Relationship skills: Communication, social engagement, relationship building, teamwork

Negotiating Conflict Constructively/Seeking and Offering Help When Needed

Grade Span	Standard 1	Skill	HECAT Content Areas and Specific Content	SEL Competency and Subcompetencies
PreK–2	1.2 1 Identify that healthy behaviors, *such as being able to resolve conflict,* affect their personal *social/emotional* health	4.2.1 Demonstrate healthy ways to express needs, wants, and feelings *when experiencing a conflict with a peer.* 4.2.4 Demonstrate ways to tell a trusted adult if threatened or harmed.	Mental/Emotional Health-Resolving conflict. — Friendships	Relationship skills: Communication, social engagement, relationship building, teamwork
3–5	1.5.1 Describe the relationship between healthy behaviors *such as using a skill to resolve conflict* and personal health.	4.5.3 Demonstrate nonviolent strategies to manage or resolve conflict *with a peer.*	Mental/Emotional Health-Resolving conflict.— Friendships	Relationship skills: Communication, social engagement, relationship building, teamwork
6–8	1.8.7 Describe the benefits of and barriers to practicing healthy behaviors *such as maintaining a healthy relationship.*	4.8.3 Demonstrate effective conflict management or resolution strategies *with peers.*	Mental/Emotional Health-Resolving conflict.— Friendships	Relationship skills: Communication, social engagement, relationship building, teamwork
9–12	1.12.1 Predict how a *healthy dating relationship* affects health status.	4.12.3 Demonstrate strategies to prevent, manage, or resolve interpersonal *dating* conflicts without harming self or others.	Mental/Emotional Health-Resolving conflict—Resolving conflict in a dating relationship.	Relationship skills: Communication, social engagement, relationship building, teamwork

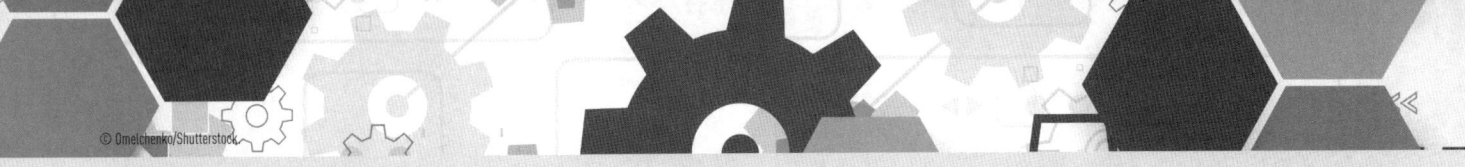
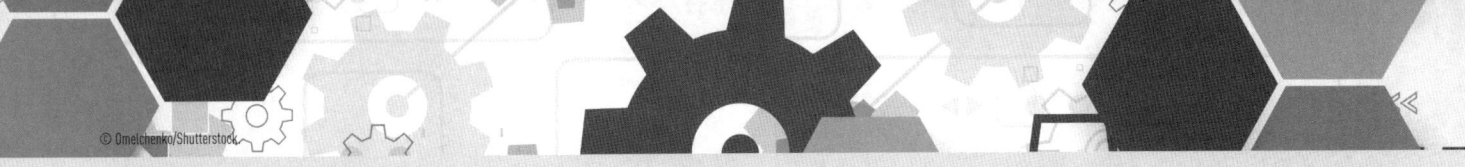

About the Author

Mary Connolly, BS, MEd, CAGS, CHES is the Program Chair of the Skills-Based Health/Social Emotional program at Cambridge College, Boston, Massachusetts, where she is responsible for delivering quality programs for students seeking a Master of Education Degree, a certificate for School and Community, and online health and physical education certificates.

She is also a health education consultant and has helped many Massachusetts districts transform their curriculum from content based to skills based.

Mary is the author of *Skills-Based Health Education*, first and second editions, published by Jones & Bartlett Learning. The texts are used to train pre-service and in-service professionals how to teach skills-based health/SEL.

Mary presents at the annual MAHPERD and SHAPE America conferences and has designed and presented several SHAPE America skills-based health education webinars. She served as the Chair of the SHAPE America Task Force on Social Emotional Learning and is a member of the SHAPE Health Education Council.

In 2020, Mary received the Joseph McKenney Award, the highest award bestowed by the Massachusetts Association of Health, Physical Education, Recreation and Dance, given to one individual each year for their distinguished service. Also in 2020, she received the SHAPE America Hall of Fame Award, given to an individual who has made educational contributions of significance and service to the profession at the national, regional, or local level.

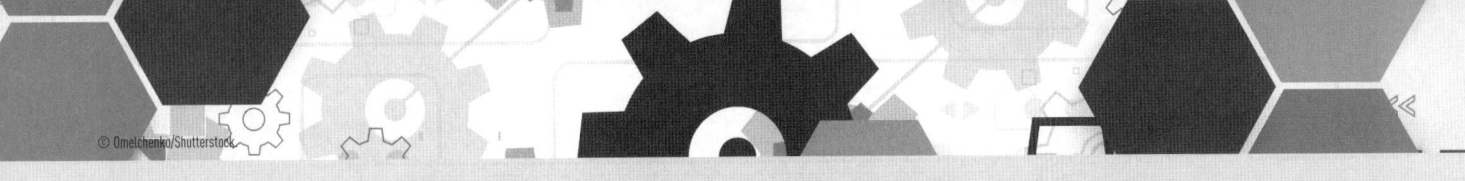

Acknowledgments

SHAPE America Acknowledgments

Thomas Lawson, SHAPE America Vice President of Marketing, Membership and Publications

SHAPE America Publications Advisory Committee

Holly Alperin, University of New Hampshire

Jayne Greenburg, US Department of Health and Human Services

Louis Harrison, The University of Texas at Austin

Brent Heidorn, University of West Georgia

Minsoo Kang, The University of Mississippi

Pamela Kulinna, Arizona State University

K. Andrew R. Richards, University of Illinois at Urbana-Champaign

Kristi Roth, University of Wisconsin-Stevens Point

Author Acknowledgments

Writing this book would have been impossible without the support of Jones & Bartlett Learning, SHAPE America, Cambridge College, colleagues, and most importantly, family. My sincere thanks and gratitude for the support each has provided.

I would like to provide a special acknowledgment to my husband, Richard, who is my greatest supporter and writing coach.

Special thanks to my children and their spouses for their support and my five grandsons who provided me with many contemporary ideas for prompts and clarification of the diverse challenges our youth face and experience as they grow and develop.

—Mary Connolly

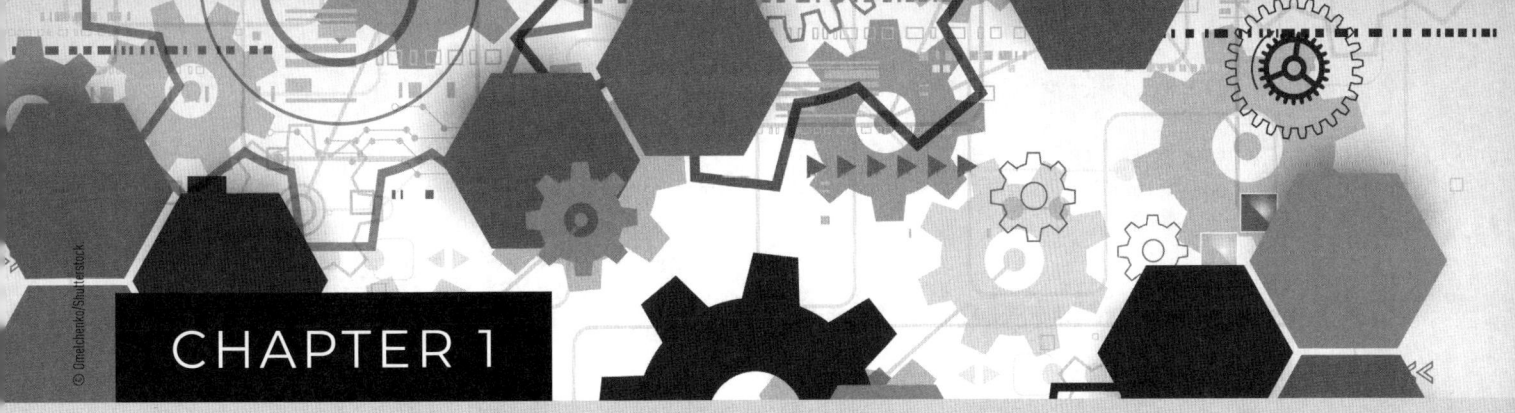

CHAPTER 1

Introduction to Social Emotional Learning

LEARNING OBJECTIVES

Upon finishing this course, students will be able to:

- Role of social emotional learning in the Every Student Succeeds Act.
- Research that supports the role of **social emotional learning (SEL)** in academic performance.
- Research that supports specific health curricula.
- National Health Education Standards (NHES).
- Alignment of the SEL competencies with the NHES.
- Contribution of CASEL.org to social emotional education.
- Contribution of the Wallace Foundation to social emotional education.
- Contribution of the Yale Center for Emotional Intelligence to social emotional education.
- Connection between SEL and the Whole School, Whole Community, Whole Child model.

KEY TERMS

Every Student Succeeds Act (ESSA)
Growth mindset

Social Emotional Learning
(SEL)

Whole School, Whole Community,
Whole Child (WSCC) Model

Social Emotional Learning and The Every Student Succeeds Act

Social Emotional Learning (SEL) is becoming more and more prevalent across the country. Although the **Every Student Succeeds Act (ESSA)** does not specifically include social emotional learning, social and emotional factors were recently included in federal policy in state accountability systems, school climate and anti-bullying initiatives, positive behavior supports, and discipline reform. (Stephanie Jones, March 2017, p. 5)

However, ESSA does include health and physical education and other disciplines that the state or local educational agency has determined are an essential part of a well-rounded education. The objective of this is to provide all students with access to a robust curriculum and educational experience. (US Department of Education, 2019) Including health education in the law elevates its status. Additionally, the legislation provides funding to develop, implement, and evaluate comprehensive, well-rounded programs to support safe and healthy students.(Connolly, 2018)

Many states have made SEL a goal and, consequently, numerous state frameworks and standards now include SEL. Districts are hiring SEL coordinators and implementing SEL throughout the district, and teachers are responsible for including SEL in their curriculum.

SEL and Academic Performance

Abundant research supports SEL efficacy in improving learning and student academic achievement.

A 2017 meta-analysis, <u>Promoting Positive Youth Development Through School-based Social and Emotional Learning Interventions: A Meta-analysis of Follow-up Effects</u>, produced evidence that SEL interventions significantly improved skills, positive attitudes, prosocial behavior, and academic performance. In addition, the programs served as protective factors against the problems of conduct, emotional distress, and drug use. The results were the same for students in different racial groups and socioeconomic statuses, domestically and internationally. Most interestingly, improving inter and intra-personal skills, such as self-regulation, problem solving, and relationship skills, enhanced academic performance and behavior. (Rebecca D. Taylor, 2017, p. 1166)

Furthermore, this research illustrates that SEL programming enhances a student's academic performance. Students who are self-aware are more confident about their ability to learn, try harder, and continue no matter which challenges face them. Students who have ambitious academic goals demonstrate self-discipline and self-motivation, manage their stress, organize their workload, study responsibly, and earn higher grades. (Durlak, January/February 2011, p. 417)

SEL Curriculum

More and more research supports the effectiveness of SEL curriculum. The Harvard Graduate School of Education, with funding from the Wallace Foundation, published an in-depth analysis of 25 SEL programs that are considered a practical resource for schools and out-of-school providers. (Stephanie Jones, March 2017) Many of the evaluated programs are traditional health education curricula. Conclusively, the curriculum research not only supports the efficacy of SEL but it also supports certain skills-based health education curricula.

The Collaborative for Academic, Social, and Emotional Learning (CASEL) is one of the SEL forerunners in the field. Its competencies and sub-competencies share a synergy with the National Health Education Standards (NHES), which embody the foundation of skills-based health education.

National Health Education Standards

The NHES and the CASEL SEL competencies, when taught together, provide the health content and personal and social skills to reinforce personal health and navigate life's challenges. (Connolly, Skills-Based Health Education, 2nd ed., 2018)

There are eight National Health Education Standards, which are divided into grade spans: PreK–2, 3–5, 6–8, and 9–12 (see **Table 1.1**). Age-appropriate performance indicators are listed in each grade span. The verbs used with the performance indicators coincide with Bloom's Taxonomy and become more complex as the grade span increases. Each performance indicator is preceded by three numbers.

Example: 1.8.7 Describe the benefits of and barriers to practicing healthy behaviors.

The three numbers identify the indicator as standard 1, performance in the 6–8 grade span, and the 7th indicator in the list for that grade span (1.8.7). (NHES, pg. 25)

Curriculum planners select a standard one performance indicator, pair it with a skills performance indicator, and align a SEL competency.

CASEL Social Emotional Learning Competencies

SEL is the process of understanding and managing emotions, setting and achieving goals, feeling and demonstrating empathy for others, building and maintaining positive relationships, and making responsible decisions. (CASEL, 2019)

The SEL competencies are aligned with standard 1 and skills performance indicators and become a part of assessment and instruction (see **Figure 1.1**). **Table 1.2** demonstrates the similarities between the standards and competencies, making it easier for the planner to align the SEL competency to the standard.

Although skills-based instruction and social emotional learning are a great pair, there are differences in teacher training and how they are implemented.

Table 1.1 National Health Education Standards

Standards	Description
Standard 1	Students comprehend concepts related to health promotion and disease prevention to enhance health.

Pre-K–Grade 2

1.2.1 Identify that healthy behaviors affect personal health.
1.2.2 Recognize that there are multiple dimensions of health.
1.2.3 Describe ways to prevent communicable diseases.
1.2.4 List ways to prevent common childhood injuries.
1.2.5 Describe why it is important to seek health care.

Grades 3–5

1.5.1 Explain the relationship between healthy behaviors and personal health.
1.5.2 Cite examples of emotional, intellectual, physical, and social health.
1.5.3 Describe how safe and healthy school and community environments can promote personal health.
1.5.4 Demonstrate how to prevent common childhood injuries and health problems.
1.5.5 Explain when it is important to seek health care.

Grades 6–8

1.8.1 Analyze the relationship between healthy behaviors and personal health.
1.8.2 Describe the interrelationships of emotional, intellectual, physical, and social health in adolescence.
1.8.3 Analyze how the environment affects personal health.
1.8.4 Describe how family history can affect personal health.
1.8.5 Describe ways to reduce or prevent injuries and other adolescent health problems.
1.8.6 Explain how appropriate health care can promote personal health.
1.8.7 Describe the benefits of and barriers to practicing healthy behaviors.
1.8.8 Examine the likelihood of injury or illness if engaging in unhealthy behaviors.
1.8.9 Examine the potential seriousness of injury or illness if engaging in unhealthy behaviors.

Grades 9–12

1.12.1 Predict how healthy behaviors can affect health status.
1.12.2 Describe the interrelationships of emotional, intellectual, physical, and social health.
1.12.3 Analyze how environment and personal health are interrelated.
1.12.4 Analyze how genetics and family history can affect personal health.
1.12.5 Propose ways to reduce or prevent injuries and health problems.
1.12.6 Analyze the relationship between access to health care and health status.
1.12.7 Compare and contrast the benefits of and barriers to practicing a variety of healthy behaviors.
1.12.8 Analyze personal susceptibility to injury, illness, or death if engaging in unhealthy behaviors.
1.12.9 Analyze the potential severity of injury or illness if engaging in unhealthy behaviors.

Standard 2	Students analyze the influence of family, peers, culture, media, technology, and other factors on health behaviors.

Pre-K–Grade 2

2.2.1 Identify how the family influences personal health practices and behaviors.
2.2.2 Identify what the school can do to support personal health practices and behaviors.
2.2.3 Describe how the media can influence health behaviors.

Grades 9–12

2.12.1 Analyze how the family influences the health of individuals.
2.12.2 Analyze how the culture supports and challenges health beliefs, practices, and behaviors.
2.12.3 Analyze how peers influence healthy and unhealthy behaviors.

(continues)

Table 1.1 National Health Education Standards (continued)

Standards	Description

Grades 3–5

2.5.1 Describe how the family influences personal health practices and behaviors.

2.5.2 Identify the influence of culture on health practices and behaviors.

2.5.3 Identify how peers can influence healthy and unhealthy behaviors.

2.5.4 Describe how the school and community can support personal health practices and behaviors.

2.5.5 Explain how media influences thoughts, feelings, and health behaviors.

2.5.6 Describe ways that technology can influence personal health.

Grades 6–8

2.8.1 Examine how the family influences the health of adolescents.

2.8.2 Describe the influence of culture on health beliefs, practices, and behaviors.

2.8.3 Describe how peers influence healthy and unhealthy behaviors.

2.8.4 Analyze how the school and community can affect personal health practices and behaviors.

2.8.5 Analyze how messages from media influence health behaviors.

2.8.6 Analyze the influence of technology on personal and family health.

2.8.7 Explain how the perceptions of norms influence healthy and unhealthy behaviors.

2.8.8 Explain the influence of personal values and beliefs on individual health practices and behaviors.

2.8.9 Describe how some health risk behaviors can influence the likelihood of engaging in unhealthy behaviors.

2.8.10 Explain how school and public health policies can influence health promotion and disease prevention.

2.12.4 Evaluate how the school and community can affect personal health practice and behaviors.

2.12.5 Evaluate the effect of media on personal and family health.

2.12.6 Evaluate the impact of technology on personal, family, and community health.

2.12.7 Analyze how the perceptions of norms influence healthy and unhealthy behaviors.

2.12.8 Analyze the influence of personal values and beliefs on individual health practices and behaviors.

2.12.9 Analyze how some health risk behaviors can influence the likelihood of engaging in unhealthy behaviors.

2.12.10 Analyze how public health policies and government regulations can influence health promotion and disease prevention.

Standard 3 — Students demonstrate the ability to access valid information and products and services to enhance health.

Pre-K–Grade 2

3.2.1 Identify trusted adults and professionals who can help promote health.

3.2.2 Identify ways to locate school and community health helpers.

Grades 6–8

3.8.1 Analyze the validity of health information, products, and services.

3.8.2 Access valid health information from home, school, and community.

3.8.3 Determine the accessibility of products that enhance health.

Grades 3–5

    3.5.1 Identify characteristics of valid health information, products, and services.

    3.5.2 Locate resources from home, school, and community that provide valid health information.

    3.8.4 Describe situations that may require professional health services.

    3.8.5 Locate valid and reliable health products and services.

Grades 9–12

    3.12.1 Evaluate the validity of health information, products, and services.

    3.12.2 Use resources from home, school, and community that provide valid health information.

    3.12.3 Determine the accessibility of products and services that enhance health.

    3.12.4 Determine when professional health services may be required.

    3.12.5 Access valid and reliable health products and services.

Standard 4	Students demonstrate the ability to use interpersonal communication skills to enhance health and avoid or reduce health risks.

Pre-K–Grade 2

    4.2.1 Demonstrate healthy ways to express needs, wants, and feelings.

    4.2.2 Demonstrate listening skills to enhance health.

    4.2.3 Demonstrate ways to respond when in an unwanted, threatening, or dangerous situation.

    4.2.4 Demonstrate ways to tell a trusted adult if threatened or harmed.

Grades 3–5

    4.5.1 Demonstrate effective verbal and nonverbal communication skills to enhance health.

    4.5.2 Demonstrate refusal skills that avoid or reduce health risks.

    4.5.3 Demonstrate nonviolent strategies to manage or resolve conflict.

    4.5.4 Demonstrate how to ask for assistance to enhance personal health.

Grades 6–8

    4.8.1 Apply effective verbal and nonverbal communication skills to enhance health.

    4.8.2 Demonstrate refusal and negotiation skills that avoid or reduce health risks.

    4.8.3 Demonstrate effective conflict management or resolution strategies.

    4.8.4 Demonstrate how to ask for assistance to enhance the health of self and others.

Grades 9–12

    4.12.1 Use skills for communicating effectively with family, peers, and others to enhance health.

    4.12.2 Demonstrate refusal, negotiation, and collaboration skills to enhance health and avoid or reduce health risks.

    4.12.3 Demonstrate strategies to prevent, manage, or resolve interpersonal conflicts without harming self or others.

    4.12.4 Demonstrate how to ask for and offer assistance to enhance the health of self and others.

Standard 5	Students demonstrate the ability to use decision-making skills to enhance health.

Pre-K–Grade 2

    5.2.1 Identify situations when a health-related decision is needed.

    5.2.2 Differentiate between situations when a health-related decision can be made individually or when assistance is needed.

Grades 3–5

    5.5.1 Identify health-related situations that might require a thoughtful decision.

    5.5.2 Analyze when assistance is needed in making a health-related decision.

    5.5.3 List healthy options to health-related issues or problems.

Grades 6–8

    5.8.1 Identify circumstances that can help or hinder healthy decision making.

    5.8.2 Determine when health-related situations require the application of a thoughtful decision-making process.

    5.8.3 Distinguish when individual or collaborative decision making is appropriate.

    5.8.4 Distinguish between healthy and unhealthy alternatives to health-related issues or problems.

    5.8.5 Predict the potential short-term impact of each alternative on self and others.

    5.8.6 Choose healthy alternatives over unhealthy alternatives when making a decision.

(continues)

Table 1.1 National Health Education Standards   *(continued)*

Standards	Description	
	5.5.4 Predict the potential outcomes of each option when making a health-related decision. 5.5.5 Choose a healthy option when making a decision. 5.5.6 Describe the outcomes of a health-related decision.	5.8.7 Analyze the outcomes of a health-related decision. **Grades 9–12** 5.12.1 Examine barriers that can hinder healthy decision making. 5.12.2 Determine the value of applying a thoughtful decision-making process in health-related situations. 5.12.3 Justify when individual or collaborative decision making is appropriate. 5.12.4 Generate alternatives to health-related issues or problems. 5.12.5 Predict the potential short-term and long-term impact of each alternative on self and others. 5.12.6 Defend the healthy choice when making decisions. 5.12.7 Evaluate the effectiveness of health-related decisions.
Standard 6	Students demonstrate the ability to use goal-setting skills to enhance health.	
	Pre-K–Grade 2 6.2.1 Identify a short-term personal health goal and take action toward achieving the goal. 6.2.2 Identify who can help when assistance is needed to achieve a personal health goal. **Grades 3–5** 6.5.1 Set a personal health goal and track progress toward its achievement. 6.5.2 Identify resources to assist in achieving a personal health goal.	**Grades 6–8** 6.8.1 Assess personal health practices. 6.8.2 Develop a goal to adopt, maintain, or improve a personal health practice. 6.8.3 Apply strategies and skills needed to attain a personal health goal. 6.8.4 Describe how personal health goals can vary with changing abilities, priorities, and responsibilities. **Grades 9–12** 6.12.1 Assess personal health practices and overall health status. 6.12.2 Develop a plan to attain a personal health goal that addresses strengths, needs, and risks. 6.12.3 Implement strategies and monitor progress in achieving a personal health goal. 6.12.4 Formulate an effective long-term personal health plan.
Standard 7	Students demonstrate the ability to practice health-enhancing behaviors and avoid or reduce health risks.	
	Pre-K–Grade 2 7.2.1 Demonstrate healthy practices and behaviors to maintain or improve personal health. 7.2.2 Demonstrate behaviors that avoid or reduce health risks. **Grades 3–5** 7.5.1 Identify responsible personal health behaviors. 7.5.2 Demonstrate a variety of healthy practices and behaviors to maintain or improve personal health.	**Grades 6–8** 7.8.1 Explain the importance of assuming responsibility for personal health behaviors. 7.8.2 Demonstrate healthy practices and behaviors that will maintain or improve the health of self and others. 7.8.3 Demonstrate behaviors that avoid or reduce health risks to self and others. **Grades 9–12** 7.12.1 Analyze the role of individual responsibility in enhancing health.

7.5.3 Demonstrate a variety of behaviors that avoid or reduce health risks.	7.12.2 Demonstrate a variety of healthy practices and behaviors that will maintain or improve the health of self and others. 7.12.3 Demonstrate a variety of behaviors that avoid or reduce health risks to self and others.

Standard 8	Students demonstrate the ability to advocate for personal, family, and community health.

Pre-K–Grade 2

8.2.1 Make requests to promote personal health.

8.2.2 Encourage peers to make positive health choices.

Grades 3–5

8.5.1 Express opinions and give accurate information about health issues.

8.5.2 Encourage others to make positive health choices.

Grades 6–8

8.8.1 State a health-enhancing position on a topic and support it with accurate information.

8.8.2 Demonstrate how to influence and support others to make positive health choices.

8.8.3 Work cooperatively to advocate for healthy individuals, families, and schools.

8.8.4 Identify ways in which health messages and communication techniques can be altered for different audiences.

Grades 9–12

8.12.1 Use accurate peer and societal norms to formulate a health-enhancing message.

8.12.2 Demonstrate how to influence and support others to make positive health choices.

8.12.3 Work cooperatively as an advocate for improving personal, family, and community health.

8.12.4 Adapt health messages and communication techniques to a specific target audience.

Reproduced from Joint Committee on National Health Education Standards. (2007). National Health Education Standards, Second Edition. SHAPE America.

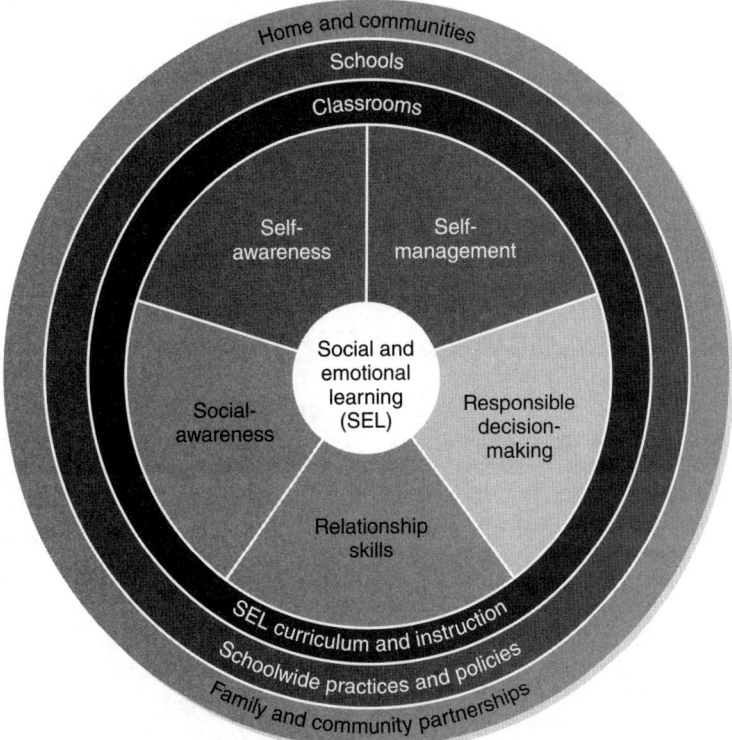

Figure 1.1 The CASEL Framework.

Table 1.2 The Alignment of NHES and CASEL Competencies

Skills-Based Health Education	Social Emotional Learning
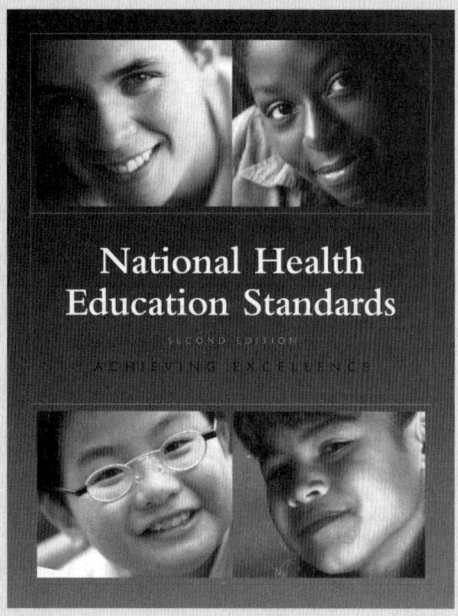 	
Standard 2 Students **analyze the influence** of family, peers, culture, media, technology, and other factors on health behaviors.	**Self-Awareness** The ability to accurately recognize emotions, thoughts, and values and how they **influence behavior**. ■ Identifying emotions ■ Accurate self-perception ■ Recognizing strengths ■ Self-confidence ■ Self-efficacy
Standard 3 Students demonstrate the ability to **access valid information and products and services** to enhance health.	**Social-Awareness** The ability to take perspective and empathize with people from diverse backgrounds and culture. The ability to understand social and ethical norms and to **recognize family, school, and community resources and supports**. ■ Perspective taking ■ Empathy ■ Appreciating diversity ■ Respect for others
Standard 5 Students demonstrate the ability to **use decision-making skills** to enhance health.	**Responsible Decision Making** The ability to make **constructive choices** about personal behavior and social interactions based on ethical standards, safety concerns, and social norms. The ability to make a realistic evaluation of consequences of various actions as well as a consideration of the well-being of self and others. ■ Identifying problems ■ Analyzing situations ■ Solving problems ■ Evaluating ■ Reflecting ■ Ethical responsibility

Standard 7 Students demonstrate the ability to **practice health-enhancing behaviors** and avoid or reduce health risks. Standard 6 Students demonstrate the ability to **use goal-setting skills to enhance health**.	Self-Management The ability to successfully regulate emotions, thoughts, and behaviors in different situations such as: **managing stress, controlling impulses, and self-motivation**. The ability to **set and work toward personal and academic goals**. ■ Impulse control ■ Stress management ■ Self-discipline ■ Self-motivation ■ Goal setting ■ Organizational skills
Standard 4 Students demonstrate the ability to use interpersonal **communication skills** to enhance health and avoid or reduce health risks. Standard 8 Students demonstrate the ability to **advocate** for personal, family, and community health.	Relationship Skills The ability to **communicate** clearly, listen, cooperate with others, resist inappropriate social pressure, negotiate conflict constructively, and seek and offer help when needed. ■ Communication ■ Social engagement ■ Relationship building ■ Teamwork
(Joint Committee on National Health Education Standards, 2007)	(Collaborative for Academic and Social Emotional Learning, 2020)

Reproduced from Joint Committee on National Health Education Standards. (2007). National Health Education Standards, Second Edition. SHAPE America.

Table 1.3 demonstrates additional similarities and a few differences.

As the skills-based health/SEL teacher plans lessons, he or she aligns the SEL competency to the standard 1 and skills performance indicators and weaves the SEL competency into the practice prompt and performance task. An authentic assessment determines if the student reached proficiency.

With training, the educator includes many of the sub-competencies in his or her assessment and instruction, thereby helping students develop their SEL skills.

The Evolution of Social Emotional Learning

Competent individuals are "those who manage well the circumstances which they encounter daily, and who possess judgment which is accurate in meeting occasions as they arise and rarely miss the expedient course of action." Socrates (Waters & Sroufe, 1983)

As early as 1983, competency was paired with having the skills to respond effectively to various situations. (Waters & Sroufe, 1983, p. 4) In looking carefully

at these early years, we uncover very contemporary ideas. For example, children who were deemed socially competent were judged by teachers to be more empathetic and able to respond positively to and sustain relationships with peers. (Waters & Sroufe, 1983, p. 10)

Also contributing to the social emotional movement is Daniel Goleman who in 1995, authored *Emotional Intelligence*. He states that emotional intelligence is the ability to be effective in all of the critical aspects of life, including school. According to Goleman, emotional intelligence is a different way of being smart. (Elias, 1997)

In 1997, character education was introduced into the schools. The goal was to help youth develop good character by acquiring positive values, such as fairness, honesty, compassion, responsibility, and respect for self and others. (Elias, 1997)

Collaborative for Academic and Social Emotional Learning

Although many people associate SEL with CASEL, it was not until 2005 that the five interrelated cognitive, affective, and behavioral competencies that we recognize today were published. (Frey, Fisher, & Smith, 2019, pp. 3–4)

Table 1.3 Alignment of SEL Competencies to the National Health Education Standards

Skills-based Health Education	Social Emotional Learning

- is a PreK-12 comprehensive, coordinated approach to teaching health education based on the National Health Education Standards.
- is taught by licensed, trained professionals and supported by district budgets and professional development. Curriculum varies by district and is sometimes integrated with other subjects.
- instruction is flexible and responds to district, state, and federal policy by implementing required curriculum.
- provides the opportunity to improve the health and well-being of students through the Whole School, Whole Community, Whole Child wellness committee.

- is a coordinating framework for educators, families, and community partners to promote students' social, emotional, and academic learning.
- is embedded in strategic plans, staffing, professional learning, and budgets.
- is implemented through direct practice as well as integrated instruction.
- drives schoolwide practices and policies. It informs how adults and students relate with each other, creating a welcoming, participatory, and caring climate for learning.
- shapes partnerships with families and community members, highlighting engagement, trust, and collaboration.

CASEL recommends integrating competencies into all content areas. The result is maintaining a cohesive and coordinated implementation. Other health curricula also recommend this implementation. A district-wide commitment to SEL involves the school board, superintendent, principals, teachers, and support staff including lunch staff, custodians, crossing guards, and bus drivers. This implementation ensures that SEL is institutionalized, taught in every classroom, and practiced in all aspects of the school.

The Wallace Foundation

The Wallace Foundation is a national philanthropic organization whose goal is to improve the lives of urban disadvantaged children and to cultivate the spirit of the arts. The foundation focuses on school leadership, after-school programming, summer learning, expanded learning, building audiences for the arts, and arts education for young people. (The Wallace Foundation, 2019)

The Wallace Foundation model proposes that acquiring social emotional skills is essential for students' development. During the first 10 years of a child's life, the skills that they learn provide the framework for the skills that the child needs at a later age. The skills that a child learns during one stage in development help the child to handle the demands that emerge and provide the foundation for the next stage.

In 2018, the Wallace Foundation organized its version of social emotional competencies into three domains **Figure 1.2**.

Cognitive Regulation

- Cognitive regulation includes attention control, inhibitory control, working memory and planning, and cognitive flexibility.

Emotional Processes

- Emotional Processes include emotion knowledge and expression, emotion and behavior regulation, and empathy or perspective taking.

Social/Interpersonal Skills

- Social/Interpersonal Skills include understanding social cues, conflict resolution, and prosocial behavior.

Figure 1.2 Wallace Foundation Social Emotional Competencies.

Reproduced from Frey, N., Fisher, D., & Smith, D. (2019). All Learning is Social and Emotional; Helping Students Develop Essential Skills for the Classroom and Beyond. Alexandria: ASCD.

Cognitive Regulation

Children use cognitive regulation skills when they need to perform tasks for which they need to concentrate, plan, solve problems, coordinate, make conscious choices over alternatives, or override a strong internal or external desire (Diamond & Lee, 2011, p. 70)—all key skills for behavioral and academic success.

Cognitive regulation includes skills that help children with basic tasks that require sequencing behavior, such as the steps of handwashing and knowing that they should put their shoes on last.

Children:

- Learn to respond appropriately to situations regardless of a more familiar but less appropriate manner. For example, choosing to stand in line to exit the classroom rather than standing with friends in a group; asking for permission to do something rather than following an impulse to act independently.
- Maintain information related to specific tasks, such as the ability to place worksheets in a particular place or finishing one assignment before beginning another.
- Resist distractions.
- Switch between task goals.
- Use functional health knowledge to make healthy decisions.
- Create rules.
- Cope with unfamiliar situations (Stephanie Jones, March 2017, p. 16).

Cognitive regulation aligns with Standard 7: Demonstrate the ability to practice health-enhancing behaviors and avoid or reduce health risks (Joint Committee on National Health Education Standards, 2007, p. 35) and Standard 1: Comprehend concepts related to health promotion and disease prevention to enhance health (Joint Committee on National Health Education Standards, 2007, p. 24)

While preparing to show how to practice healthy behaviors during a practice prompt or performance assessment, students practice cognitive regulation by paying attention and controlling their impulses in order to meet the performance task requirements. They use the functional health knowledge that they learned in the unit to collaboratively plan a demonstration of content and skills.

Emotional Processes

Emotional processes are a set of skills and understandings that help children recognize, express, and regulate their emotions as well as being able to see things from the perspective of others. (Stephanie Jones, March 2017, p. 16) The skills are essential when developing positive social interactions and establishing relationships with other peers and adults. Children use these skills to cope with tasks that require emotional, behavioral, and interpersonal responses. They learn how different situations affect their feelings and how to respond in positive ways. (Stephanie Jones, March 2017, p. 16)

These processes are closely aligned to the CASEL SEL competency of Self-Awareness and Standard 2: Students analyze the influence of family, peers, culture, media, technology, and other factors in health behaviors.

The skills-based health/SEL teacher addresses these processes by intertwining them into the practice prompts after he or she has defined and explained the skill and modeled it. The teacher then gives the students time to practice while he assesses the students' progress and proficiency.

Social and Interpersonal Skills

Once a child has developed the personal skills of cognitive regulation, he or she has the foundation to learn about others and to develop social/interpersonal skills. These skills include understanding social cues, conflict resolution, and positive social behavior. These skills fortify emotional knowledge and processes and help students to accurately interpret the behavior of others, effectively navigate social situations, and interact successfully with peers and adults. (Stephanie Jones, March 2017, p. 16)

These skills align with Standard 4 of the National Health Education Standards (see **Table 1.4**). (Joint Committee on National Health Education Standards, 2007, p. 30)

The skills-based health educator skillfully places the competencies into prompts and challenges students to demonstrate healthy emotional language and verbal and nonverbal skills, understand the behavior of others, respond to a situation that may be threatening or dangerous, negotiate, resolve conflict, and request help.

Example

Jeremy tried his older brother's vape. He liked the taste, how it made him feel, and the fact that his parents could not smell any cigarette smoke. The next day, he took the vape to school and asked his friend Ben if he wanted to try it.

Ben knows his friend tries to impress people, but he was surprised, curious, and annoyed and said, "No. I don't want to try it." Ben said, "Why did you take your brother's vape? You know he will be mad and will tell your parents!

If you get caught with it in school, you will be in a lot of trouble." Jeremy's shoulders slumped and he stepped back. He didn't think of that. Ben told Jeremy to put the vape in his locker and keep it there until dismissal.

At the end of the day, Ben went to Jeremy's house and helped him put the vape back where he found it.

Table 1.4 Example of SEL Alignment to a Prompt and Review Questions

Questions to Clarify Social and Interpersonal Skills	Response
1. When did the boys exhibit social cues?	■ Ben was surprised when Jeremy asked him to try the vape. ■ Jeremy's shoulders slumped and he stepped back when Ben told him he could get in a lot of trouble.
2. How did Ben take perspective of the situation?	■ Ben realized immediately that Jeremy made a mistake bringing the vape to school and asking him if he wanted to try the vape.
3. Which communication skills did Ben demonstrate?	■ Refusal skills ■ Conflict resolution
4. Which SEL competency did Ben demonstrate?	■ Relationship skills • Communication • Teamwork
5. What skills from the Wallace Foundation did Ben demonstrate?	■ Ben knew that Jeremy likes to impress people. ■ Resolved conflict ■ Solved a social problem ■ Coexist peacefully with his friend.
6. How did Ben resolve this conflict?	■ He convinced Jeremy to put the vape into his locker and keep it there until dismissal.
7. What prosocial behavior did you observe in the prompt?	■ Ben helped his friend realize that he should not have brought the vape to school and to put it into the locker until dismissal.
8. How did Ben navigate the situation and still interact positively with Jeremy?	■ Ben refused the vape and helped Jeremy realize that he should not have brought the vape to school and to put it into the locker until dismissal.

Character

Over the years, the concept of character has evolved from teaching about positive and negative values to skills, values, and habits that help children live and work with others as friends, families, and citizens. (Stephanie Jones, March 2017, p. 17) The core values of understanding and demonstrating ethical values, such as respect, justice, citizenship, and responsibility, continue to be valued and embraced.

Perseverance, diligence, and self-control are now also considered essential to being a good worker and to help the individual to reach his potential. However, character does not mean simply having core values; it also means acting on them and following through when faced with a difficult situation. Character means speaking up when a difficult decision is necessary, being tolerant of others and civically responsible, persevering when facing a challenge, and following through on commitments as well.

Mindset

As with the CASEL competencies, the Wallace Foundation encourages a "**growth mindset**," which is important in coping with daily challenges. A mindset consists of the attitudes and beliefs held about oneself, others, and personal circumstances. A person with a "growth mindset" believes that success happens because of hard work rather than innate ability. When a person manages frustration and discouragement, solves interpersonal conflict, and perseveres in difficult situations, he or she is demonstrating a "growth mindset." (Stephanie Jones, March 2017, p. 17)

The Yale Center for Emotional Intelligence—RULER Model

The Yale Center for Emotional Intelligence conducts research and designs educational approaches that support people of all ages in developing emotional intelligence and the skills to flourish and contribute to society. (Yale Center for Emotional Intelligence, 2019)

The **RULER** model for social emotional intelligence/learning contains skills of **R**ecognizing emotions in oneself and others, **U**nderstanding the causes and consequences of emotions, **L**abeling emotions with accurate words, **E**xpressing emotions differently depending on context, and **R**egulating emotions with helpful strategies. (Yale Center for Emotional Intelligence, 2019)

Results of the model, based on research from several publications, include:

- Students
  - Have better academic performance, leadership skills, and attention.
  - Are less likely to bully other students.
- Teachers
  - Have more solid relationships with students.
  - Burn out less frequently.
  - Maintain better relationships with administration.
  - Remain positive about teaching. (Yale Center for Emotional Intelligence, 2019)
- RULER
  - Improves school atmosphere.
  - Increases students' emotional intelligence and social skills.
  - Decreases anxiety and depression.

The RULER implementation plan integrates social and emotional learning into all aspects of learning and school life to provide a safe place for students to learn and grow. To accomplish this, the school community, including superintendents and school boards, are engaged. Teachers are trained and use anchor tools (Mood Meter, Meta-Moment, Charter, Blueprint) (Yale Center for Emotional Intelligence, 2019) to introduce skills into classroom routines, academics, and throughout the school that are associated with emotional intelligence.

Whole School, Whole Community, Whole Child Connection to Social Emotional Learning

Collaboration

The effectiveness of skills-based health/SEL is increased when members of the school and community work together to minimize student risk factors and maximize academic achievement.

The Wellness Team represents the school and community, and its structure stems from the **Whole School, Whole Community, Whole Child Model** designed by the Centers for Disease Control and Prevention (CDC) and the Association for Supervision and Curriculum Development (ASCD). The Wellness Team recommends, reviews, and implements district policies regarding school nutrition, nutrition education, physical activity, and relevant issues that affect student health. (Massachusetts

Department of Public Health, 2020) Additionally, the team analyzes youth risk behavior data, health district data, and disciplinary data and designs interventions or supportive programming in response.

Districts organize the teams in numerous ways. For example, some districts have a district team composed of the district leaders of each component while others provide wellness teams in each building. Some districts include both models. With SEL as a component of the team, the representative has a voice in implementing SEL within the school and district.

When health educators specifically teach the SEL competencies, students learn them. Acquiring these additional skills helps students to develop positive attitudes, positive social behavior, conduct, levels of distress, and academic performance. (Frey, Fisher, & Smith, 2019, p. 10) The hope is that once the students learn the competencies, they will use those skills to handle challenging situations outside of school. Although the intent of the implementation plan for SEL is to be integrated into every classroom, the health educator and the wellness team have a unique and comprehensive role in the implementation.

In 2017, the USDA established guidelines for wellness policies that often serve as the foundation for district wellness committees. According to the guidelines, the team:

- Including parents, students, food service members, physical education teachers, health professionals, the school board, school administrators, and the general public work together to develop, implement, review, and update the local wellness policy.
- Identifies a leader with the authority and responsibility to ensure compliance and gather all of the necessary components.
- Informs and updates the public regarding the content and implementation of the wellness policy.
- Reviews and considers evidence-based strategies that help establish specific goals for nutrition promotion and education, physical activity, and other school-based activities that promote student wellness.
- Establishes nutrition policies for all foods and beverages offered for sale or available during the school day for parties, classroom snacks, and food brought by parents or given as incentives; policies that limit food and beverage marketing and advertising only to Smart Snacks according to the School Nutrition Standards.
- Provides a description of public involvement, updates, policy leadership, and an evaluation plan.

(USDA, 2020)

The structure and components of the WSCC Model and the CASEL SEL Wheel are similar and may serve a related purpose. Both have a center and components surrounding them and are connected to school and community affiliations, thereby facilitating alignment and collaboration (see **Table 1.5**).

In **Figure 1.3**, lines connect the similar components of each model.

Table 1.5 Comparison of the Structure and Components of the WSCC Model and the SEL Competencies

CASEL SEL Model	CDC/ASCD WSCC Model
Center SEL	**Center** Youth who are healthy, safe, engaged, supported, and challenged.
Components Self-Awareness Self-Management Social-Awareness Responsible Decision Making Relationship skills	**Components** Health education Physical education & Physical activity Nutrition Environment & Services Health services Social & emotional climate Counseling & psychological & social services Physical environment Employee wellness Family engagement Community involvement
Wrap arounds SEL Curriculum and instruction School wide practices and policies Family & community partnerships	**Wrap arounds** Improving learning and improving health Coordinating policy, process, & practice Community

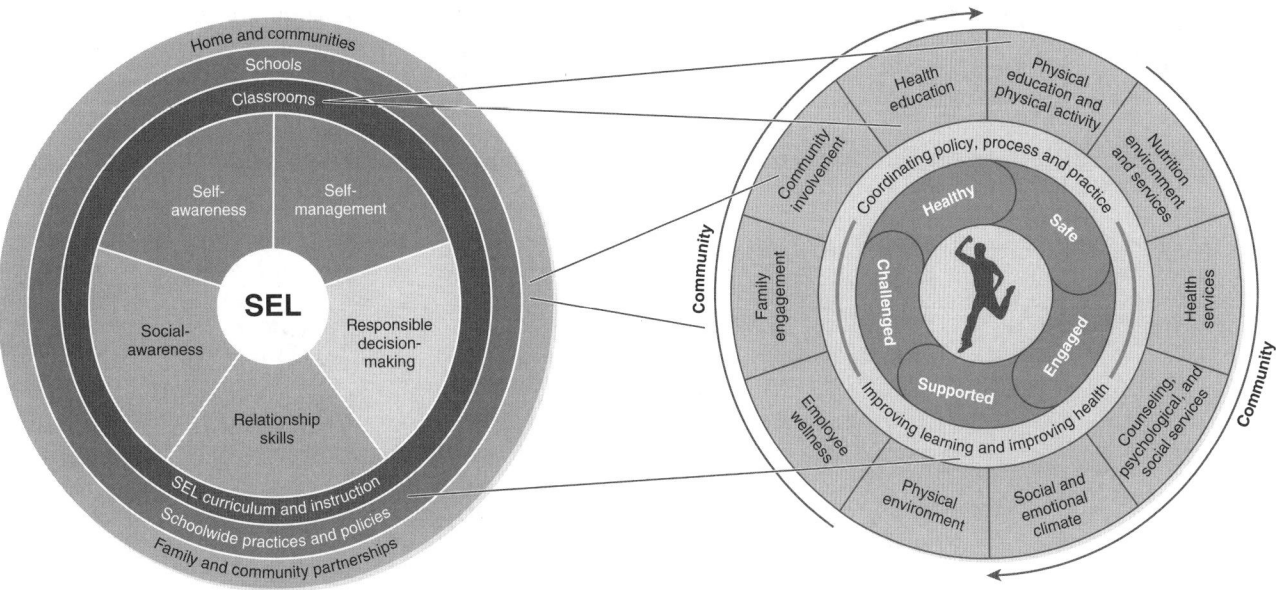

Figure 1.3 Comparison of the WSCC Model and the SEL Competency Wheel.

Whether we embrace the CASEL competencies, the Wallace Foundation model, the Yale RULER model, WSCC, or any other competencies, content, skill, and SEL acquisition, taught by licensed and trained professionals are fundamental to developing and maintaining healthy relationships and behaviors.

Chapter Review Questions

1. How does The Every Student Succeeds Act support health education?
2. What evidence supports SEL efficacy in improving student academic achievement?
3. How are the National Health Education standards organized?
4. What do the numbers on the performance indicators indicate?
5. When planning, how do teachers connect performance indicators with SEL competencies?
6. Explain how the CASEL competencies are aligned with the National Health Education Standards.
7. Explain the evolution of SEL from 1983 to the present.
8. Describe the social emotional competencies of the Wallace Foundation.
9. Describe the Yale Center for Emotional Intelligence RULER model.
10. Compare and contrast the WSCC model and the CASEL SEL Competency Wheel.

References

Armstrong, T. (2019). *Mindfulness in the Classroom*. Alexandria: ASCD.

Brackett, M. A. (2018). The emotional intelligence we owe students and educators. *Educational Leadership, 76*(2), 13–18.

Centers for Disease Control and Prevention, CDC Healthy Schools. (2020). *Whole School, Whole Community, Whole Child (WSSC)*. Retrieved from Centers for Disease Control and Prevention, CDC Healthy Schools: https://www.cdc.gov /healthyschools/wscc/index.htm

Collaborative for Academic and Social Emotional Learning. (2020). *CASEL Competencies*. Retrieved from CASEL: https://casel.org/wp-content/uploads/2019/12/CASEL -Competencies.pdf

Collaborative for Academic, Social and Emotional Learning. (2020). *What is SEL?* Retrieved from CASEL.org: https://casel .org/what-is-sel/

Connolly, M. (2018). *Skills-based health education* (2nd ed.) Burlington: Jones and Bartlett.

Elias, M. J. S. (1997). *Promoting social and emotional learning.* Alexandria: ASCD.

Frey, N., Fisher, D., & Smith, D. (2019). *All learning is social and emotional; helping students develop essential skills for the classroom and beyond.* Alexandria: ASCD.

Joint Committee on National Health Education Standards. (2007). *National health education standards,* (2nd ed.) SHAPE America.

PIco, I. (2019). *The Wheel of Emotion by Robert Plutchick.* Retrieved from PsicoPico: https://psicopico.com/en/la-rueda -las-emociones-robert-plutchik/

Taylor, R. D., Oberle, E., Durlak, J. A., & Weissberg, R. P. (2017). Promoting positive youth development through school-based social and emotional learning interventions: A meta-analysis of follow-up effects. *Child Development, 88,* 1156–1171.

Jones, S., Brush, K., Bailey, R., Brion-Meisels, G., & McIntyre, J. (2017). *Navigating SEL from the inside out. Looking inside and across 25 leading SEL programs: A practical resource for schools and OST Providers.* Boston: Harvard Grduate School of Education with Funding from the Wallace Foundation.

U.S. Department of Education. (2020). *Every Student Succeeds Act (ESSA).* Retrieved from The US Department of Education https://www.ed.gov/ESSA

The Wallace Foundation. (2019). *A Brief History.* Retrieved from The Wallace Foundation: https://www.wallacefoundation .org/about-wallace/pages/history.aspx

US Department of Education. (2019). *Every Student Succeeds Act of 2015.* Retrieved from US Department of Education: https://www.ed.gov/ESSA

Waters, E., & Sroufe, A. L. (1983). Social competence as a developmental construct. *Developmental Review, 3*(1), 79–97.

Yale Center for Emotional Intelligence. (2019). *Mission & Vision.* Retrieved from Yale Center for Emotional Intelligence: http://ei.yale.edu/who-we-are/mission/

Yale Center for Emotional Intelligence. (2019). *Staff Development.* Retrieved from RULER: http://ei.yale.edu/ruler/staff -development/

Yale Center for Emotional Intelligence. (2019). *The Anchor Tools.* Retrieved from RULER: http://ei.yale.edu/ruler/the-anchor -tools/

Yale Center for Emotional Intelligence. (2019). *What is RULER.* Retrieved from RULER: ei.yale.edu/ruler/results

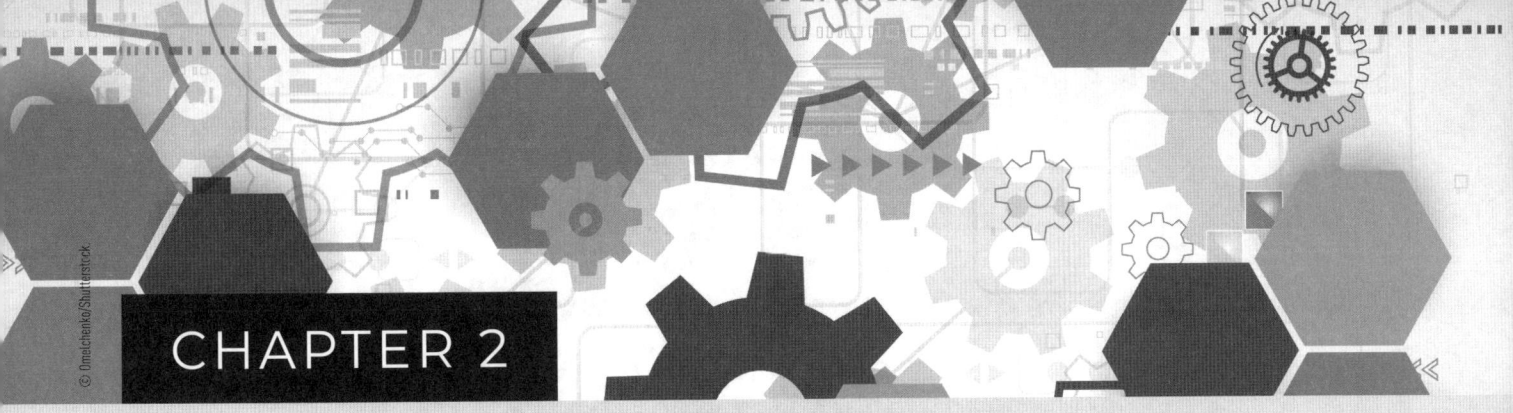

CHAPTER 2

Pedagogical Practices

LEARNING OBJECTIVES

Upon finishing this course, students will be able to:

- Plan skills-based health (SBH)/SEL based on the developmental growth of the students.
- Use the SAFE (sequenced, active forms of learning, focused time for skill development, explicit learning goals) approach to plan SBH/SEL instruction.
- Use neuroscience to plan effective SBH/SEL instruction.
- Design and utilize formative and summative assessments.
- Use the alignment of the National Health Education Standards (NHES) and the CASEL competencies to design assessment and instruction.
- Use backwards design to plan assessment and instruction.
- Use effective SBH/SEL strategies when planning activities.

KEY TERMS

Authentic assessment
Backwards design
Infused performance indicators

Neuroplasticity (neuroplastic response)
Neuroscience

Pedagogy
Performance task

Developmental Considerations

When we examine how social emotional learning (SEL) skills develop over time, we discover that some skills are the foundation for those that develop later and, therefore, should be taught first during certain grades or grade spans. (Stephanie Jones, March 2017)

Cognitive regulation skill development (attention control, inhibitory control, working memory and planning, and cognitive flexibility) occurs during the ages from 4 to 6 years. Concurrently, the prefrontal cortex of the brain is expanding during this time.

During preschool, pre-Kindergarten, and Kindergarten, if the cognitive regulation skills are developed, they prepare the child for the more difficult skills of long-term planning, decision making, and coping skills.

During the early elementary grades, children are challenged to plan, organize, and set goals. As they begin to understand the needs of others, they need to learn how to develop empathy, social awareness and perspective taking. During the later elementary years and middle school, students benefit from learning how to develop friendships, engage in prosocial and ethical behavior, and resolve conflicts. (Stephanie Jones, March 2017)

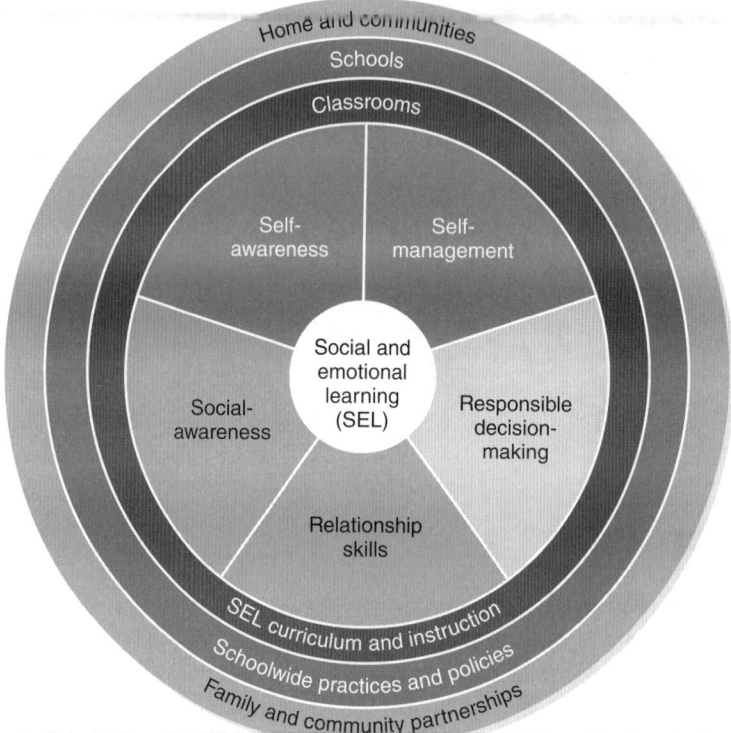

Figure 2.1 The CASEL Framework.

Knowing how SEL competencies develop helps the curriculum planner align them with the grade span performance indicators and design an age-appropriate scope and sequence (**Figure 2.1**).

Implementation of the social and emotional competencies may include processing, integrating, and applying them in appropriate ways. This type of instruction, like skills-based health education, is very engaging and interactive, allowing students to make contributions to class, school, and community and thereby increase their sense of satisfaction, belonging, and motivation. Students also develop social-emotional skills when the teacher establishes safe, caring learning environments,

involves peers and families, uses effective classroom management and teaching strategies, and implements activities that include the whole school, whole community, whole child. (Durlak, January/February 2011, p. 407)

SAFE is an effective four-pronged approach to implementing skills-based health/social emotional programs. The program is **S**equenced and provides a step-by-step implementation, uses **A**ctive forms of learning, **F**ocused time for skill development, and has **E**xplicit learning goals. (Durlak, January/February 2011, p. 408)

Table 2.1 illustrates how skills-based health/SEL meet these criteria.

Table 2.1 SAFE Plan and Skills-based Health/SEL Implementation

SAFE Plan	SBH/SEL Implementation
Sequenced	Skills-based health/SEL is sequenced from PreK–12. The grade span performance indicators generate the assessment and instruction.
	The SEL competencies are aligned with the content and skill performance indicators and are assessed either concurrently (goal setting, decision making, communication skills) or separately.
Active forms of learning	Skills-health/SEL is engaging and interactive. Instructors begin by explaining the five steps of teaching a skill.
	1. Why the skill/competency is important.
	2. Explain the steps of completing the skill/competency.
	3. Model the steps.

	4. Provide time for students to practice. 5. Formatively assess while students practice, providing effective feedback. (Joint Committee on National Health Education Standards, 2007) During each class, students demonstrate the content, skill, and SEL competency through practice prompts and a variety of class activities. Students collaborate to demonstrate proficiency either through the design and implementation of a graphic organizer for standard 1 or a role play or other interactive modalities for the skills standards.
Focused time for skill development	In the elementary school, under the direction of the elementary health specialist, time is scheduled for direct instruction. Additional time is allocated for classroom teacher follow-up lessons either prepared by the health educator or scheduled from the prepared curriculum. According to the National Health Education Standards , health knowledge begins to increase after 15 hours of instruction, particularly in grades 4–7. Forty-five to 50 hours of instruction are needed to affect attitudes and practices. Maximum learning and attitude or behavior change occurs after 60 hours of instruction in one school year. (Joint Committee on National Health Education Standards, 2007, p. 63)
Explicit learning goals	The aligned SEL competency and the infused performance indicators of the National Health Education Standards serve as the explicit learning goals.

Understanding by Design Meets Neuroscience and Skills-based Health/Social Emotional Learning

Neuroscience research reveals how the classroom environment, activating prior knowledge, using attention getting techniques and graphic organizers result in sensory information being transformed into understanding. (McTighe & Judy Willis, 2019, p. 3) These strategies are all used in skills-based health/SEL assessment and instruction.

Before a skills-based health/SEL teacher activates prior knowledge, she implements a pre-test to determine the extent of that knowledge. With the results, the educator learns the status of content, skills, and SEL competency learned and measures the change in acquisition over time with the post-test. Also, once the brain has stored knowledge, it is easier to link new knowledge and skill with it. (McTighe & Judy Willis, 2019, p. 9) Consequently, the teacher scaffolds what is known with what is new to enhance the knowledge, skill, and SEL competency of the student.

When the teacher begins class and conducts a review, preview, introduces risk behavior data, or other attention-getting information, the student is engaged and the teacher has the interest of the student. Targeted feedback maintains engagement with the students because it occurs several times in each class and provides students with suggestions on how

to meet the lesson objectives. As the student makes the adjustment, the teacher revisits the student and continues the cycle. As the class concludes, the teacher instructs students to pack up their belongings then reviews all the content, skill, and SEL competencies taught during class.

Standard 1 **infused performance indicators** challenge the students to demonstrate what they know and are able to do. Graphic organizers are an effective tool for students, including special needs students and English learners, to demonstrate what they learned. Faced with a blank organizer and information about a health topic, students are challenged to read, interpret, analyze, and arrange information, then explain their work to a larger group. This strategy provides the student with additional SEL training that includes organization, teamwork, and relationship skills.

When students are reluctant to try, it may be a result of previous failures and the belief that there is no point in trying again because they will only fail again. This is called a "fixed mindset." In a skills-based/SEL classroom, the teacher learns to interrupt this pattern by frequently using formative assessment and providing effective feedback. This gentle attention, in small doses, increases self-confidence and provides a road map to success and a challenge to the "fixed mindset." Learning that effort, perseverance, and trying different strategies controls the outcome of the efforts to meet expectations and results in the development of a "growth mindset." (McTighe & Judy Willis, 2019, pp. 7–8)

The brain grows neuropathways when it experiences something new. This is called the neuroplastic response. (McTighe & Judy Willis, 2019, p. 12) Those pathways are strengthened when the same activity is repeated over time. However, if the activity is not repeated, the neuro connections dissolve so, we either "use it or lose it!" In a PreK–12 skills-based health/SEL curriculum, students learn to demonstrate their learning through a variety of modalities. Examples include but are not limited to: graphic organizers, video, music, poetry, role plays, and presentations to younger children, peers, or adults. This consistent yet varied pedagogical practice contributes to **neuroplasticity (neuroplastic response)** by strengthening the current neural pathways and growing new ones.

In our classrooms, we facilitate neural growth by establishing consistent and repetitive teaching practices from greeting the students in the hall to the end-of-class review and exit ticket. When used, these practices also promote growth and learning of functional health knowledge, skills, and SEL competencies. (Davidson, 2020)

A well-designed and thoughtful classroom environment is crucial for students to learn content, skill, and SEL competency. If students enter class anxious, sad, hungry, angry, frustrated, bored, or alienated, or if the teacher is struggling physically, intellectually, socially, or emotionally, teaching and learning are much more difficult. (McTighe & Judy Willis, 2019, p. 140)

Being aware of one's social emotional status is beneficial when teaching a class. Often, the mood of the teacher impacts the mood of the class. (McTighe & Judy Willis, 2019, p. 140) A self-assessment helps students take stock of how they are feeling and provides an opportunity to adjust their attitude in order to be more receptive to learning.

The following are examples of neuro-friendly teaching practices that enhance teaching and learning:

- *Welcoming routines and rituals*. Using rituals and routines in the classroom makes the student feel safe and more comfortable in taking an academic risk. Standing at the classroom door and greeting the students may seem like a simple practice but in fact, when the students see the teacher in the same place and wearing the same pleasant smile, it brings a sense of safety and predictability. Other routine examples include the daily explanation of the agenda, a structure to pass out and pass in work, conducting the end-of-class review, filling out an exit ticket, and lining up to exit the class. Rituals such as demonstrating respect for each member of the class, responding appropriately to

student questions and behaviors, collaboratively setting classroom norms, and providing time for students to connect with one another to develop a sense of belonging, also contributes to a safe learning environment. A healthy and safe learning environment with established routines also decreases behaviors that interfere with learning. (Massachusetts Department of Elementary and Secondary Education, 2019, p. 26)

- *Engaging **pedagogy***. Engaging instructional practices are also brain-compatible strategies and promote relationships, cultural acceptance, responsiveness, empowerment, and collaboration. (Davidson, 2020) Skills-based health/SEL embraces the pedagogical practice of engaging students. During each lesson, content is taught through the skill and SEL competency. Students show proficiency by working in groups to complete a graphic organizer and demonstrate proficiency of content and skill through a practice prompt challenge. To engage the students socially and emotionally, the teacher takes the SEL pulse by asking a variety of questions. Students respond anonymously either by putting their heads down, using emojis, or placing sticky notes on a feelings wheel. The teacher may decide to change the lesson plan if he detects there is a general problem in the group. Addressing the problem makes it public and gives the teacher the opportunity to teach positive coping strategies. Once the anxiety level subsides, the planned lesson resumes. When detecting student energy is low, the teacher engages the students by implementing a movement break. Movement to music; a fun, quick movement game; a stand and stretch; belly breathing, a yoga exercise; or anything that gives the brain a little rest and re-energizes the body and brain is an excellent way to spend a few minutes. Productivity may increase because the students are refreshed physically and mentally.

- *Optimistic Closure*. (Davidson, 2020) At the end of each SBH/SEL lesson, the teacher instructs the students to put away their belongings and participate in an end-of-class review. During this time, students are asked questions about the content, skill, and SEL competencies taught. Students may refer to their notes and information on the board or any other available resource. This practice brings the students back to the infused performance indicators and SEL competency that serve as the lesson objectives. It is a way for the teacher to reinforce the lesson content and determine the

Table 2.2 Pedagogical Practices to Help the Student Brain Learn

Pedagogical Practice	Implementation
Explain unit goals.	When introducing a new skills unit, provide the data that explain why the unit is being taught, introduce the Standard 1, skills performance indicators, and SEL competency/subcompetency as the goals of the unit.
Ensure the performance task challenge (authentic assessment) is achievable by all.	Explain the performance task (authentic assessment) and the steps to completion so that each student understands, with hard work and determination ("growth mindset"), they will succeed.
Provide frequent formative assessments with specific feedback.	During instruction, demonstrating SEL competency, skill practice, and while students are planning and practicing their authentic assessment, formatively assess and provide specific feedback so they target working toward proficiency.
Acknowledge student progress and achievement throughout the unit.	During the unit, provide a procedure to track progress such as a graphic, an arrow, a self-check, daily written progress reflection, etc.

Data from McTighe, J., & Judy Willis, M. (2019). Upgrade Your Teaching, Understanding by Design Meets Neuroscience. Alexandria: ASCD, p. 16.

extent of student learning. In addition to the end-of-class review, provide time for the students to answer an exit ticket. The ticket question may challenge the student to think of how they plan to use the content, skill, and SEL competency in their daily lives.

As a new unit begins, help the student brain learn by implementing the pedagogical practices shown in **Table 2.2**.

Assessment

The word assess is derived from Latin and means "to sit" with the student. Therefore, to assess students, we monitor learning and the practice of demonstrating knowledge of content and competency in demonstrating the skill and SEL competency.

Assessment improves teaching and learning. Effective classroom assessment occurs over time, includes a variety of formative and summative assessments, effective feedback, and a record of achievement shared with students, parents, and administration.

Before starting a new unit, teachers administer a pre-test to determine prior knowledge and skill levels. Because new learning is scaffolded to previous learning, it is important to assess what students know in order to design an effective, interesting, and engaging new unit. Preassessments inform the teacher of skill gaps or a student's incorrect understanding of content, skill, and competency. The information gathered helps the teacher plan and accommodate for different levels of student knowledge and skill. (McTighe & Judy Willis, 2019, p. 71)

At the beginning of a unit, the teacher explains the performance indicators and SEL competencies, how to demonstrate proficiency, the assessments and grading. During instruction, the teacher uses formative assessment and provides feedback to inform students of progress in reaching the performance indicators and SEL competency.

If assessment indicates the students are not learning, the teacher reteaches or reviews and assesses again. Students practice and revise their performance or product prior to the summative assessment. As the teacher analyzes the formative and summative assessments, she improves upon the delivery of content, skill, and SEL instruction. This assessment cycle results in improvements to teaching and learning. (Connolly, 2018, p. 73)

Data drives the skills-based health/social emotional learning (SBH/SEL) program. The planner accesses youth risk behavior data and designs assessments and instruction to reduce the risk factor data. Assessment results determine the scope of learning and in turn, informs adjustments to curriculum.

The verbs of the infused performance indicators of the National Health Education Standards and the aligned SEL competencies determine assessment and instruction. Rather than a chapter test, skills-based health/SEL utilizes a **performance task** that is an **authentic assessment**. In this practice, students demonstrate the content, skill, and SEL competency learned. For example, see **Table 2.3**.

When planning assessment and instruction, SBH/SEL teachers use youth risk behavior data to decide which Standard 1, skills standard, and SEL competency best reduces the risk behavior.

Table 2.3 Examples of Authentic Assessment that Includes National Standards and SEL Competencies

Assessment Example	National Health Education Standard	SEL Competency
Students highlight the positive and negative influences of emotions on the components of personal health.	Standard 1: Content Standard 2: Analyzing Influences	Self-Awareness
Access valid and reliable information	Standard 1: Content Standard 3: Accessing Information	Social-Awareness
Demonstrate refusal and negotiation skills	Standard 1: Content Standard 4: Interpersonal Communication	Relationship Skills
Demonstrate decision-making skills	Standard 1: Content Standard 5: Decision Making	Responsible Decision Making
Demonstrate the steps of handwashing; the steps of putting on a bicycle helmet	Standard 1: Content Standard 7: Practicing Healthy Behaviors	Self-Management
Write and perform public service announcements.	Standard 1: Content Standard 8: Advocacy	Relationship skills

Teachers are mindful to design prompts and challenges that are developmentally appropriate, culturally relevant, diverse, reflective of their audience, and have multiple opportunities to succeed. Assessment measures student proficiency in content, skill, and SEL competency. Instruction provides the functional health information for students to be successful on the assessment and at the same time, it accommodates for the range of abilities and languages found in the SBH/SEL classroom. (Assessment Work Group, 2019)

Formative Assessment

Assessment *for* learning is formative. It measures the student's progress toward achieving the content, skill, and SEL competencies. By using a variety of formative assessment tools and strategies, the teacher discovers how the class or the individual student is progressing. The teacher then determines if she needs to review, reteach, or continue the instruction. Researchers discovered that when teachers use an abundance of formative assessments that students learn in in several months what classrooms with fewer assessments achieve in one year. (Connolly, 2018, p. 75)

Formative assessment is not graded and occurs during instruction, observations, conversations, and self-assessments. When providing student feedback, the teacher comments on the evidence in terms of how it meets or does not meet the infused performance indicators and SEL competency rather than just the comments of "Excellent!," "Well-done," or "Great Job," where the student feels terrific with

such positive comments from the teacher but doesn't really know why his work was so good. Formative assessment helps the teacher determine if he should continue with instruction or pause and revise or review previous instruction. (Connolly, 2018, p. 73)

Formative assessment is interactive. After assessing, the teacher provides specific targeted feedback that compares what was observed with the infused performance indicators and SEL competency. The teacher provides specific suggestions and resources for improvement. This type of feedback results in students having a better understanding of their status and what they need to do to improve, if needed. Formative assessment is not a "one and done." Students may revise their work and resubmit. With continuous effective formative assessment, students improve their performance and attain the lesson and unit objectives. (Connolly, 2018, p. 76)

Assessment tools may be formative, summative, or both, depending on how they are used. If the tool is an analytical rubric and used to monitor progress and is not graded, it is formative. When the tool is used during the presentation of the authentic assessment for a grade, it is summative.

Other examples of formative assessment include:

- Preclass questions and answers to determine current knowledge
- Self-assessments
- Presentations for practice
- Examination of a portfolio to examine learning progress (Connolly, 2018)

There are a variety of formative assessments strategies to implement during a unit. Be adventuresome and try several. Over time, favorites emerge that provide students and the teacher with valuable information about teaching and learning.

Formative Assessment Tools

Formative tools have a variety of uses. Some tools provide general information to the teacher and are helpful to assess group progress. The same assessment, when given to individual students, provide specific information and is very helpful in monitoring progress in achieving the infused performance indicators and SEL competency. Below are some examples of formative tools (**Table 2.4**) but let your

imagination be your guide to design and develop new and innovative tools!

Summative Assessment

Summative assessment is assessment *of* learning and occurs at the end of a unit as the result of a performance task and generates a grade. In the context of SBH/SEL, the SEL competencies are aligned, integrated, and assessed with the infused performance indicators.

Using the **backwards design** model for planning, the teacher knows, before she begins teaching, what the students should accomplish by the end of the unit to demonstrate proficiency. (Connolly, 2018, p. 85) At the beginning of the

Table 2.4 Formative Assessment Tools

Formative Assessment	Example
Thumbs up, down, sideways	When the teacher asks a variety of questions, students put their thumb up, down, or sideways. This strategy provides the teacher with a general idea of the student's status.
	If each student has a set of thumbs and he places his status thumb on the desk, this provides the teacher with specific information about the status of this student and an opportunity to "check in."
	This check in is used to assess the social emotional status of the students at a given time, the progress in a group activity, or whether the students are ready for the teacher to continue instruction. This activity aligns with but is not limited to the SEL competencies of Self-Awareness and Social-Awareness.
Five fingers 	Checking for understanding may include asking for the number of steps in a procedure or the number of facts known about content. For example, the teacher asks, "How many steps are involved in fitting a bicycle helmet?" This provides general information but no guarantee that the students know the steps.
	Another strategy is to ask, "How many decision-making steps do you feel confident to demonstrate?" This questioning technique results in more individual information and more opportunities for the teacher to provide targeted feedback.
	This activity aligns with but is not limited to the SEL competency of Self-Awareness.
Red/yellow/green circles	Students place the red circle up if they do not know what to do; the yellow circle up if they have a question; and the green circle up if they do not need any help.
	When asking True/False preview or review questions, students raise the red circle for False; the yellow circle if they are not sure; and the green circle for True.
	When determining whether to continue with instruction or wait, students raise the red circle if they need more time; the yellow if they are almost finished; and the green if they are finished with their work and do not need any more time.
	This activity aligns with but is not limited to the SEL competency of Self-Awareness.

(continues)

Table 2.4 **Formative Assessment Tools**

(continued)

Formative Assessment	Example
Learning continuum	During group work, students place a group mark on the continuum to indicate progress toward completing the performance task. The mark indicates group progress but does not explain why the mark was placed on a certain point. The teacher visits the group to learn more about the project and provides targeted feedback. During individual work, each student has his own continuum and marks individual progress. With this strategy, the teacher has a better idea of how to provide targeted feedback to help the student progress. This activity aligns with but is not limited to the SEL competencies of Self-Awareness and Social-Awareness.
Bull's eye/target	During group work, students place a group mark on the target to indicate progress toward completing the performance task. The mark indicates group progress but does not explain why the mark was placed on a certain point. The teacher visits the group to learn more about the project and provides targeted feedback. During individual work, each student has his own target and marks individual progress. With this strategy, the teacher has a better idea of how to provide targeted feedback to help the student progress. This activity aligns with but is not limited to the SEL competencies of Self-Awareness and Social-Awareness.
Cubes Assertive / "I" messages	Cubes are used to review terms, clarify steps in a process, or any pairing exercise. For example, place terms on one cube and the definitions on the other. In pairs, one student rolls the term cube, or the definition cube, and then matches to the other cube. The partner checks the response against the answer sheet. Students take turns. This activity aligns with but is not limited to the SEL competencies of Self-Awareness and Social-Awareness.
Sticky notes	Sticky notes are used in a variety of ways to check for understanding or transfer of skill. • A question is place on the board and students write the response on the sticky note then "splash" the response under the question. As students place their notes, the teacher reads the response and knows the extent of learning and determines if the content/skill/ SEL competency needs to be reviewed, retaught, or if she can continue instruction. • Students write a response to an exit ticket question and either leave the note on the desk or place it on the doorway as they exit class. This is a good tool to check for understanding or ask how the student plans to use the content/skill/SEL competency after they leave class. This activity aligns with but is not limited to the SEL competencies of Self-Awareness and Social-Awareness.
Letter card responses B B D A C E F T ?	When previewing or reviewing, prepare questions that assess content, skill, and SEL competency. Prepare sets of index cards that contain the symbols: A, B, C, D, E, T, F, and ? Place the cards in a plastic bag so they are ready to use. After asking the question, students respond by holding up the card that responds to the answer they think is correct. The questions may require a True/False answer or a letter answer for a multiple choice. The question mark is used when the student is not sure of the answer. This activity aligns with but is not limited to the SEL competencies of Self-Awareness: Self-confidence.

Graphic Organizers	
Formative Assessment	**Example**
Bow tie 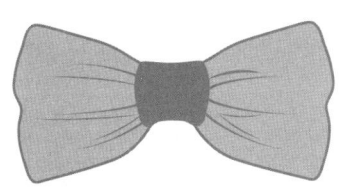	The bow tie is a good tool to use for Standard 1 when students are challenged to compare and contrast information. The topic is placed in the knot. One student writes the "benefits of" the challenge on one side and another student writes the "barriers to" on the other. For example: What are the benefits of and barriers to wearing a bicycle helmet? This activity aligns with but is not limited to the SEL competencies of Self-Awareness and Social-Awareness.
Graphic wheel 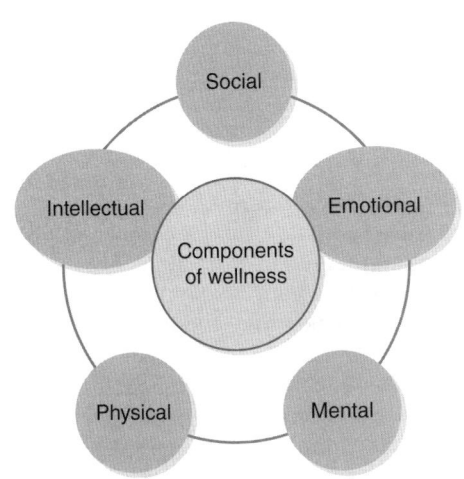	The wheel is often used with the performance indicator. 1.8.2 Describe the interrelationships of emotional, intellectual, physical, and social health in adolescence. (Joint Committee on National Health Education Standards, 2007) When paired with Standard 2 and the SEL competency, self-awareness, students write, draw, or place pictures of emotions next to the component of wellness to explain the effect of positive and negative influences on their emotions and personal wellness. This activity aligns with but is not limited to the SEL competencies of Self-Awareness and Social-Awareness.

Comparison sort
 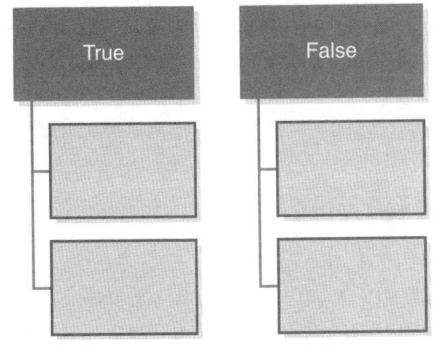
	Sorts can be used in a variety of ways.
	 ■ True false
	   • Prepare questions about content, skill, and SEL competencies.
	   • Cut the questions into strips and place the graphic organizer and strips of paper in a plastic bag.
	   • Distribute the bags and provide time for the students to sort the statements.
	   • Formatively assess as the students sort.
	
	 This activity aligns with but is not limited to the SEL competencies of Self-Awareness and Social-Awareness.

Sequencing sort
 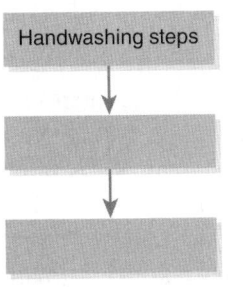
	Sorts can be used in a variety of ways.
	 ■ Sequencing (use words or pictures)
	   • Place the steps of handwashing pictures; steps to properly fitting a bicycle helmet; steps of putting on a condom; steps of CPR, Heimlich, rescue breathing, etc.; on strips of paper.
	   • Include SEL competencies as choices for alignment.
	   • Place the graphic organizer and strips of paper in a plastic bag.
	   • Distribute the bags and provide time for the students to sort the steps.
	   • Formatively assess as the students sort.
	
	 This activity aligns with but is not limited to the SEL competencies of Self-Awareness and Social-Awareness.

(continues)

Table 2.4 **Formative Assessment Tools**   *(continued)*

Formative Assessment	Example
Positive and negative effects on personal health 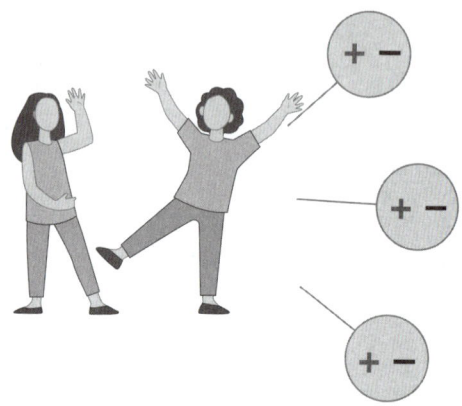	To analyze the positive and negative influences on personal health, this graphic organizer allows the students to write down the impact of influences on youth. Students then examine the positive and negative effects of the influences. This activity aligns with but is not limited to the SEL competency of Self-Awareness: Identifying emotions.
Carousel	Group students and use large sticky paper for a variety of group activities: ■ After reading a challenge prompt, students use the steps of decision making to solve a problem. This activity aligns the SEL competency of Responsible Decision Making to Standard 5, Decision making. ■ After reading an engaging prompt about how a teen changed as a result of a life experience, students write down how perspective changed. This activity aligns with but is not limited to the SEL competency Social-Awareness: Perspective taking or Self-Awareness: Accurate self-perception to Standard 2, Analyzing Influences. ■ Students respond to a prompt by using the goal setting steps to set a goal and track progress. This activity aligns with but is not limited to the SEL competency Self-Management: goal-setting with Standard 6 Goal setting.

unit, the teacher introduces the content, skill, and SEL competencies and the requirements for the summative assessment. All daily lessons provide time to become proficient in the content, skill, and SEL competency to ensure success on the summative assessment.

Summative assessment for SBH/SEL is authentic. Students demonstrate the content, skill, and SEL competency learned by meeting the criteria of the performance task prompt challenge. A summative assessment rubric is used to compare the evidence to the performance indicators and SEL competency and generate a grade. Because the SEL competencies are not standards, they are assessed separately on the rubric, and the grade becomes a percentage of the overall grade generated by the rubric. For example, the standards portion of the authentic assessment may be established as 95% and the SEL competency at 5%.

Performance Task

We propose that the goals of understanding and transfer are most appropriately assessed through performance assessment tasks that ask students to apply their learning to a new situation and provide an explanation or justification. (McTighe & Judy Willis, 2019, p. 79)

A performance task is a summative assessment and the preferred pedagogical practice to measure achievement and learning. It is distributed after all the content, skill, and SEL competencies are taught. The performance task includes prompts, the unit rubric, self-check, and backup information the student uses to successfully complete the challenge. The task is based on the National Health Education Standards and SEL competencies and presented through a prompt.

For example, an interpersonal communication unit on pregnancy prevention may include the pros and cons of types of birth control (1.12.7) and negotiating or collaborating on the use (4.12.2). The SEL competency is Relationship skills—Communication and Teamwork.

Students utilize the content and skills learned in class to resolve the challenge then present the project or performance to the class to demonstrate their proficiency of the performance indicators and SEL competency.

Performance tasks are examples of authentic assessment because students demonstrate their proficiency of content, skill, and SEL competency. This type of assessment is grounded in real a world, age-appropriate prompt. It requires the student to use knowledge and skills to solve a problem and asks the students to explore ways of solving a problem rather than merely reciting content taught in class. Performance tasks place the students in realistic situations, similar to their personal lives, where they must resolve a situation by using knowledge and skills to resolve a complicated task. They require time to practice, consult resources, and improve performance or product based on the teacher formative assessment feedback. (Connolly, 2018, p. 99)

> *Performance tasks that are authentic in terms of both real world applications and personal interests can increase students' motivation, their willingness to apply effort, and their receptiveness to the associated lessons that will prepare them for the task.* (McTighe & Judy Willis, 2019, p. 82)

Students have a certain amount of days to work together to design how they will present their task. As the students work, the teacher formatively assesses and provides targeted feedback. When ready, students present to the class and are graded with a summative evaluation tool. Feedback is written on the tool, so the students better understand the grade and have a foundation of criteria to discuss with the teacher.

In scoring performance tasks, there are a variety of summative assessment rubrics available such as an analytical rubric, structured observation guides, rating scale, holistic rubric, and a checklist rubric. (Connolly, 2018, pp. 88–98) The rubric contains criteria based on the infused performance indicators of Standard 1 (content), the skills-infused performance indicator(s), and the SEL competency. The most common rubrics are the holistic and the analytical. The holistic rubric gathers all the content criteria into one description and provides the same

for the skill criteria. It provides an overall impression of a student's work. (McTighe & Judy Willis, 2019, p. 86) An analytical rubric scores each infused performance indicator separately. The SEL competencies are scored in the nonstandard portion of the rubric. This score is an average of the grades and the SEL competency is scored separately or as a percentage of the standards grade.

Using the Backwards Design to Plan Assessment and Instruction

Sound pedagogical practice enhances the teaching and learning of SEL in the skills-based classroom. The four steps of backwards design are aligned with and support the teaching of SBH/SEL **Figure 2.2**.

When planning SBH/SEL, use backwards design to examine data; target content, skills, and SEL competencies; plan assessment and instruction.

The Steps of Backwards Design

Step 1: Data Analysis

The first step in backwards design is to examine youth risk behaviors. The Centers for Disease Control and Prevention provides excellent data on their Youthonline website. (Centers for Disease Control and Prevention, 2020) The site provides the results of high school and middle school youth risk behavior surveys. The high school surveys are conducted across the country, biannually. The middle school data is recorded by state and major cities.

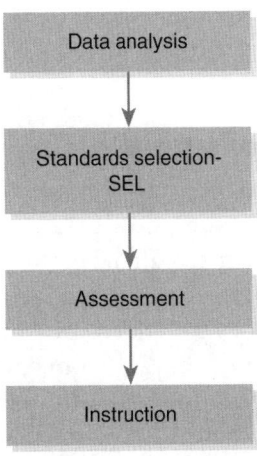

Figure 2.2 Backwards Design.

Once the data is collected, it serves as rationale for the development of SBH/SEL units. With limited health education time, addressing the needs of youth is an efficient and effective way to design curriculum. With periodic curriculum updates and revisions, the SBH/SEL curriculum stays current and meets the needs of the district youths.

Step 2: Standards/SEL Selection

Once the data is analyzed, the planner selects a Standard 1 performance indicator and a skills performance indicator to reduce the risk factor. In making the selection, the planner considers the students and their needs because any skill is appropriate to address a risk factor. For example, if the planner thinks the student needs more skill in analyzing influences, this is the skill selected for the unit. For the same risk factor, the planner may believe that the students need the skill of accessing valid and reliable information and, instead, select Standard 3, Accessing Information. There is no right or wrong. The choice is made by the planner based on his knowledge of the scope of student skill acquisition or gaps in skill.

The SEL competencies are aligned with the National Health Education Standards:

- Self-Awareness pairs with Standard 2, Analyzing influences, and Standard 1, functional health knowledge
- Social-Awareness pairs with Standard 1, functional health knowledge, and Standard 3, Accessing information
- Responsible Decision-Making pairs with Standard 5, Decision Making
- Self-Management pairs with both Standard 7, Practicing healthy behaviors, Standard 6, Goal setting, and Standard 1, functional health knowledge
- Relationship Skills pairs with Standard 4, Interpersonal communication, Standard 8, Advocacy, and Standard 1, functional health knowledge.

Step 3: Assessment

During this step, the planner asks the assessment question, "What must my students do to demonstrate they are proficient in the performance indicator and SEL competency?" (Connolly, 2018, p. 74)

Assessment is generated by the performance indicator verb and the SEL competency. The verb informs what the student does to demonstrate proficiency. If the verb is to explain, the student "gives the reason for or cause of something." (Merriam Webster, 2020) For example, the student may be challenged to explain how the perception of norms influence healthy and unhealthy behaviors. (Joint Committee on National Health Education Standards, 2007, p. 27)

The SEL assessment depends on the performance indicator with which it is paired. Responsible decision making does not need a separate assessment when it is paired with Standard 5, decision making. Self-management includes stress management and does not need a separate assessment when paired with the infused Standard 7 performance indicator 7.5.2 Demonstrate a variety of healthy practices and behaviors, *such as stress management*, to maintain or improve personal health, because both are assessed through Standard 7. The Relationship Skills subcompetency, Communication, does not need a separate assessment when paired with Standard 4, Interpersonal communication or Advocacy because it is assessed through the standard.

The remaining SEL competencies are woven into practice prompts and the performance task. Students demonstrate proficiency in a variety of ways.

- Watch the YouTube video of Susan Boyle's audition on Britain's Got Talent and write a reflection on how the perception of the contestant changed from the beginning of the video to the end of the performance (Social-Awareness: Perspective taking). (YouTube—Britain Has Talent, 2020)
- Comment on recognizing the strengths in self or others how a character developed self-confidence and self-efficacy. (Self-Awareness)
- Examine how a character demonstrated empathy, appreciation of the diversity, and respect of others. (Social-Awareness)
- Analyze how a character demonstrated impulse control, self-discipline, self-motivation, or organizational skills. (Self-Management)
- Demonstrate social engagement, relationship building, and teamwork. (Relationship Skills).

Step 4: Instruction

During this step, the planner asks the instruction question, "What do I need to teach in order for my students to be successful on the performance task?" (Connolly, 2018, p. 74) In looking at the assessment, the planner bullets everything that she needs to teach to help the students meet proficiency. For example, teach:

- The definition of the verbs, SEL competency, and other vocabulary associated with the performance task.
- The content of the infused Standard 1 performance indicator.
- The skills of the infused skill performance indicator.
- The steps of teaching the skill.

Planning instruction also includes a well-planned lesson that includes

- Review of the previous lesson or a preview of the lesson of the day.
- Review of the class agenda.
- Explain the SEL competency aligned with the lesson.
- Review/teach the steps of teaching a skill.
- Introduce new content based on the infused performance indicator.
- Provide a prompt for student practice.
- Formatively assess while the students are practicing and provide effective feedback.

- Review the content/skill/SEL competency taught in class.
- Provide an exit ticket to further assess student understanding. (Connolly, 2018)

Backwards Design Example

The following is a Grade 8 practicing healthy behaviors example of backwards design with the content of vaping.

Step 1: Data Analysis

Table 2.5 shows high school vaping risk behavior data used for this example of backwards design.

Step 2: Standards Selection

Identify the desired results (McTighe & Judy Willis, 2019, pp. 28-29) by selecting Standard 1, Standards 2–8 skill(s), and SEL competencies to reduce the risk factor.

Steps 3 and 4 are first described for standard 1 then the skills performance indicator.

Table 2.5 Youth Risk Behavior Data

High School Youth Risk Behavior Survey 2019 Currently used an Electronic Vaping Product Including e-cigarettes, e-cigars, e-pipes, vape pipes, vaping pens, e-hookahs, and hookah pens, on at least one day during the 30 days before the survey.			
	Total	Female	Male
United States	32.7 (30.7–34.8) 12,767	33.5 (30.9–36.1) 6,464	32.0 (29.7–34.3) 6,183

High School Youth Risk Behavior Survey 2019 Currently frequently used an Electronic Vaping Product Including e-cigarettes, e-cigars, e-pipes, vape pipes, vaping pens, e-hookahs, and hookah pens, on 20 or more days of the 30 days before the survey.			
	Total	Female	Male
United States	10.7 (9.5–11.9) 12,767	9.7 (8.6–10.9) 6,464	11.6 (10.0–13.4) 6,183

High School Youth Risk Behavior Survey 2019 Currently used Vaping Products Daily Including e-cigarettes, e-cigars, e-pipes, vape pipes, vaping pens, e-hookahs, and hookah pens, on 20 or more days of the 30 days before the survey.			
	Total	Female	Male
United States	7.2 (6.2–8.3) 12,767	6.4 (5.4–7.6) 6,464	7.9 (6.7–9.4) 6,183

Data from Centers for Disease Control and Prevention. (2020, September 4). 2019 High School YRBS, Currently Frequently Used Electronic Vapor Products. Retrieved from Centers for Disease Control and Prevention: https://nccd.cdc.gov/youthonline/App/Results.aspx?TT=B&OUT=0&SID=HS&QID=QNDAYEVP&LID=LL&YID=RY&LID2=&YID2=&COL=&ROW1=&ROW2=&HT=&LCT=&FS=&FR=&FG=&FA=&FI =&FP=&FSL=&FRL=&FGL=&FAL=&FIL=&FPL=&PV=&TST=&C1=&C2=&QP=&DP=&VA=CI&CS=Y&SYID=&EYID=&SC=&SO=

Steps 3 and 4: Assessment and Instruction for Standard 1

In this step, the planner determines acceptable evidence. (McTighe & Judy Willis, 2019, p. 29) and **Step 4 Instruction**. In this step, the planner designs learning experiences and instruction. (McTighe & Judy Willis, 2019, p. 30)

Step 3: Standard 1 Assessment. During this step, the planner asks the assessment question, "What can the students do to show me they are proficient in the performance indicators and SEL competency?" (Connolly, 2018, p. 74)

The verb of the performance indicator informs the assessment and instruction. For example, the verbs compare and contrast the performance indicator 1.12.7 Compare and contrast the benefits of and barriers to practicing a variety of healthy behaviors, (Joint Committee on National Health Education Standards, 2007, p. 25) generates the assessment and instruction. Because the verbs are "compare" and "contrast," the assessment consists of the students comparing and contrasting the benefits of and barriers to practicing a variety of healthy behaviors.

The planner then infuses the performance indicator with content and includes specific criteria for the assessment.

> 1.12.7 Compare and contrast *three* benefits of and *three* barriers to practicing a variety of healthy behaviors, *such as quitting vaping*. (Joint Committee on National Health Education Standards, 2007, p. 25)

For this performance indicator, the competency of Self-Awareness: self-confidence is a good alignment. The SEL assessment consists of a reflection question, how does comparing and contrasting the benefits of and barriers to quitting vaping increase a person's self-confidence to quit?

The planner now has a clear vision of the assessment and begins to plan the instruction.

Step 4: Standard 1 Instruction. This redesigned, infused performance indicator allows the planner to teach about the benefits of not vaping, the barriers to not vaping, and the development of self-confidence to quit.

This performance indicator lends itself to the use of a Venn diagram or T bar. Students fill in the graphic organizer with content and are assessed when they present the content on the poster or during role play or other assessment modalities. On the graphic organizer,

the teacher can add a text box and ask the reflection question, "How does the information on the poster increase a teen's self-confidence to quit vaping?"

Steps 3 and 4: Assessment and Instruction for Standard 7

Step 3: Standard 7 Assessment. The Standard 1 performance indicator is paired with a skills performance indicator. Performance indicator 1.12.7 with the content of quitting vaping, pairs nicely with 7.12.2 Demonstrate a variety of healthy practices and behaviors that maintain or improve the health of self and others. (Joint Committee on National Health Education Standards, 2007, p. 35) The competency of Self-Awareness: self-confidence subcompetency aligns well with this performance indicator also.

When infused with vaping content and specific criteria, the performance indicator reads:

> 7.12.2 Demonstrate a variety of healthy practices and behaviors *such as three quitting vaping strategies* that maintains or improves the health of self and others.

The verb of this performance indicator is to demonstrate. The assessment, therefore, requires the students to demonstrate three strategies to quit vaping. Include the assessment for the SEL competency by demonstrating how learning quitting strategies increases the self-confidence to quit.

Strategies to demonstrate include role play, video, simulated meeting with a cessation specialist, etc.

Let your imagination be your guide along with the verb demonstrate!

Step 4: Standard 7 Instruction. The instruction includes strategies for quitting vaping and how learning the strategy increases the self-confidence to be able to quit:

- Set your quit date.
- Know what challenges to expect.
- Imagine your vape-free self.
- Build your team. (National Institutes for Health, 2020)

Delivery of Skills-Based Health/SEL

Health content, skills, and social emotional competencies are delivered in a variety of ways. In the elementary school, they may be integrated into all subjects, taught separately by a health specialist, or taught as a special topic by the classroom teacher. At the middle- and high-school levels, the skills are integrated or taught by a licensed health education professional. Regardless, research has proven that school staff effectively delivers SEL programs. (Durlak, January/February 2011, p. 417)

In a skills-based lesson, the content (functional health information) is taught each day through the skill. Units are designed by skill, providing the opportunity to teach content across a variety of skills.

Effective SBH/SEL Teaching Strategies

Effective teaching strategies are paramount to pedagogical practice. Below are several practices that have proven to be effective in teaching skills-based health/SEL.

Skill Practice

Since practicing helps reinforce and retain skills, students practice SEL skills as they practice the skills of analyzing influences, accessing information, communication skills, refusal skills, decision making, goal setting, and advocating. Often, practice occurs during a role play but may also include a variety of modalities such as a song, a poem, a public service announcement, etc.

To reinforce speaking and listening skills, students paraphrase what their partner says to demonstrate good listening skills. To demonstrate calming down strategies, students use emotion/behavior regulation strategies. (Stephanie Jones, March 2017, p. 20)

Role Play

For younger children, use puppets to demonstrate how to role play. Older students may role play in pairs at their seat or in groups in front of the class. Scenarios include a demonstration of functional health knowledge, skill, and SEL competency. Role playing may be used to act out emotions, demonstrate skills such as emotion regulation strategies, problem-solving, or how to manage conflict and interpersonal challenges. (Stephanie Jones, March 2017, p. 20)

Discussion

Discussions in the SBH/SEL classroom occur in pairs, small groups, or as a whole class. Discussion questions challenge the student to demonstrate content knowledge, a skill, and the SEL competency.

Discussion is used to:

- Introduce an SEL theme aligned with functional health knowledge and a skill.
- Pose questions to students regarding how a person may feel or act in a given practice prompt or authentic assessment.
- Facilitate conversation about how an SEL theme, health content, and targeted skill relate to student life.
- Describe how a SEL theme, health content, and targeted skill are related to books they read and movies they watch. (Stephanie Jones, March 2017, p. 19)

Book/Story

To use a book, story, or article to teach skills-based health/SEL, the teacher selects a passage that incorporates targeted information, a skill, and SEL competency. Students identify the content, skill, and SEL components then discuss the passage. The teacher assesses by asking the students to design a comic strip, companion prose, poem, role play, demonstration, or graphic organizer that illustrates proficiency of the performance indicators and SEL competency. (Stephanie Jones, March 2017, p. 19)

Teaching Skills

The steps of teaching a skill include the following:

1. Explain why the skill is important.
2. Explain the steps
3. Model the skill
4. Provide practice time
5. Formatively assess and provide effective feedback. (Connolly, 2018, p. 134)

To enhance learning, the teacher defines the terms associated with the performance indicators and the SEL competencies (**Figure 2.3**).

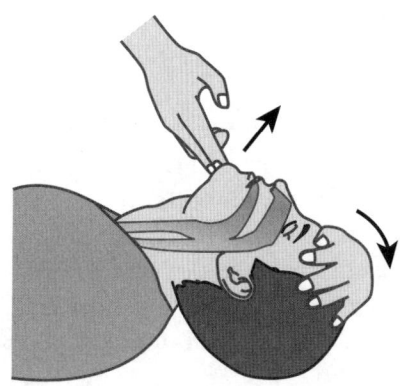

Figure 2.3 Teaching a Skill.

The verb of the performance indicator generates the assessment and instruction. To reach proficiency, students must demonstrate their knowledge, skill, and SEL competency. In order to do this, they must understand the meaning of the words.

Vocabulary

For English Learners (ELs) a word wall is very helpful, labeled pictures, and pairing an EL with a peer with higher levels of English skills and comprehension. This is strategy is appropriate for English learners and students with special needs. (Connolly, 2018)

SBH/SEL Tools and Handouts

Use of a tool or material to promote SBH/SEL strategies helps students visualize concepts in a concrete way. For example, use a conflict escalator to explore how certain choices worsen or improve a conflict, using a feelings thermometer to talk about emotions, setting up a problem box to collect class problems for future discussion, or using student handouts such as planning templates. (Stephanie Jones, March 2017, p. 19)

Writing

Ask students to write about experiences related to a SBH/SEL theme or to the record the experiences of others. For example, students write about a time they were angry with someone, what they did, how they resolved the problem, and how it felt.

Writing activities may also be collaborative, such as a team composing a poem with a health/SEL theme. At younger ages, students draw pictures that depict an experience or event. (Stephanie Jones, March 2017, p. 19)

Drawing

Students draw an activity rather than an event or experience. Drawing activities are different from writing exercises because they focus on artistic expression rather than a narrative experience.

For example, ask students to draw a picture of something that makes them happy rather than drawing about a specific time they felt happy. Reflect by asking targeted questions about content, skills, or SEL competency to connect it to instruction. (Stephanie Jones, March 2017, p. 19)

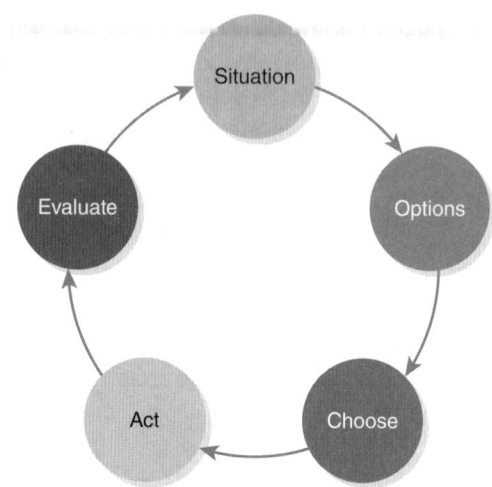

Figure 2.4 Visual Display.

Art/Creative Project

Design an art or creative project related to a SBH/SEL theme. For example, students use clay to make faces that show different emotions, figures that show different ways to communicate, a road map to the nurse's office, etc. (Stephanie Jones, March 2017, p. 20)

Visual Display

Students design charts, posters, or other visual displays to demonstrate a standard 1, skill, or SEL competency. For example, the student draws a DECIDE chart, the wellness components and how emotions influence each, stress management skills, and mindfulness activities (**Figure 2.4**). (Stephanie Jones, March 2017, p. 20)

Video

Video the students role playing content, skill, and SEL competency. Standard 8, Advocacy, and the SEL competency Relationship skills: communication, lends themselves nicely to this form of assessment.

Video a challenging situation (discussion around emotions, conflict resolution, and appropriate behaviors). Stop the video and brainstorm how to resolve the problem using functional health knowledge, skills, and SEL competencies. (Stephanie Jones, March 2017, p. 20)

Song

Use songs (and music videos or sing-songy chants) to reinforce an SBH/SEL theme. Students may include dances, hand movements, and/or strategy practice.

For example, students design a song that leads them through the steps of belly breathing or problem-solving. (Stephanie Jones, March 2017, p. 20)

Game

Games are used to reinforce content, skill, and SEL competencies; build relationships; or transition students to the next unit. For example, play charades to teach about emotions and social cues. Use Simon Says to practice cognitive regulation skills. (Stephanie Jones, March 2017, p. 20)

While the above strategies are effective, use your imagination to meet the needs of your students. You know your students better than anyone. Use that knowledge to target your knowledge/skill/SEL competency instruction. Have fun!

References

American Institutes for Research. (2019, October 5). *ED School Climate Surveys*. Retrieved from National Center on Safe Supportive Learning Environments https://safesupportivelearning.ed.gov/edscls

Armstrong, T. (2019). *Mindfulness in the classroom: Strategies for promoting concentration, compassion, and calm.* Alexandria: ASCD.

Assessment Work Group. (2019). *Student social and emotional competence assessment.* Chicago: Collaborative for Academic, Social, and Emotional Learning.

Association for Supervision and Curriculum Development. (2019). Brian Coleman on Showing Up Authentically. *Educational Leadership*, 12–13.

Association for Supervision and Curriculum Development. (2019). Making school a safe place. *Educational Leadership*.

CASEL. (2019). *What is SEL?* Retrieved from CASEL https://casel.org/what-is-sel/

Centers for Disease Control and Prevention & Association for Supervision and Curriculum Development. (2020). *Whole School, Whole Community, Whole Child (WSCC).* Retrieved from Centers for Disease Control & Prevention https://www.cdc.gov/healthyschools/wscc/index.htm

Centers for Disease Control and Prevention. (2020). *High School YRBS.* Retrieved from Centers for Disease Control and Prevention https://nccd.cdc.gov/youthonline/App/Default.aspx

Centers for Disease Control and Prevention. (2020). *2019 High School YRBS, Currently Frequently Used Electronic Vapor Products.* Retrieved from Centers for Disease Control and Prevention https://nccd.cdc.gov/youthonline/App/Results.aspx?TT=B&OUT=0&SID=HS&QID=QNDAYEVP&LID=LL&YID=RY&LID2=&YID2=&COL=&ROW1=&ROW2=&HT=&LCT=&FS=&FR=&FG=&FA=&FI=&FP=&FSL=&FRL=&FGL=&FAL=&FIL=&FPL=&PV=&TST=&C1=&C2=&QP=&DP=&VA=CI&CS=Y&SYID=&EYID=&SC=&SO=

Collaborative for Academic and Social Emotional Learning. (2020). *CASEL Competencies.* Retrieved from CASEL https://casel.org/wp-content/uploads/2019/12/CASEL-Competencies.pdf

Connolly, M. (2018). *Skills-based health education*, (2nd ed.). Burlington: Jones and Bartlett Learning.

Davidson, D. R. (2020). *3 Signature SEL Practices.* Retrieved from Washoe County School District https://www.washoeschools.net/Page/11083

Durlak, J. A., Weissberg, R. P., Dymnicki, A. B., Taylor, R. D., & Schellinger, K. B. (2011). The impact of enhancing students' social and emotional learning: A meta-analysis of school-based universal interventions. *Child Development, 82*(1), 405–432.

Elias, M. J.-S. (1997). *Promoting social and emotional learning.* Alexandria: ASCD.

Frey, N., Fisher, D., & Smith, D. (2019). *All learning is social and emotional; helping students develop essential skills for the classroom and beyond.* Alexandria: ASCD.

Joint Committee on National Health Education Standards. (2007). *National health education standards*, (2nd ed.). American Cancer Society.

Massachusetts Department of Elementary and Secondary Education. (2019). *Guidelines for the candidate assessment of performance; assessment of teacher candidates.* Malden, MA: Massachusetts Department of Elementary and Secondary Education.

Massachusetts Department of Public Health. (2020). *105 CMR 215: Standards for school wellness committees (PDF 24.84 KB).* Retrieved from https://urldefense.com/v3/__https://www.mass.gov/doc/105-cmr-215-standards-for-school-wellness-committees/download__;!!NCEDZeEw!r8jQoGXfdcWXveuvNzyQeDZv9qr9PhUFC3QQzWngbSFd_vlF7DcY7Ye3wroOTyayTFecHgm4VgU$

McTighe, J., & Judy Willis, M. (2019). *Upgrade your teaching, understanding by design meets neuroscience.* Alexandria: ASCD.

Merriam Webster. (2020). *Explain.* Retrieved from Merriam Webster: https://www.merriam-webster.com/dictionary/explain

Merriam Webster. (2020). *Neuroscience.* Retrieved from Merriam Webster: https://www.merriam-webster.com/dictionary/neuroscience

Merriam Webster. (2020). *Pedagogy.* Retrieved from Merriam Webster: https://www.merriam-webster.com/dictionary/pedagogy

National Institutes for Health. (2020). *How to quit vaping.* Retrieved from National Institutes for Health: https://teen.smokefree.gov/quit-vaping/how-to-quit-vaping

Stephanie Jones, K. B.-M. (March 2017). *Navigating SEL from the inside out looking inside & across 25 learning SEL programs: A practical resource for schools and OST providers.* Boston: Harvard Grduate School of Education with Funding from the Wallace Foundation.

USDA Food and Nutrition Service. U.S. Department of Agriculture. (2019). Retrieved from USDA Food and Nutrition Service; US Department of Agriculture https://www.fns.usda.gov/tn/local-school-wellness-policy

Waters, E., & Sroufe, A. L. (1983). Social competence as a developmental construct. *Developmental Review, 3*(1), 79–97.

YouTube Britain Has Talent. (2020, February 8). *Susan Boyle, first audition.* Retrieved from You Tube https://www.youtube.com/watch?v=jca_p_3FcWA

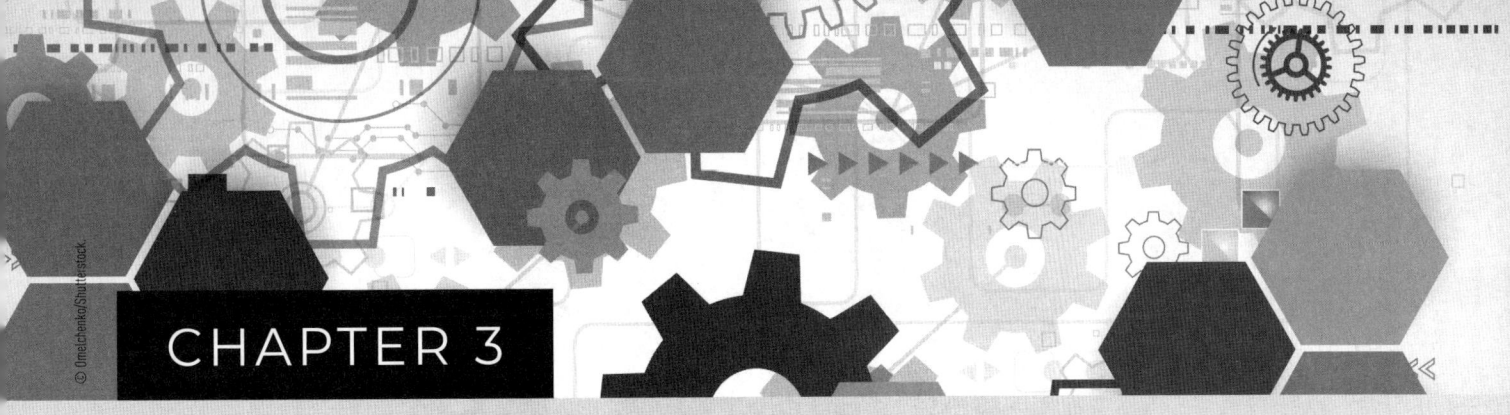

CHAPTER 3

Teaching Self-Awareness

LEARNING OBJECTIVES

Upon finishing this course, students will be able to:

- Plan skills-based health (SBH)/SEL lessons using backwards design and practice prompts.
- Incorporate the sub-competencies of self-awareness into assessment and instruction.

KEY TERMS

Emotions	Personal strengths	Self-efficacy
Fixed mindset	Self-awareness	Self-perception
Growth mindset	Self-confidence	

Social and Emotional Learning (SEL) Competencies*

- SELF-AWARENESS **Figure 3.1**
  - *The ability to accurately recognize one's own emotions, thoughts, and values and how they influence behavior. The ability to accurately assess one's strengths and limitations, with a well-grounded sense of confidence, optimism, and a growth mindset. (CASEL, 2019)*

Introduction

The competencies of Self-Awareness and Self-Management are linked because they are skills that regulate **emotions**, thoughts, values, and behavior.

They help us assess our strengths, allow us to goals, manage, and motivate ourselves with a sense of confidence.

Self-awareness is developed as youth learn to identify their emotions, develop an accurate **self-perception**, increase their **self-confidence**, develop their **self-efficacy**, and move from a **fixed mindset** to a **growth mindset**.

Teachers help students to develop self-awareness through numerous resources, activities, assessments, and reflections. At the beginning of the class, teachers often check SEL status. Younger students identify their emotions or those of a character in a prompt by pointing to pictures of faces expressing a range of emotions. English learners refer to an "emotional word/emoji wall" that lists the emotions in English and other languages. For older students, an SEL

---

*A scope and sequence document is included as an appendix at the end of this chapter.

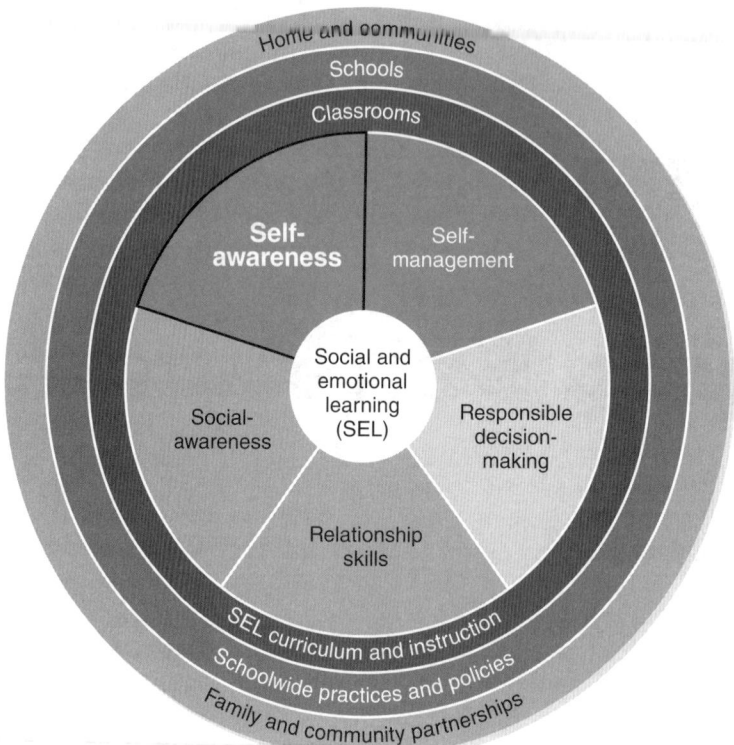

Figure 3.1 The CASEL Framework—Competency on Self-Awareness.

check-in consists of a written, graphic, or kinesthetic show of SEL status.

Strategies to help PreK-2 children develop self-awareness:

- Provide a picture word wall of the performance indicator verbs and the SEL competency and subcompetencies.
- Teach and practice mindfulness.
- Design a Cue Wall that shows pictures of physical and emotional cues. Use the pictures in various situations such as when identifying cues in stories or role plays. (Collaborative for Academic Social Emotional Learning, 2020)
- Use reading materials to identify the dimensions of health and how they are affected by behavior.
- Design prompts that challenge the student to identify an influence on the character's behavior and determine if it is positive or negative. Ask the students to identify the cues of an emotion. For example, students identify an emotional cue that helps them know if they are angry, happy, sad, etc. (Collaborative for Academic Social Emotional Learning, 2020)
- Read a sentence starter relating to how family or friends influence personal health and ask a student to complete the sentence. Encourage the children to identify the emotion, recognize how

it affected a dimension of health, and identify if there was a positive or negative influence and what they could do about it.
  - I was mad when my brother….because……
    I can feel better by……
  - I was happy when my mom……because….
  - I didn't like it when my friend……because…..
    I can feel better by……
- As students enter the classroom, they take an index card and write or draw how they are feeling. The teacher reviews the entrance tickets privately or walks from desk to desk to assess the emotional well-being of the students and how aware they are of their status. (Jones, 2018) The teacher provides feedback and coping skills to help and encourage the students. When she thinks the students are ready, she proceeds with the class.
- Students use a self-check during practice to remind them of the content, skill, and SEL competency requirements. During practice, the teacher determines the extent of student proficiency of content, skill, and SEL competency by observing and examining the self-check. She provides targeted feedback, when necessary.
- As students prepare to exit the class, the teacher provides an exit ticket that asks how the class

helped them be more self-aware. This technique is an excellent way to assess the acquisition of the content, skills, and SEL competencies.

Plutchik's Wheel of Emotion is a tool that helps identify feelings and how they relate to one another. (PsicoPico, 2019) **Figure 3.2**. Ways to use the wheel to enhance self-awareness include:

- Share a practice prompt and refer to the Wheel of Emotions to identify the emotion in the story.
- Use a personal Wheel of Emotion to identify feelings at the beginning or end of the class.
- Identify emotions when practicing Mindfulness.

The skills-based/SEL educator designs student engaging, age-appropriate instruction with targeted formative assessments and effective feedback. As students learn content and practice skills and SEL competencies, they become more self-aware and develop self-confidence.

When planning lessons, teachers use practice prompts as the daily vehicle to demonstrate and reinforce content, skill, and SEL competencies. The practice prompt includes how the characters are feeling to help students identify feelings in others and, thereby, become more aware of their own feelings. The teacher then challenges the student to determine how feelings influence behavior. If the influence is identified as positive, the student learns to reinforce the influence. If negative, he learns healthy coping strategies.

Providing effective feedback to students as they practice helps guide and direct the student to become proficient in the performance indicator and SEL competency. Successful completion of a skill practice gives the student the self-confidence to learn other skills, develop self-efficacy, and ultimately a growth mindset. (Frey, Fisher, & Smith, 2019, p. 29)

Table 3.1 describes the alignment of Self-Awareness to Standard 2 of the National Health Education Standards: Students analyze the influence of family, peers, culture, media, technology, and other factors on health behaviors. (Joint Committee on National Health Education Standards, 2007)

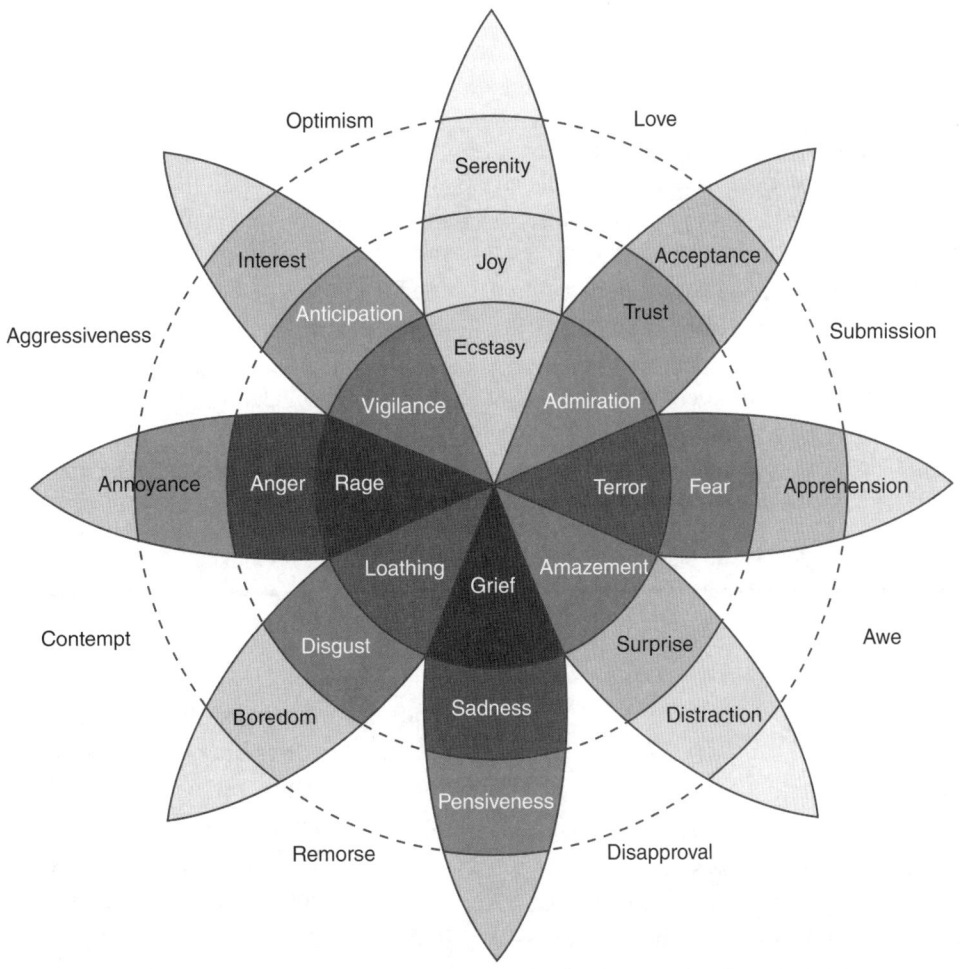

Figure 3.2 Plutchik's Wheel of Emotion.

Table 3.1 Alignment of Self-awareness to Standard 2 of the National Health Education Standards

Competency	Description	Subcompetencies
Self-Awareness	The ability to accurately recognize emotions, thoughts, and values and how they influence behavior. The ability to accurately assess strengths and limitations, with a well-grounded sense of confidence, optimism, and a "growth mindset." (Collaborative for Academic and Social Emotional Learning, 2020)	■ Identifying emotions ■ Accurate self-perception ■ Recognizing strengths ■ Self-confidence ■ Self-efficacy

When a person is self-aware, she is able to realistically assess strengths and shortcomings and have the confidence to embrace the strengths and know how to overcome short comings with effort or help. Skills-based health/SEL educators use prompts, based on infused performance indicators, to help students become self-aware and demonstrate proficiency in content, skill, and SEL competency.

For example:
Infused performance indicators:

- 1.5.1 Describe the relationship between healthy behaviors *such as not vaping* and personal health. (Joint Committee on National Health Education Standards, 2007, p. 24)
- 2.5.3 Identify how peers influence unhealthy behaviors *about vaping*. (Joint Committee on National Health Education Standards, 2007, p. 26)
- SEL: Self-awareness: Identifying emotions, accurate self-perception, recognizing strengths, self-confidence, self-efficacy, and growth mindset.

Shakina joined peer leadership and wants to teach the elementary students about vaping because her older sister tried vaping to look attractive and is now addicted. (1.5.1) The team is preparing a field trip to grade 5 to teach a lesson about how *peers influence each other to try vaping.* (2.5.3)

In groups, the 5th graders are taught to positively influence their peers by making public service announcements about the dangers of vaping and include information taught by the team. (2.5.3)

The problem is Shakina believes she cannot get up in front of the 5th graders and teach a lesson.

The advisor assured Shakina that the team would practice until the lesson was ready to present.

The advisor was right! The team practiced and practiced. As time went on, Shakina became more confident and was looking forward to working with the younger children. (SEL: Self-awareness: Identifying emotions, accurate self-perception, recognizing strengths, self-confidence, self-efficacy, growth mindset.)

In this example, the lesson taught to the 5th grade students included the relationship between not vaping and personal health as well as a plan to influence others not to vape through a public service announcement. Shakina increased her self-awareness by identifying her emotions, established an accurate self-perception, recognized her strengths, gained self-confidence and self-efficacy, and developed a "growth mindset."

Preview

Unit Plan

In a skills-based/SEL unit, the planner accesses and analyzes data then selects a standard 1 and skills performance indicator to reduce the risk factor and infuses them with content. The SEL competency and sub-competency are aligned with the infused performance indicators. Once established, the instructor plans the assessment and instruction.

Once the content, skill, and competency are taught, the teacher distributes the performance task, which consists of the unit prompt(s), the scoring rubric, back-up materials needed such as supplemental content, self-checks, and any other information the students need to show proficiency in the performance indicators and SEL competency. The students organize and practice for a few days and present their work to the class. This summative assessment is scored with an analytical rubric.

Skills-Based Lesson Plan

The skills-based/SEL lesson plan contains an agenda, the lesson objectives (infused standard 1 performance indicator and skills indicator, and the SEL competency/sub competency), a review/preview, the standard 1 content, the skill, competency, a student engaging practice prompt, clarifying questions relating to the prompt and learning objectives, a lesson review, and an exit ticket.

Skills-Based Lesson Infrastructure

The following sections present infrastructure for a lesson, not a unit. The infrastructure guides the teacher without interfering with individual creativity. Each lesson begins with an overview, data (when available), and a list of resources. Following the overview, a table initiates backwards design. It consists of the infused performance indicators and SEL competencies as the lesson objectives. Assessments are designed for each of the performance indicators and SEL competency. The prompt and the review questions engage the learner and help the teacher determine if the students met the lesson objectives. An exit question concludes the lesson infrastructure and provides an opportunity for students to reflect on how to use what was taught.

When reading, let your imagination guide your planning. You may need more or fewer lessons to teach the material. You may like an idea and modify it to meet the needs of your students. You may find the worksheets valuable or may prefer to edit them.

When modifying, maintain the integrity of the backwards design. Teach content, skill, and SEL each day. If the lesson infrastructure contains too much material, plan an additional day(s) but maintain the integrity of aligning SEL and teaching content through the infused performance indicators. Refer to the sample lessons at the end of each chapter to understand how to align SEL and teach content through the skill.

Organization

The learning activities for the core competency of self-awareness are divided into two sections:

- Recognizing emotions, thoughts and values, and how they influence behavior.
- Accurately assessing one's interests, strengths, and limitations, and possessing a well-grounded sense of self-efficacy and optimism.

Table 3.2 Self-Awareness by Subcompetencies

Identifying emotions	Self-confidence
Accurate self-perception	Self-efficacy
Recognizing strengths	

Each section below contains background information about the sub-competency followed by lesson suggestions and resources.

The National Health Education Standards (NHES) are grouped according to the grade spans PreK–2, grades 3–5, grades 6–8, and grades 9–12. The examples below follow that structure. The classroom examples may require the teacher to be creative and adjust instruction to accommodate the age and abilities of the students.

The headings of each section represent a self-awareness subcompetency (**Table 3.2**). The practice prompt is aligned with the competency and the infused performance indicators of the National Health Education Standards. State SEL standards from across the country also influence the design of the prompt.

Being self-aware is a fundamental life skill that develops with our cognitive development. (Randy M. Page., 2015, p. 52)

Section 1. Recognizing Emotions, Thoughts, and Values and How They Influence Behavior

(Collaborative for Academic Social Emotional Learning, 2020)

Recognizing/Identifying Emotions

How do we help a child recognize his own emotions, thoughts, and values? Standard 2 of the National Health Education Standards provides infrastructure for the development of self-awareness by analyzing the influence of family, peers, culture, media, technology, and other factors on health behaviors. The performance indicators challenge youth to examine the positive and negative influences they experience as well as clarifying personal values, beliefs, and perceived norms. (Joint Committee on National Health Education Standards, 2007, p. 26)

The steps of backwards design lesson instruction begin with the standards and SEL competency then progresses to assessment and instruction.

Through a variety of content taught through standard 1, the skills of standard 2, and the SEL competency, skills-based health/SEL educators help youth recognize how their own emotions, thoughts, and values influence their behavior.

PreK–2: Self-Awareness: Identifying Emotions

Lesson Overview: How the Family Influences Emotions.
Students learn the dimensions of wellness, how a family influences its children, and how to identify emotions.

Resources:

- Feel Wheel: https://media.centervention.com/pdf/Feel-Wheel-Worksheet-v2.pdf
- The Feelings Song: https://media.centervention.com/pdf/The-Feelings-Song-Worksheet.pdf
- Emotion regulation, Lesson 2-Degrees of Emotions: https://media.centervention.com/pdf/Emotion-Regulation-2-Degrees-of-Emotions.pdf
- Feelings Scavenger Hunt: www.centervention.com/

Materials needed:

- Emojis, wellness model, smiley and frowny faces, and pictures of a child expressing different emotions.
- **Worksheet 3.1 Identifying Feelings**

Table 3.3 provides an overview of the lesson objectives, assessment, and instruction for this lesson.

Step 3 – Instruction

1. Define
   a. Recognize: To identify a person or thing because there is a history of having seen or interacted with that person or thing in the past.
   b. Identify: To recognize a particular person or an object.
   c. Emotion: Human feelings, including love, happiness, anger, and fear, which also often involves a physical reaction.
2. 1.2.2 Recognize that there are multiple dimensions of health *affected by the positive or negative effects of emotion*
   a. Show the children several photos/emojis of faces that express different feelings. Ask the children which emotion the person is expressing.
   b. Caution the children that looks (body language) may be deceiving. A person may appear angry but may be just tired or sick.
   c. Introduce the physical, social, intellectual, and emotional components of wellness by describing the four circles on the board that depict the components of wellness: emotional, intellectual, social, and physical health. Above each circle, place a happy face and a

---

Table 3.3 Lesson Objectives, Assessment, and Instruction

Step 1 – Lesson Objectives	Step 2 – Assessment
The verb of the *infused* performance indicator and the SEL competency generate the assessment and instruction.	Design the assessment based on the objectives. Ask yourself the question, "What can my students do to show me they have met the standard?"
1.2.2 Recognize that there are multiple dimensions of health *affected by the positive or negative effects of emotion.* (Joint Committee on National Health Education Standards, 2007, p. 24)	1.2.2 Students recognize the multiple dimensions of health by placing *one* picture of an emotion from the practice prompt beside the component then determine if the emotion has a positive or negative effect on it.
2.2.1 Identify how the family influences personal health practices and behaviors *of their children.* (Joint Committee on National Health Education Standards, 2007, p. 26)	2.2.1 Students identify *two* examples of how the family's personal health practices and behaviors.
SEL-Self-Awareness: Identifying emotions, self-confidence	Students identify pictures of emotions from a story, categorize them as positive or negative influences on behavior, and discuss how their self-confidence changed as a result.

Step 3 – Instruction	
Design the instruction so that students learn the content, skill, and competency to be successful on the assessment. Ask yourself the question, "What do I need to teach so that the students will be successful when assessed?"	

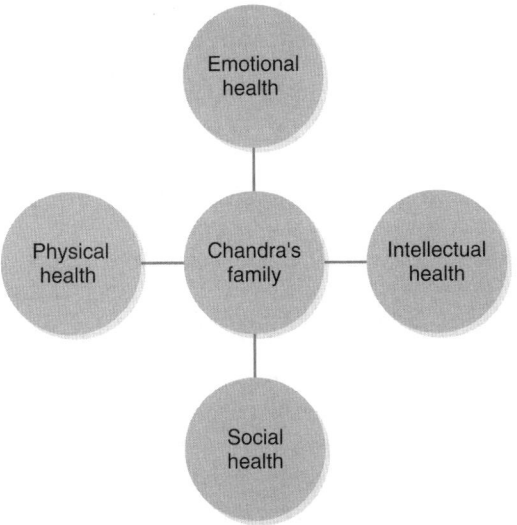

Figure 3.3 Chandra's Health as Related to her Emotions and her Family.

sad face. The graphics guide the children to categorize an emotion as having a positive or negative effect on that component of health.

   d. Read the story about Chandra (below) then show pictures of emotions that Chandra experienced in the story. Ask for volunteers to identify the component of wellness the picture represents. Help the student figure out if the emotion has a good or bad effect on Chandra's health. Place the picture near the component's happy or sad face (**Figure 3.3**). (SEL-Self-Awareness: iIdentifying emotions, self-confidence)

3. 2.2.1 <u>Identify</u> how the family influences personal health practices and behaviors *of their children*.
   a. Provides positive social interaction with each other and other families.
   b. Is a positive influence and support to their children and each other.
   c. Take care of one another when ill or upset.

4. Read the practice prompt, have students answer the reflection questions, and discuss.

Practice Prompt: Chandra

Chandra is in 2nd grade. She is a happy child and has several good friends. They like the same things she likes, and they have lots of fun together. The families know each other and often spend Saturdays together going on picnics or biking. She and her friends work hard in school and help one another with homework or when someone is having a bad day.

Her family supports one another when happy or sad, takes care of each other when illness occurs, encourages each child to do his or her best in

school and to make friends with peers who have the same family values they have.

Chandra tries hard to do what her family expects but sometimes she doesn't. When that happens, she feels sick, doesn't want to go to school, gets very quiet, and doesn't want to be around her family or her friends. One day, the family saw that Chandra was upset and they asked her, "What is wrong?" Chandra explained that she had an argument with her best friend, Lilly, and then Lilly wouldn't play with her during recess, the family gave her a few suggestions about how to handle the situation.

Chandra felt much better when she knew what to do to solve the problem. She looked forward to going to school, talking to Lilly, and being with her friends again. Her belly ache went away, and she was able to concentrate on her schoolwork.

5. To help the children accurately recognize emotions, thoughts, and values, ask the questions shown in **Table 3.4**.

6. End of class review. Ask the students to put away their materials then ask review questions.
   a. What is the name of one dimension of health? (1.2.2)
   b. How did Chandra's family help her when she was upset? (2.2.1)
   c. SEL-Self-Awareness: Identifying emotions.
      1) How did you identify emotions from the story?
      2) Once you identified the emotions, how did you figure out the effect on health?

7. Exit ticket (self-Awareness: identifying emotions)
   a. Draw a picture of an emotion you experienced in class.

   In addition to using prompts to help children recognize emotions, thoughts, and values and how they influence behavior, **Worksheet 3.1 Identifying Feelings** is a simple strategy to help children identify their feelings. The worksheet may serve as a SEL formative assessment and provide the teacher with valuable information regarding the status of the child. The child may need intervention to settle down in order to cope with a problem or an exciting situation.

Grades 3–5: Self-Awareness: Identifying Emotions
Lesson Overview: Reducing Screen Time. Students are challenged to self-assess their screen time, identify the feelings associated with unlimited and limited screen time, identify feelings

Table 3.4 The Effect of Emotions on the Components of Health and the Influences of Family on Children: How Emotions Change

Question	Answer
What were the effects of resolving Chandra's problem on her components of health? Were they positive or negative? (1.2.2)	**Chandra's emotional health** ■ Happy: *Positive influence* ■ Family is supportive: *Positive influence* ■ Family takes care of each other when illness occurs: *Positive influence* ■ As a result of having an argument with Lilly, she got quiet: *Negative influence* ■ When her family gave her suggestions about solving the problem with Lilly, Chandra felt better: *Positive influence* **Chandra's intellectual health** ■ Works hard in school: *Positive influence* ■ Help each other with homework: *Positive influence* ■ Family encourages each child to do their best in school: *Positive influence* ■ As a result of having an argument with Lilly, she didn't want to go to school: *Negative influence* ■ When her family gave her suggestions about solving the problem with Lilly, Chandra looked forward to going to school: *Positive influence* ■ When her family gave her suggestions about solving the problem with Lilly, Chandra was able to concentrate on her school work: *Positive influence* **Chandra's social health** ■ Has several good friends: *Positive influence* ■ Friends have fun together: *Positive influence* ■ Families know each other and have fun together: *Positive influence* ■ Help each other if one is having a bad day: *Positive influence* ■ Family encourages her to make friends with peers who have the same family values they have: *Positive influence* ■ As a result of having an argument with Lilly, she didn't want to be around her family or her friends: *Negative influence* ■ When her family gave her suggestions about solving the problem with Lilly, Chandra looked forward to going to school and being with her friends again: *Positive influence* **Chandra's physical health** ■ Sometimes Chandra does not do what her family expects, and she feels sick: *Negative influence* ■ When her family gave her suggestions about solving the problem with Lilly, Chandra's belly ache went away: *Positive influence*
What are two examples of how Chandra's family helped her? Did Chandra's family affect her health? (2.2.1)	■ Chandra's family recognized that Chandra was upset. ■ When her family learned what was bothering Chandra, they made suggestions on how to solve the problem. ■ Chandra felt much better when she knew how to solve the problem with Lily.
Did Chandra's emotions remain the same or did they change depending on the situation? (SEL Self-awareness: Identifying emotions)	Chandra's emotions changed depending on the situation. Most of the time, she was happy but sometimes things bothered her and she felt sick. When she felt this way, she did not want to be around her friends or go to school.

Emotional health — Physical health — Chandra's family — Intellectual health — Social health

| SEL-Self-Awareness: Identifying emotions, Self-confidence | The emotions identified in the story include: happy, sad, sick, quiet, upset. Chandra felt better when she knew what to do to solve the problem between Lily and herself. |

associated with being active, and consider ways to replace screen time with active time.

Between 40.9% and 51.2%, middle school students played video or computer games or used a computer three or more hours a day. (Center for Disease Control and Prevention, 2020) Screen time is associated with increased weight, decreased school performance, and an interference in friend and family relationships. (KidsHealth from Nemours, 2020)

Materials needed:

- Headings: Computer, mobile device, television, video games or **Worksheet 3.2 Self-awareness—Identifying Emotions—Screen Time**

   Table 3.5 provides an overview of the lesson objectives, assessment, and instruction for this lesson.

Step 3 – Instruction

1. Define
   a. Describe: To use words that help others envision the physical attributes of a person, place, or·thing.

   b. Emotion: Human feelings, including love, happiness, anger, and fear, which also often involves a physical reaction.
   c. Screen time: The amount of time a person spends watching television, playing electronic games, or on some other device(s). **Table 3.6** lists positive and negative effects of screen time.
2. 2.5.6. Describe ways that technology, *especially screen time,* influences thoughts, feelings, and health behaviors
   a. Place the following headings on the board: Computer, mobile device, television. (Kids Health from Nemours, 2020) As an alternative or small group work, use **Worksheet 3.2 Self-awareness—Identifying Emotions—Screen Time**
   b. On a sticky note, ask the students to write down the number of hours, each day, they spend in front of each of the above categories. Video games may be included in each category. Average the group time. Students place the

Table 3.5 Lesson Objectives, Assessment, and Instruction

Step 1 – Lesson Objectives	Step 2 – Assessment
The verb of the *infused* performance indicator and the SEL competency generate the assessment and instruction.	Design the assessment based on the objectives. Ask yourself the question, "What can my students do to show me they have met the standard?"
1.5.1 <u>Describe</u> the relationship between healthy behaviors *such as screen-free fun activities* and personal health. (Joint Committee on National Health Education Standards, 2007, p. 24)	1.5.1. <u>Describe</u> *two screen-free fun activities and* how they affect personal health.
2.5.6. <u>Describe</u> ways that technology, *especially screen time*, influences thoughts, feelings, and health behaviors. (Joint Committee on National Health Education Standards, 2007, p. 26)	2.5.6. <u>Describe</u> *two* ways that technology, *especially screen time*, influences thoughts, feelings, and health behaviors.
SEL-Self-Awareness: Identifying emotions.	Students identify the emotions experienced when screen time is limited or unlimited and when participating in screen free activities.
Step 3 – Instruction	
Design the instruction so that students learn the content, skill, and competency to be successful on the assessment. Ask the question, "What do I need to teach so that the students will be successful when assessed?"	

Table 3.6 Positive and Negative Effects of Screen Time

Positive Effects of Playing Video Games	Negative Effects of Screen Time
Improve eye–hand- coordination.	Spending a lot of time playing video games may limit active play time and lead to weight gain. (KidsHealth from Nemours, 2020)
Improve problem-solving skills.	How young people use their screens determines the result. Watching television and playing video games leads to poorer academic performance but interacting on social media sited does not. (The Bronfenbrenner Center for Translational Research (BCTR), 2020)
Improve the mind's ability to process information. (KidsHealth from Nemours, 2020)	Screen time interferes with relationships with friends and family. (KidsHealth from Nemours, 2020)

sticky notes under the headings. Discuss. (Amounts will vary by child, by school day, and weekday).

c. For each of the experiences, draw a T-bar. On one side write, "Unlimited Time" and on the other side, "Limited Time."

d. Ask the children to write down an emotion they feel when they have unlimited screen time as compared to limited screen time. (*You may want to provide emojis to limit the variety of responses.*) (2.5.6) SEL-Self-Awareness: Identifying emotions.

e. Ask the children to describe why they experience that emotion in that circumstance.

3. 1.5.1 <u>Describe</u> the relationship between healthy behaviors *such as screen-free fun activities* and personal health.

a. To overcome the negative influence of too much screen time on personal health, ask the children to identify three screen-free fun activities they would like to try and draw a picture of each.

b. Write down the emotion that the students feel when participating in the fun activities. (SEL-Self-Awareness: Identifying emotions) (KidsHealth from Nemours, 2020)

4. Read the practice prompt, students answer the reflection questions, and discuss.

Practice Prompt: Mateo

Mateo is in 3rd grade. He goes right home after school and waits for his older sister to come home. It is lonely being home alone. While waiting, he has a few cookies, does his homework then plays his video games. He knows he is putting on weight from eating too much and not being active. He doesn't like that.

When his sister Anna gets home, she also snacks, does her homework, and checks her social media. They don't have much to say to each other. He doesn't like that either.

Mateo and Anna's parents learned that playing video games may get in the way of doing well in school, so they decided to limit the afternoon screen time of both children and asked them to think of screen-free fun things to do together until they get home. Mateo and Anna became very grumpy about having their screen time limited.

However, they got a great idea!

The children decided to put on some music and walk around the house and go up and down the stairs for 15 minutes. After walking, they wrote a letter to their parents about where they wanted to go for vacation and exercised for another 15 minutes to music.

At first, they didn't like the idea of not being able to use their screens, but they found that their time together was fun. They didn't eat cookies and could begin to think about vacation. Being together and having fun was much better than sitting alone playing video games.

5. To help the children accurately identify emotions, thoughts, and values, ask the questions shown in **Table 3.7**.

6. End of class review. Ask the students to put away their materials then ask review questions.

a. How does being in front of a screen affect weight? Why? (1.5.1)

b. How does being in front of a screen affect relationships? Why? (1.5.1)

c. Does all screen time interfere with school performance? Explain (1.5.1)

d. What are two screen-free fun activities to do at home? (2.5.6)

e. What are some emotions felt when screen time is unlimited or limited and when children

Table 3.7 Screen-Free Fun Activities and the Influence of Screen Time on Thoughts, Feelings, and Health Behaviors: Identifying Emotions

Question	Answer
What were *two screen-free fun activities Mateo and his sister designed?* How did those activities affect their personal health? (Joint Committee on National Health Education Standards, 2007, p. 24) (1.5.1)	Mateo put on some music and he and his sister walked around the house and up and down the stairs. Mateo and his sister wrote a letter to their parents about where they would like to go on vacation.
What were *two* ways technology, *especially screen time*, influenced Mateo's thoughts, feelings, and health behaviors? (Joint Committee on National Health Education Standards, 2007, p. 26). (2.5.6.)	Mateo doesn't like putting on weight from being inactive. Mateo feels lonely. Mateo doesn't like that his sister doesn't pay much attention to him because after doing her homework, she goes on social media. Mateo was grumpy when his parents limited his screen time. When Mateo and Anna did screen-free activities, he enjoyed moving to music, spending time with his sister, and writing down their ideas for vacation.
How did Mateo and Anna identify their emotions? (SEL-Self-awareness: Identifying emotions)	Mateo was grumpy when his parents limited his screen time. At first, they didn't like the idea of not being able to use their screens, but they found their time together was fun. They didn't eat cookies, and they could begin to think about vacation. Being together and having fun together was much better than sitting alone playing video games.
SEL-Self-Awareness: Identifying emotions What were the emotions Mateo experienced when screen time was limited or unlimited and when participating in screen-free activities?	The emotions Mateo experienced in the story include: Being lonely, grumpy, enjoyed having fun with his sister.

are involved in fun screen-free activities? (SEL-Self-Awareness: Identifying emotions)

7. Exit ticket (Self-Awareness: Identifying emotions)

   Write down one feeling that is experienced when enjoying a physically activity.

Grades 6–8: Self-Awareness: Identifying Emotions

Lesson Overview: Effects of Bullying; Role of Peers, and the School in Prevention. This lesson identifies the emotions that children feel being bullied, how peers influence healthy and unhealthy behavior, and how the school contributes to a healthy and safe environment.

17.4% to 28.3% of middle school students report they were "Ever electronically bullied" including texting, Instagram, Facebook, and other social media. Girls were bullied more than twice as much as boys. (Center for Disease Control and Prevention, 2020)

31.9% to 47.6% report being "Bullied on school property." Girls were more frequently bullied on school property than boys. (Centers for Disease Control and Prevention, 2020)

Materials needed:

- Newsprint, markers, **Worksheet 3.3 The Effects of Bullying on the Components of Health**

   Table 3.8 provides an overview of the lesson objectives, assessment, and instruction for this lesson.

Table 3.8 Lesson Objectives, Assessment, and Instruction

Step 1 – Lesson Objectives	Step 2 – Assessment
The verb of the *infused* performance indicator and the SEL competency generate the assessment and instruction.	Design the assessment based on the objectives. Ask yourself the question, "What can my students do to show me they have met the standard?"

(continues)

Table 3.8 Lesson Objectives, Assessment, and Instruction *(continued)*

Step 1 – Lesson Objectives	Step 2 – Assessment
1.8.2 <u>Describe</u> the interrelationships of emotional, intellectual, physical, and social health in adolescence *when being bullied.* (Joint Committee on National Health Education Standards, 2007, p. 25)	1.8.2 <u>Describe</u> *three* interrelationships of emotional, intellectual, physical, and social health in adolescence *when being bullied.*
2.8.3 <u>Describe</u> how peers influence health and unhealthy behaviors *about bullying.* (Joint Committee on National Health Education Standards, 2007, p. 26)	2.8.3. <u>Describe</u> *one way* peers influence healthy behaviors and *one way peers influence* unhealthy behaviors *about bullying.*
2.8.10 <u>Explain</u> how the school and public health policies influence health promotion and disease prevention. (Joint Committee on National Health Education Standards, 2007, p. 26)	2.8.10 <u>Explain</u> *three* ways the school influences health promotion.
SEL-Self-Awareness: Identifying emotions	Students identify the three emotions experienced when being bullied and three emotions experienced when peers intervene to help.

Step 3 – Instruction
Design the instruction so that students learn the content, skill, and competency to be successful on the assessment. Ask the question, "What do I need to teach so that the students will be successful when assessed?"

Step 3 – Instruction

1. Define
   a. Describe: To use words that help others envision the physical attributes of a person, place, or thing.
   b. Emotion: Human feelings, including love, happiness, anger, and fear, which also often involves a physical reaction.
   c. Bullying: The act of intimidating, harassing, manipulating, and/or hurting a vulnerable person.
2. 1.8.2 <u>Describe</u> the interrelationships of emotional, intellectual, physical, and social health in adolescence *when being bullied.*
   a. Review the **Worksheet 3.3 The Effects of Bullying on the Components of Health.** Bullying information is found on the reverse of the graphic organizer.
   b. Place students in groups at their desks or at newsprint stations around the room.
   c. If grouping students using newsprint, refer to **Worksheet 3.3 The Effects of Bullying on the Components of Health** as a model. Draw a Venn diagram that contains four circles labeled Physical, Emotional, Social, and Intellectual on the newsprint. Follow the directions on the worksheet to complete the assignment.
   d. Provide each group with one of the prompts below and ask the students to write down

the effects of bullying on the character in the story in the appropriate circle.
   i. Place a + sign next to positive effects and a – sign next to the negative effects.
   ii. On the bottom of the paper, write down one way peers influence healthy behaviors and one way peers influence unhealthy behaviors about bullying. (2.8.3)
   iii. Circle three emotions experienced when being bullied and three emotions experienced when peers/school intervene to help. (SEL-Self-awareness: Identifying emotions)
   e. Effects of bullying (1.8.2)
   i. Depression
   ii. Anxiety
   iii. Future delinquent and aggressive behavior
   iv. Low self-esteem
   v. Alcohol and drug use into adulthood (National Academies of Sciences, 2016, pp. 6, 13, 126)
   vi. Sadness
   vii. Loneliness
   viii. Isolation
   ix. Sleep disturbance
   x. Heart disease
   xi. Eating disorders
   xii. Slumping academic performance (stopbullying.gov, 2020)

f. Bullying prompts
  i. Ellie is a little chubby. During physical education, some of her peers make fun of her and call her names. She tries to pretend the name calling doesn't bother her, but she feels anxious and depressed that peers don't like her just because of the way she looks. They don't even know her! Ellie often tells the teacher she doesn't feel well and asks to go to the nurse. She is always glad when she is back in the classroom because she feels safe, but she has trouble concentrating on her work because she is in class with the same bullies. Gennie, Ellie's classmate, saw what happened during PE and told the teacher. She also volunteered to stay with Ellie during class. The teacher thanked Gennie and during the next class reminded the group about the school bullying rule and that bullying will not be tolerated. Ellie is happy she has a new friend and that the teacher is going to do something about the bullying.
  ii. Darren is rather small for his age. The older boys often make fun of him. When in the lavatory, the bigger boys laugh at him. He feels humiliated! In the halls, the boys trip him and sometimes call him, "gay." Lately, Darren does not want to go to school. He tells his parents he doesn't feel well or stays in the bathroom so he will miss the bus. He is miserable! Darren's sister is a year older and heard about what is happening to her brother. She told her teacher, Mr. Dunlop, and asked him what can be done. Mr. Dunlop told the lav monitors to watch for Darren and make sure he can use the bathroom safely. He also told the assistant principal and he asked the peer leaders to make a public service announcement about bullying. The lave monitor and PSAs made a big difference. The bullies didn't want to get caught so they stopped. Darren feels happy and more confident and is grateful to his sister for helping him. (Connolly, 2018, p. 261)

3. 2.8.3 <u>Describe</u> how peers influence healthy and unhealthy behaviors *about bullying*.
  a. Use the second page of **Worksheet 3.3 The Effects of Bullying on the Components of Health** to examine the role of the bystander (2.8.3) and the school in preventing bullying. (2.8.10)

b. The role of friendships and characteristics of the bystander. (2.8.3)
  i. School friendships are a protective factor.
  ii. Bystanders have
    1) Empathy for the victim.
    2) Self-efficacy and believe that he or she has the skill to handle the situation.
    3) A sense of moral responsibility. (National Academies of Sciences, 2016, p. 77)
c. 2.8.10 <u>Explain</u> how the school and public health policies influence health promotion and disease prevention.
  i. Schools implement a survey to measure how students feel about bullying. When a schoolwide survey demonstrates overwhelming disapproval of bullying, there is less reported bullying.
  ii. Schools implement fair discipline practices.
  iii. Teachers provide a climate of support and empathy.
  iv. Schools provide students with connections to others such as having one trusted and supportive adult. (National Academies of Sciences, 2016, pp. 78, 79, 82, 85, 86)
4. Read Practice Prompt 1: Damien. Have students answer the reflection questions and discuss.

Read Practice Prompt 2: Marina. Have students answer the reflection questions and discuss.

Practice Prompt 1: Damien

Damien is in the 7th grade. He is smaller than the other boys and they make fun of him in physical education. In the halls, he gets pushed by some of the bigger boys when they are changing classes. He enjoys music, so he joined chorus, but the boys make fun of that activity, too. It seems everything he does and everywhere he goes, someone is taunting him.

Lately he doesn't want to go to school and isn't sleeping very well. His stomach hurts in the morning, so he doesn't eat. He sits by himself on the bus so no one will bother him. He feels very alone and stressed. He goes to the nurse's office before class ends and gets a late pass to the next class just so he doesn't have to be in the hall with the other kids. He is thinking of quitting chorus even though he enjoys it. He is having trouble concentrating and his grades are slipping.

Devin, one of his friends from chorus, saw Damien being bullied and felt very bad for him and wanted to help. Devin is the star of many of the theater productions and everyone knows and likes him. He knew what to do because he was bullied

(continues)

Practice Prompt 1: Damien   *(continued)*

when he was younger. He walked over to Damien and said, "Come on, you are going to be late for practice. Let's go!" Damien left with Devin and the other boys said nothing.

Devin told the chorus director what happened, and she made sure Damien felt safe during practice. Later, she told the principal and they decided they needed to learn more about bullying in the school. The following week, all students took a survey that asked questions about bullying. The results showed that most students don't like bullying and want the school to do something about it.

As a result, each classroom teacher talked about bullying and the effects on the victim and on the bully. Everyone was encouraged to report bullying when they saw it. Bullying reports went down.

Damien felt safe again and was feeling happy and well. He loves singing in the chorus and has made many friends with the other members. His grades are improving and he now looks forward to going to school.

Practice Prompt 2: Marina

Marina is in the 7th grade. She is very pretty and the boys like her. Roberto used to hang out with Nina and her friends but now he likes Marina.

Nina started rumors about Marina. She takes pictures of her when she isn't looking and puts them on Instagram with text that lies about her and Roberto. Marina doesn't know what to do. She thinks everyone is staring at her and talking about her.

Her sister Karena has noticed that something is wrong. They usually have fun together, but lately Marina always looks sad and stressed. She goes straight to her room after school. She tells Karena she is doing homework but she is actually checking social media to see if there are any more posts about her. She doesn't eat much at supper or have much to say.

In school, she doesn't socialize because she doesn't know whom to trust. She is feeling very anxious and dreads going to school. Her friends think she doesn't like them anymore. Her stomach hurts and she isn't sleeping well. She cannot concentrate on schoolwork and her grades are going down.

One afternoon, Karena went into Marina's room and saw that she wasn't doing homework but was on social media. She asked what was going on. Karena couldn't hold it in anymore and told her sister everything. Karena felt really bad for her sister. What was happening to her was wrong and she knew she had to tell their parents.

Karena's mom called the principal and asked her to do something about cyberbullying. During morning announcements, the principal reminded students that

bullying of any type is hurtful and against school policy and state law. She encouraged students to tell an adult as soon as they learn about any form of bullying.

The bulling finally stopped because someone told the principal about some bullying that was happening in the bathroom. The student was caught and that made other bullies stop. They didn't want to get caught.

Things are better now for Karina. Her friends understand why she stayed away but told her they would have helped if she had told them. Karina is friendly toward Roberto, and Nina doesn't care because she has another boyfriend.

5. To help the children accurately identify emotions, thoughts, and values, ask the questions shown in **Table 3.9**.
6. End of class review. Ask the students to put away their materials then ask review questions.
   a. What is one component of health and how does bullying affect it? (1.8.2)
   b. What is *one way* peers influence healthy behaviors about bullying? (2.8.3)
   c. What is *one way* peers influence unhealthy behaviors about bullying? (2.8.3)
   d. How can the school help stop bullying? (2.8.10)
7. Exit ticket (Self-Awareness-SEL: Identifying emotions)
   How does identifying emotions and values increase self-awareness?

Grades 9–12: Self-Awareness: Identifying Emotions

Lesson Overview: Body Image. Students think about the benefits of and barriers to maintaining a healthy weight and how their values influence maintaining a healthy weight.

Overweight teenagers may feel frustrated, angry, sad, embarrassed, depressed, worried about what other people think, be afraid of being judged and bullied, and lose self-esteem. Being aware of these emotions is the first step in coping with feelings that are connected to being overweight. (TeensHealth from Nemours, 2020)

32.4% of high school students report being slightly or very overweight. (36.1% of girls and 28.7% of boys). (Centers for Disease Control and Prevention, 2020)

Materials needed:

- **Worksheet 3.4 Bow Tie**
- **Worksheet 3.5 Strategies to Maintain a Healthy Weight**

Table 3.9 The Effect of Bullying on Emotional, Intellectual, Physical, and Social Health—Influences of Peers and the School: Emotions Experienced When Being Bullied

Question	Answer
What are *three* interrelationships of emotional, intellectual, physical, and social health in adolescence *when being bullied*? (1.8.2)	Emotional: The victim: ■ Feels anxious ■ Feels lonely ■ Is afraid to be with others Intellectual: The victim: ■ Doesn't want to go to school ■ Cannot concentrate ■ Grades are going down Physical: The victim: ■ Cannot sleep ■ Has a stomachache ■ Feels stressed Social: The victim: ■ Sits alone on the bus ■ Is afraid to be with others ■ Goes to the nurse to prevent passing in the halls to classes with other students
What is *one way* peers influence healthy behaviors and *one way peers influence* unhealthy behaviors *about bullying*? (2.8.3)	Peers influencing healthy behaviors ■ A peer can make the victim feel safe by guiding him or her away from the bully and telling a trusted adult. Peers influencing unhealthy behaviors ■ Pushing younger, smaller peers. ■ Taunting other peers. ■ Spreading rumors. ■ Posting false statements on social media.
What are *three* ways the school influenced health promotion? (2.8.10)	■ Implemented a survey to measure how students feel about bullying. ■ Implemented fair discipline practices. ■ Provided a climate of support and empathy. ■ Reminded all students that bullying is not the norm and not acceptable among peers, teachers, administrators, and families.
Self-Awareness-SEL: Identifying emotions Identify the three emotions experienced when being bullied and three emotions experienced when peers/family/school intervene to help.	Students identify the three emotions experienced when being bullied: 1. Anxiety 2. Loneliness 3. Fear Students identify the three emotions experienced when peers/family/school intervene to help. Damien ■ Relief ■ Safe ■ Positive ■ Friendship ■ Being able to do the things he enjoys such as singing in the chorus Nina ■ Relief ■ Safe ■ Positive ■ Friendship ■ Family ■ Being able to socialize without being afraid

Table 3.10 Lesson Objectives, Assessment, and Instruction

Step 1 – Lesson Objectives	Step 2 – Assessment
The verb of the *infused* performance indicator and the SEL competency generate the assessment and instruction.	Design the assessment based on the objectives. Ask yourself the question, "What can my students do to show me they have met the standard?"
1.12.7 <u>Compare and contrast</u> the benefits of and barriers to practicing a variety of healthy behaviors *such as maintaining a healthy weight.* (Joint Committee on National Health Education Standards, 2007, p. 25)	1.12.7 <u>Compare and contrast</u> *three* benefits of and *three* barriers to practicing a variety of healthy behaviors *such as maintaining a healthy weight.*
2.12.8 <u>Analyze</u> the influence of personal values and belief on individual health practices and behaviors *such as maintaining a healthy weight.* (Joint Committee on National Health Education Standards, 2007, p. 27)	2.12.8 <u>Analyze</u> two influences of personal values and beliefs on individual health practices and behaviors *such as trying to maintain a healthy weight.*
SEL-Self-Awareness: Identifying emotions	Students identify five emotions that they feel when overweight.

Step 3 – Instruction
Design the instruction so that students learn the content, skill, and competency to be successful on the assessment. Ask the question, "What do I need to teach so that the students will be successful when assessed?"

Table 3.10 provides an overview of the lesson objectives, assessment, and instruction for this lesson.

Step 3 – Instruction

1. Define
   a. Propose: To present a new idea for serious consideration and discussion by other people.
   b. Overweight: The state of being heavier than a normal, healthy weight.
   c. Emotion: Human feelings, including love, happiness, anger, and fear, which also often involves a physical reaction.
2. 1.12.7 <u>Compare and contrast</u> the benefits of and barriers to practicing a variety of healthy behaviors *such as maintaining a healthy weight.*
   a. Brainstorm the emotional problems associated with being overweight:
      i. Frustration
      ii. Anger
      iii. Sadness
      iv. Embarrassment
      v. Depression
      vi. Worry about what other people think
      vii. Fear of being judged and bullied
      viii. Loss of self-esteem. (TeensHealth from Nemours, 2020)
   b. Brainstorm how exercise affects emotions and overall health:
      i. Decreases
         a) Stress

         b) Anxiety
         c) Depression
      ii. Increases blood flow to the brain resulting in improved:
         a) Memory
         b) Creativity
         c) Problem-solving skills
         d) Body conditioning (Linda Meeks, 2011, p. 98)
   c. Compare and contrast the benefits of and barriers to practicing a variety of healthy behaviors *such as maintaining a healthy weight.*
      i. Using **Worksheet 3.4 Bow Tie**, place students in pairs. On the knot of the bow tie, write "Healthy Weight." On one of the bows write, "Benefits of maintaining healthy weight" and on the other, "Barriers to maintaining healthy weight." **Figure 3.4**
      ii. On the bottom of the page, identify the emotions associated with having a healthy weight on the left side of the continuum and the emotions associated with not having a healthy weight on the right.
      iii. Review student work and encourage the students to understand that although the barriers may interfere in maintaining a healthy weight, they can overcome them.
3. 2.12.8 <u>Analyze</u> the influence of personal values and belief on individual health practices and behaviors *such as maintaining a healthy weight.*
   a. Examine the BMI index shown in **Table 3.11** and explain how to read it.

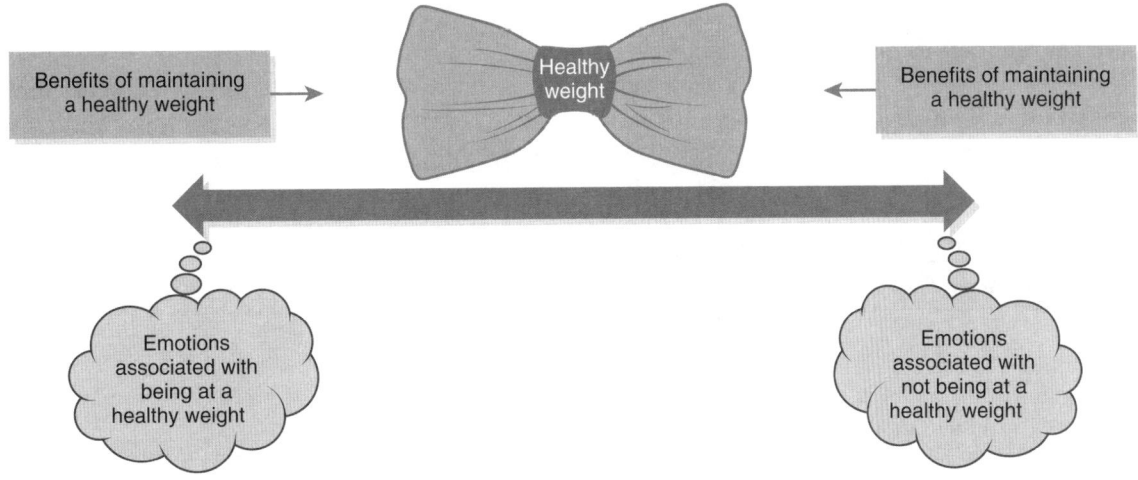

Figure 3.4 The Bow Tie.

Table 3.11 Body Mass Index

BMI	19	20	21	22	23	24	25	26	27	28	29	30	31	32	33	34	35
Height (inches)	Body Weight (pounds)																
58	91	96	100	105	110	115	119	124	129	134	138	143	148	153	158	162	167
59	94	99	104	109	114	119	124	128	133	138	143	148	153	158	163	168	173
60	97	102	107	112	118	123	128	133	138	143	148	153	158	163	168	174	179
61	100	106	111	116	122	127	132	137	143	148	153	158	164	169	174	180	185
62	104	109	115	120	126	131	136	142	147	153	158	164	169	175	180	186	191
63	107	113	118	124	130	135	141	146	152	158	163	169	175	180	186	191	197
64	110	116	122	128	134	140	145	151	157	163	169	174	180	186	192	197	204
65	114	120	126	132	138	144	150	156	162	168	174	180	186	192	198	204	210
66	118	124	130	136	142	148	155	161	167	173	179	186	192	198	204	210	216
67	121	127	134	140	146	153	159	166	172	178	185	191	198	204	211	217	223
68	125	131	138	144	151	158	164	171	177	184	190	197	203	210	216	223	230
69	128	135	142	149	155	162	169	176	182	189	196	203	209	216	223	230	236
70	132	139	146	153	160	167	174	181	188	195	202	209	216	222	229	236	243
71	136	143	150	157	165	172	179	186	193	200	208	215	222	229	236	243	250
72	140	147	154	162	169	177	184	191	199	206	213	221	228	235	242	250	258
73	144	151	159	166	174	182	189	197	204	212	219	227	235	242	250	257	265
74	148	155	163	171	179	186	194	202	210	218	225	233	241	249	256	264	272
75	152	160	168	176	184	192	200	208	216	224	232	240	248	256	264	272	279
76	156	164	172	180	189	197	205	213	221	230	238	246	254	263	271	279	287

National Heart, Lung, and Blood Institute. Body Mass Index Table 1. https://www.nhlbi.nih.gov/health/educational/lose_wt/BMI/bmi_tbl.htm. Accessed September 10, 2020.

b. Use underweight, healthy weight, and over weight numbers as hypothetical examples.

c. Discuss personal positive values (honesty, integrity, truthfulness, caring about self and others, etc.)

i. Establish that it is important to value personal health.

ii. Provide newsprint or **Worksheet 3.5 Strategies to Maintain a Healthy Weight Table 3.12**. Discuss the five strategies and

Table 3.12 Strategies to Maintain a Healthy Weight

Strategies to Maintain a Healthy Weight	Examples/Suggestions
Exercise. Physical activity burns calories, builds muscles, and helps to manage weight. To burn more calories, increase the intensity of the exercise. Add strength exercises to build muscle. The more muscle you have the more calories you burn.	Walking the dog, bicycling
Reduce Screen Time. The inactivity of sitting in front of a screen is linked to being overweight. Set limits on screen time and snack healthy while in front of the screen. Plan for exercise each day (60 minutes) and get 8–10 hours sleep.	Screen time includes television, playing video games, using computers, phones, and tablets not related to schoolwork.
Portion Distortion. Large portions include extra calories. If not balanced with exercise, weight increases. Soda, juice drinks, sports drinks are empty calories and contribute to being overweight.	Choose smaller portions or share a meal. Drink water or low-fat milk instead of soda.

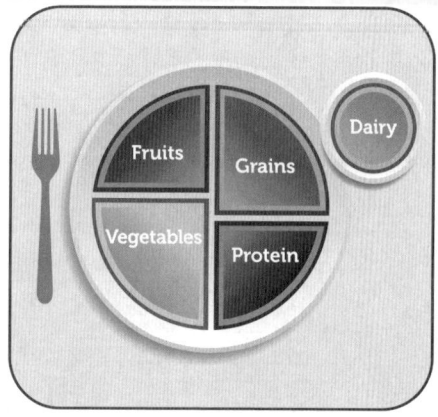
USDA Choose MyPlate, US Department of Agriculture, 2020. Retrieved from https://www.choosemyplate.gov/resources/myplate-graphic-resources
 	
Eat five servings of fruits and vegetables each day. Fruits and vegetables have the vitamins and minerals your body needs to grow. They contain fiber that makes you feel full.
	Vegetable Recommendation:
	■ Boys aged 14–18: Three cups of vegetables a day
	■ Girls aged 14–18: 2.5 cups
	   (USDA Choose MyPlate, US Department of Agriculture, 2020)
	
	Fruit Recommendation:
	■ 1–2 cups per day
	   (Choose MyPlate, US Department of Agriculture, 2020)

Eat breakfast. Breakfast provides the nutrients your body needs to start the day. Without breakfast, the person feels hungry sooner and may overeat, leading to overweight. People who skip breakfast have a higher BMI than those who do not.
 	
(TeensHealth from Nemours, 2020)
	■ Get up early enough to eat breakfast.
	■ Prepare breakfast the night before.
	■ Ask the person who does the grocery shopping to buy easy-to-eat-and-go foods:
	   • Small containers of milk or 100% juice
	   • Yogurt
	   • String cheese
	   • Cereal in individual boxes or portioned into baggies.
	   • Fresh, whole fruit
	   • Bagels
	   • Hard-boiled eggs
	   • Cold sandwich
	      (Alyssa Tucci, 2020)

provide time for the students to discuss and write down how to use the strategies in their lives or to help someone else. Also identify the emotion felt when implementing a strategy to maintain a healthy weight.

4. Read Practice Prompt 1: Charise. Have students answer the reflection questions and discuss.

    Read Practice Prompt 2: Liam. Have students answer the reflection questions and discuss.

5. To help the students accurately identify emotions, thoughts, and values, ask the questions shown in **Table 3.13**.

6. End-of-class review. Ask the students to put away their materials then ask review questions.

    a. Why is it important to compare and contrast when determining how to maintain health? (1.12.7)

    b. Why is it important to examine one's personal values and beliefs when determining how to maintain health? (2.12.8)

Practice Prompt 1: Charise

Charise has always struggled with her weight but now that she is older, it is even more difficult. When she was younger, her weight was just right, and she felt good about herself. Her clothes fit well, and she felt attractive. She would like to feel that way again.

She is frustrated because she cannot participate in after-school activities that help her control her weight because she babysits her younger brother when he gets home from first grade. Her younger brother is also a little overweight. She is a little embarrassed when she meets the bus because she feels like everyone is looking at them because they are overweight.

Lately, she is feeling a little lonely. When feeling this way, she likes to have a snack and go on social media to see what her friends are doing. She was shocked to read that someone made comments about her weight! She couldn't believe it! These are her friends! How could they say something like that about her! Maybe they won't want to hang out with her anymore! Time for a snack!

Her health teacher, Mrs. Fitwell, is teaching a unit on wellness. She started it by showing the numbers of high school students who consider themselves overweight. It was over 30%! This statistic shouldn't have made Charise feel better, but it did because now she knows she is not alone. Mrs. Fitwell challenged the class to examine the five ways to maintain a healthy weight on **Worksheet 3.5 Strategies to Maintain a Healthy Weight.**

After looking at the strategies to maintain a healthy weight, Charise decided that she and her brother could try to do something to manage their weight. When her brother comes home, instead of looking at social media, they will walk around the neighborhood to get some physical activity. If it is bad weather, they can make a game of walking around the house. Instead of snacking high calorie foods, she asked her mom to buy some fruit and flavored soda water. The water has no calories and tastes good. Because her mom is so busy in the morning, Charise is prepares breakfast foods she and her brother can eat so they don't get hungry before lunch.

After a few weeks, she started to see a difference. She feels better, her clothes are not so tight, and she has more energy.

Thank you, Mrs. Fitwell!

Practice Prompt 2: Liam

Liam works at a fast-food restaurant after school and on weekends. He goes to work right from school and is very hungry when he gets there. He has a few minutes before his shift begins so he grabs a cheeseburger and a soda. Although he is on his feet for his shift, he is not getting much exercise. When he gets home, he has a late supper. His mom makes great sauce, so he often has a dish of spaghetti. It is easy to make and is filling. After spending time with his family, he does his homework and checks social media. Before he knows it, it is time for bed.

When he was younger, Liam's weight was just right, and he felt good about himself. His clothes fit well, and he felt attractive. He would like to feel that way again.

Lately, his clothes are getting tighter, and it is not because he is growing! He is becoming self-conscious around his peers and is beginning to hear comments about his weight and his burger waist.

(continues)

Practice Prompt 2: Liam   *(continued)*

Liam doesn't like the way he looks and wants to do something about it. No one in his family is overweight. The family has always enjoyed time together that involves fun activities. He is missing those times with his family because he is working so many hours.

His health teacher, Mrs. Fitwell, is teaching a unit of wellness. She started the unit by showing the numbers of high school students who consider themselves overweight. It was over 30%! This statistic shouldn't have made him feel better but it did because now he knows he is not alone. Mrs. Fitwell challenged the class to examine the five ways to maintain a healthy weight on **Worksheet 3.5 Strategies to Maintain a Healthy Weight.**

After looking at the strategies to maintain a healthy weight, Liam decided that he would try to do something to manage his weight. Instead of eating high-calorie foods when he gets to work, he packs an extra lunch and eats healthy. To get exercise, he joined the before-school physical activity club. The teacher provides fun activities that get his heart and lungs working hard. Instead of eating a big dish of spaghetti for supper, he is trying to eat a variety of foods in the right portion. He is even taking time in the morning to eat breakfast.

Everything is making a difference. He feels better, his clothes are not so tight, and he has more energy. Thank you, Mrs. Fitwell!

Table 3.13 Benefits of and Barriers to Maintaining a Healthy Weight, Influences on Maintaining a Healthy Weight, and Emotions Experienced when Overweight

Question	Answer
What were *three* benefits of and *three* barriers that challenged Charise and Liam when trying to practice a variety of healthy behaviors *such as maintaining a healthy weight*? (1.12.7)	Three benefits of maintaining a healthy weight: ■ Feel better ■ Look better ■ Feel more confident Three barriers to maintaining a healthy weight: ■ No time to exercise ■ Unhealthy snacking ■ Eating when tired or distressed
What were two influences of Charise and Liam's personal values and beliefs on individual health practices and behaviors *such as wanting to maintain a healthy weight*? (2.12.8)	The worksheet Mrs. Fitwell used in class gave five excellent suggestions to maintain weight. Their responsibilities interfered with eating healthy and exercising.
Self-Awareness: Identifying emotions Identify five emotions experienced when overweight.	Five emotions experienced when overweight: ■ Frustration ■ Anger ■ Sadness ■ Embarrassment ■ Worry about what other people think ■ Feelings of loss due to a decrease in self-esteem (Linda Meeks, 2011, p. 98)

Data from TeensHealth from Nemours. (2020, February 21). Dealing With Feelings When You're Overweight. Retrieved from TeensHealth from Nemours: https://teenshealth.org/en/teens/feelings-overweight.html

c. How does eating healthy and exercising to maintain a healthy weight influence emotions? (Self-Awareness: Identifying emotions)

7. Exit ticket (Self-Awareness: Identifying emotions) What is one thing you can do to maintain a healthy weight? How does that decision make you feel?

Section 2. Accurately Assessing One's Interests, Strengths and Limitations, and Possessing a Well-grounded Sense of Self-efficacy and Optimism and a "Growth Mindset."

(Collaborative for Academic Social Emotional Learning, 2020)

Assessing interests, strengths, limitations, and developing self-efficacy, optimism, and a growth mindset requires introspection. A self-assessment is useful when gauging personal characteristics. The result of the assessment helps students discover their strengths and limitations and provides a window into how they perceive themselves. How we see ourselves and how others perceive us, however, may not be the same. The challenge to help youth become self-aware includes the discovery of an accurate perception of self.

Self-Perception is influenced by the media, family, friends, and teachers. (Randy M. Page., 2015, p. 58) If the influence is positive, the skills-based health/SEL educator encourages the students to embrace the influence and nurture it. If negative, we teach the coping skills necessary to overcome it.

The skills-based health/SEL instructor helps students gain self-confidence by teaching content, skills, and competencies step by step until the student reaches proficiency. This strategy helps students identify their strengths and learn to cope with their limitations in a healthy way. With self-confidence, students believe they are able to face challenges, set and achieve goals, and increase their self-efficacy. When children find ways to achieve goals, it brings a sense of optimism to their perception of self.

Example of Self-Efficacy and Growth Mindset

Although Mary has never competed in cross country, she believes she will do well in the meet. She practices hard, takes suggestions from her coach on how to improve her performance, watches other teammates who score well, and studies the videos of professional competitors. She knows something may happen beyond her control but she is prepared for the challenge. She has worked hard and is ready. Mary is demonstrating self-efficacy and a growth mindset.

When a student accurately assesses her interests, strengths and limitations, and possesses a well-grounded sense of self-efficacy and optimism, she may also exhibit a growth mindset.

Accurate Self-Perception/ Recognizing Strengths

PreK–2: Self-Awareness: Accurate Self-perception/Recognizing Strengths

Lesson Overview: Bicycle Safety. Students learn how to prevent injuries to the head and appreciate the influence parents have on their safety.

Between 26.3% (Vermont) and 80.4% (Kentucky) of middle school students rarely or never wear a bicycle helmet. (Center for Disease Control and Prevention, 2020) In this lesson, PreK–2 students advocate for bicycle safety and learn how to properly fit a helmet. The prompt demonstrates self-perception may change in response to different events and that children have strengths they did not know they possessed.

Materials needed:

- Bicycle helmet
- **Worksheet 3.6 Strengths, Weaknesses, and Asking for Help**

Table 3.14 provides an overview of the lesson objectives, assessment, and instruction for this lesson.

Table 3.14 Lesson Objectives, Assessment, and Instruction

Step 1 – Lesson Objectives	Step 2 – Assessment
The verb of the *infused* performance indicator and the SEL competency generate the assessment and instruction.	Design the assessment based on the objectives. Ask yourself the question, "What can my students do to show me they have met the standard?"

(continues)

Table 3.14 Lesson Objectives, Assessment, and Instruction (continued)

Step 1 – Lesson Objectives	Step 2 – Assessment
1.2.4 <u>List</u> ways to prevent common childhood injuries *to the head*. (Joint Committee on National Health Education Standards, 2007, p. 24)	Students <u>list</u> one way to prevent common childhood injuries *to the head*.
2.2.1 <u>Identify</u> how the family influences personal health practices and behaviors *about bicycle safety*. (Joint Committee on National Health Education Standards, 2007, p. 26)	Students <u>identify</u> three ways the family influences bicycle safety.
Self-Awareness: Accurate Self-perception, Recognizing strengths	▪ Students explain how self-perception changes in different situations. ▪ Students explain how a peer recognizes a personal strength he didn't know he had.

Step 3 – Instruction
Design instruction so that students learn the content, skill, and competency to be successful on the assessment. Ask the question, "What do I need to teach so that the students will be successful when assessed?"

Step 3 – Instruction

1. Define
   a. List: A number of related elements that appear one after another in a group.
   b. Demonstrate: To show how something is accomplished.
   c. Encouragement: Providing support to someone that facilitates the completion of a behavior.
   d. Self-perception: The complete understanding that a person has of who they are as a whole (physically, emotionally, mentally, and psychologically).
2. 1.2.4 List ways to prevent common childhood injuries *to the head*.
   a. Ask the children
      1) Who enjoys riding a bicycle?
      2) What safety equipment should we wear when we ride a bicycle? (helmet)
      3) What can happen if you don't wear a bicycle helmet?
      4) Is there a proper way to wear a bicycle helmet?
         a. **Fit:** Measure your head to get the right size.
         b. **Position:** Place the helmet level on your head and low on your forehead, one or two finger widths above your eyebrows.
         c. **Side Straps:** Adjust the straps so they make a "V" under and in front of the ears. Lock the clasp.

   d. **Buckles:** Center the buckle under the chin by adjusting the straps.
   e. **Final fitting:**
      • Yawn. The helmet should pull down on your head.
      • If the helmet moves forward or backward more than two fingers, adjust the straps.
      • Roll the rubber bands down to the buckle so the straps do not move. (National Highway Transportation Safety Association, 2020)
   5) Students practice how to properly fit a bicycle helmet to protect the head.
3. 2.2.1 <u>Identify</u> how the family influences personal health practices and behaviors *about bicycle safety*.
   a. Establish family bicycle safety rules, "No helmet, no wheels."
   b. Parents ride bicycles with their children and model how to properly fit a bicycle helmet.
4. To assess a child's accurate self-perception and their own strengths, ask
   a. Would you be comfortable asking a friend to wear a helmet when riding bikes? Why? Why not? (SEL-Self-awareness: Accurate self-perception)
   b. Is asking a friend to wear a helmet a sign of strength in your relationship? (SEL-Self-awareness: Recognizing strengths)
5. Read the practice prompt. Students answer the reflection questions and discuss.

Practice Prompt: Davide

Davide's family loves to go bike riding. His mom and dad showed him how to properly fit his helmet and won't let him ride without it. His mom says, "No helmet, no wheels!"

He rides his bicycle to school when the weather is good, and his mom walks beside him. Some of the children in the "Walking School Bus" do not wear helmets. Some children can't afford them, and others wear them on the back of their heads or don't clasp them.

Davide is not comfortable speaking up when he sees someone doing something that isn't safe because he doesn't want anyone to get mad at him. However, one day, his friend Mike, who never wears a helmet, rode over a hole in the sidewalk. He lost control, fell off his bike, and hit his head. His head starting bleeding, and he didn't wake up. His mother dialed 911 and the ambulance took him to the hospital. He had a concussion!

At lunch, the principal told the students that Mike was going to be okay but would be absent for a while until his concussion went away. Davide feels really bad that he didn't talk to Mike about wearing a helmet. He has an extra one and could have given it to him. Maybe Mike wouldn't have a concussion if he did!

Davide's mom is a member of the parent council and he asked her if they could organize a bicycle safety program. Part of the program would be to ask for helmet donations and distribute them to students who need them. Another part of the program would be a demonstration by the local bicycle shop owner about how to properly fit a helmet. The parent council loved the idea and the principal asked Davide to explain the program to the school during the morning announcements.

Because he saw his friend get hurt, Davide found the strength to speak up. After the announcements, all his friends and teachers complimented him. Although he didn't think he would be comfortable speaking up, Davide discovered that he could because he wanted to help his school mates be safe when riding a bicycle.

6. To help the students understand accurate self-perception and recognize strengths, ask the questions shown in **Table 3.15**.
7. Ask the students to put away their materials then ask review questions.
   a. Who can give an example of listing something? (1.2.4)
   b. Who can show me how to properly fit a helmet? (7.2.2)
   c. Who can give an example of how to encourage a friend to make a healthy choice? (Self-Awareness: Recognizing strengths)
   d. Give an example of a peer who has an accurate perception of themselves and another who does not. (SEL-Accurate self-perception)
   e. Give an example of how a friend can recognize his or her own personal (not physical) strengths. (SEL-Personal strengths)
8. Exit ticket (Self-Awareness: Accurate self-perception, recognizing strengths)
   a. Draw a picture of yourself wearing a bicycle helmet.
   b. Write down one personal strength (not physical) you have.

Table 3.15 Ways to Prevent Injuries to the Head, Influence of Family on Bicycle Safety, Speaking Up, and Self-Perception

Question	Answer
What is one way to prevent common childhood injuries *to the head*? (1.2.4)	Wear a bicycle helmet.
What are three ways Davide's family influences personal health practices and behaviors *about bicycle safety*? (2.2.1)	■ Davide's family taught him how to properly fit a bicycle helmet. ■ Davide's family will not let him ride his bike unless he wears a helmet. ■ Davide's mom is on the Parent Council and she organized a Bicycle Safety Program
Self-Awareness: Accurate Self-perception, Recognizing strengths How did speaking up about bicycle safety help Davide change how he felt about himself? How did Davide recognize a personal strength he didn't know he had?	Because he saw his friend get hurt, he decided he needed to speak up. After the announcements, all his friends and teachers complimented him and that made him feel good. Although Davide didn't think he had the personal strength to speak up, he realized he did because he wanted to help his school mates be safe when riding a bicycle.

In addition to using prompts to help children identify emotions, thoughts, and values and how they influence behavior, **Worksheet 3.6 Strengths, Weaknesses, and Asking for Help,** is a self-assessment that provides space for children to draw their strengths, weakness, and who they would approach if they needed help. The worksheet may serve as a SEL formative assessment and be used to inform assessment and instruction.

Grades 3–5: Self-Awareness: Accurate Self-Perception/Recognizing Strengths

Lesson Overview: Sun Safety. Students learn the relationship between sun safety and personal health and influence that peers have regarding sun safety.

57.2% of middle school students report having a sunburn in the last 12 months prior to the Youth Risk Behavior survey (YRBS). In this lesson, students learn how to protect themselves from the sun and how their self-perception can change with education.

Materials needed:

- Sunscreen
- Wide-brimmed hat
- Umbrella
- Sunglasses

Table 3.16 provides an overview of the lesson objectives, assessment, and instruction for this lesson.

Step 3 – Instruction

1. Define
   a. List: A number of related elements that appear one after another in a group.
   b. Describe: To use words that help others envision the physical attributes of a person, place, or thing.
   c. Self-perception: The complete understanding that a person has of who they are as a whole (physically, emotionally, mentally, and psychologically).
2. 1.5.1 <u>Describe</u> the relationship between healthy behaviors, *such as practicing sun safety,* and personal health.
   a. Ask the children:
      i. Who enjoys playing in the sun?
      ii. How do you protect yourself from the sun?
      iii. Show pictures of
         a) Wide-brimmed hat
         b) Sunscreen with an SPF (Sun Protection Factor) of 30 or more
         c) Sunglasses
         d) Umbrella
         e) Shade tree (**Figure 3.5**)

Table 3.16 Lesson Objectives, Assessment, and Instruction

Step 1 – Lesson Objectives	Step 2 – Assessment
The verb of the *infused* performance indicator and the SEL competency generate the assessment and instruction.	Design the assessment based on the objectives. Ask yourself the question, "What can my students do to show me they have met the standard?"
1.5.1 <u>Describe</u> the relationship between healthy behaviors, *such as practicing sun safety,* and personal health. (Joint Committee on National Health Education Standards, 2007, p. 24)	1.5.1 <u>Describe</u> *two* relationships between healthy behaviors, *such as practicing sun safety,* and personal health.
2.5.3. <u>Identify</u> how peers influence healthy and unhealthy behaviors *about sun safety.* (Joint Committee on National Health Education Standards, 2007, p. 35)	2.5.3. <u>Identify</u> *two ways* that peers influence healthy and unhealthy behaviors *about sun safety.*
Self-Awareness: Accurate Self-perception/recognizing strengths	Students explain how self-perception changes in different situations. Students explain how a peer recognizes a personal strength he didn't know he had.

Step 3 – Instruction
Design the instruction so that students learn the content, skill, and competency to be successful on the assessment. Ask yourself the question, "What do I need to teach so that the students will be successful when assessed?"

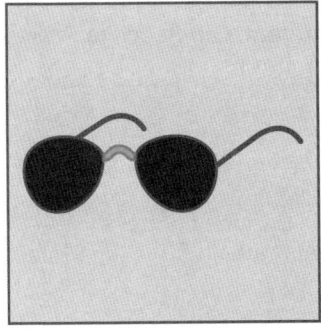 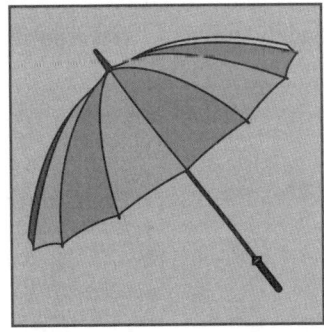 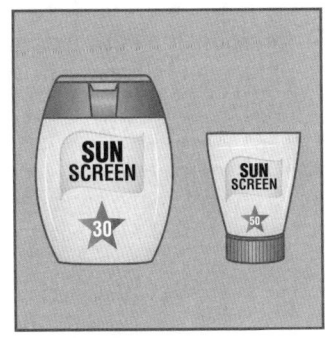

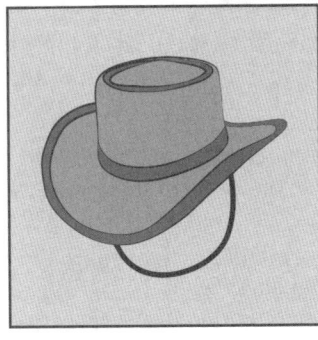 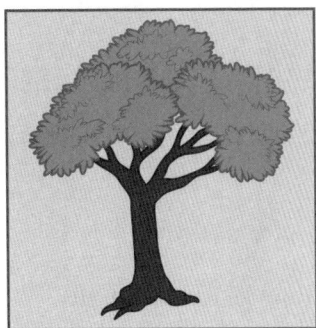

Figure 3.5 Ways to Practice Sun Safety.

b. Watch: George The Sun Safe Superstar-AXA-PPP Healthcare: https://www.youtube.com/watch?v=EwyqaLnsi5Q
c. Can dark-skinned people get sunburn?
   i. Dark-skinned people turn a darker brown.
   ii. Even if a dark-skinned person doesn't get a sunburn, their skin is still damaged by the sun. (American Academy of Dermatology, 2020)
   iii. (SEL-Self-Awareness: recognizing strengths)
3. 2.5.3 Identify how peers influence healthy and unhealthy behaviors *about sun safety*.
   a. **Worksheet 3.7 Sun Safety**
   i. Draw a picture of one peer influencing another peer to practice sun safety.
   ii. Draw a picture of one peer influencing another peer to not practice sun safety. How could you change that negative influence to a positive one?
4. Read the practice prompt. Students answer the reflection questions and discuss.

Practice Prompt: Carmella

Carmella lives in a sunny southern state. She has brown skin and has many friends with different shades of skin. She and her friends are always outside when it is not too hot out. She knows about sun safety but has never gotten a sunburn, so she doesn't worry about it. She thinks her brown skin protects her from the harmful rays of the sun.

Her family joined the community pool and now she is in the sun much more. The other day, the family settled under a tree and Carmella and her sister went swimming. They had a great time. When they weren't swimming, they were playing on the playground. When the family got home, Carmella saw that she had a sunburn. It hurt! The family was so excited about their first day at the pool that they forgot to put on sunscreen! She also didn't put on her hat, her long-sleeved T-shirt, or sunglasses when she was on the playground.

The next weekend, Carmella invited her friends to the pool. She was ready this time. She now knows she can get sunburn and plans to protect herself and her friends. Before her mother and father picked up her friends, she told them to put on sunscreen, bring a wide-brimmed hat, a cover-up, and sunglasses. She doesn't usually tell her friends what to do but she learned a lesson and didn't want them to get a sunburn.

Everyone had a great time swimming and playing and no one got burned!

5. To help the students understand accurate self-perception and recognize strengths, ask the questions in **Table 3.17**.
6. Ask the students to put away their materials then ask review questions.
   a. What are two ways to protect yourself from the harmful effects of the sun? (1.2.4)

Table 3.17 Relationship between Sun Safety and Personal Health, Influence on Peers to Practice Sun Safety, and Changes in Self-Perception

Question	Answer
<u>What were</u> *two* relationships between healthy behaviors, *such as practicing sun safety* and personal health, that Carmella discovered? (1.5.1)	Carmella practiced four sun safety tips to prevent sunburn and skin damage by ■ Wearing a wide-brimmed hat ■ Using sunscreen with an SPF (Sun Protection Factor) of 30 or more ■ Wearing sunglasses ■ Using an umbrella
<u>What were</u> *two ways* that Carmella influenced healthy behaviors *about sun safety*? (2.5.3)	Carmella invited her friends to the pool but told them to wear a hat, a cover-up, and bring sunglasses and sunscreen.
Self-Awareness: Accurate self-perception, recognizing strengths How did Carmella's self-perception change in different situations? How did Carmella recognize a personal strength she didn't know she had?	Carmella thought her brown skin protected her from the sun but realized it didn't when she got a sunburn from being in the sun for a long time without protection. Carmella doesn't usually tell her friends what to do but she didn't want them to get sunburn, so she told them what to bring to the pool to protect themselves.

    b. How can you be a positive influence about sun safety? (7.2.2)

    c. What is an example of a peer who has an accurate perception of him- or herself about sun safety and another peer who does not? (SEL-Accurate self-perception)

    d. What is an example of how to take action and demonstrate/recognize a personal strength? (SEL—recognizing strengths)

7. Exit ticket (self-awareness: Accurate self-perception, recognizing strengths)

Draw a picture of each way to protect yourself from the sun.

Did your perception of sun safety change after this lesson? Why? Why not?

Grades 6–8: Self-awareness: Accurate self-perception/recognizing strengths

Lesson Overview: Interests and Strengths. In this lesson, students identify their interests and strengths and build on them to improve their personal health. This lesson is a good way to introduce all the resources, clubs, and activities of the school.

Materials needed:

● Worksheet 3.8 Identifying Strengths and Matching to School Activities

Table 3.18 provides an overview of the lesson objectives, assessment, and instruction for this lesson.

Table 3.18 Lesson Objectives, Assessment, and Instruction

Step 1 – Lesson Objectives	Step 2 – Assessment
The verb of the *infused* performance indicator and the SEL competency generate the assessment and instruction.	Design the assessment based on the objectives. Ask yourself the question, "What can my students do to show me they have met the standard?"
1.8.1 <u>Analyze</u> the relationship between healthy behaviors, *such as identifying interests and strengths*, and personal health. (Joint Committee on National Health Education Standards, 2007, p. 25)	1.8.1 <u>Analyze</u> *two* relationships between healthy behaviors *such as identifying interests and strengths*, and personal health.
2.8.4 <u>Analyze</u> how the school and community affect personal health practices and behaviors *by helping students identify and connect their interests and strengths with academics, school clubs, and activities.* (Joint Committee on National Health Education Standards, 2007, p. 27)	2.8.4 <u>Analyze</u> *two* ways the school affects personal health practices and behaviors *by helping students identify and connect their interests and strengths with academics, school clubs, and activities.*

Self-Awareness: Accurate self-perception/Recognizing strengths	Students explain how self-perception changes in different situations.
	Students explain how a peer recognizes a personal strength he didn't know he had.

Step 3 – Instruction

Design the instruction so that students learn the content, skill, and competency to be successful on the assessment. Ask yourself the question, "What do I need to teach so the students will be successful when assessed?"

Step 3 – Instruction

1. Define
   a. Analyze: To scrutinize something or someone in order to understand how it or they work(s).
   b. Self-perception: The complete understanding that a person has of who they are as a whole (physically, emotionally, mentally, and psychologically).
2. 1.8.1 <u>Analyze</u> the relationship between healthy behaviors, *such as identifying interests and strengths*, and personal health.
   a. Ask the students
      i. Why is it important to understand your interests and strengths?
      ii. How does knowing your interests and strengths affect your personal health?
   b. Construct an interest and strength chain. Adapted from 2017 Understood for All. https://assets.ctfassets.net/p0qf7j048i0q /uvqC72wUOXlmeeSapX3Y6/7c0fcc7b 9271d4374c7a9afdcabd8b08/Strengths _Chain_Understood.pdf
3. 2.8.4 <u>Analyze</u> how the school and community affect personal health practices and behaviors *by helping students identify and connect their interests and strengths with academics, school clubs, and activities*.
   a. Ask the students how the school connect student interests and strengths with academics, clubs, and activities?
   b. Use **Worksheet 3.8 Identifying Strengths and Matching to School Activities** to help students identify their strengths and connect them to school.
4. Read the practice prompt. Students answer the reflection questions and discuss.

Practice Prompt: Spencer

Spencer is new to the middle school. His family moved from the city to the suburbs, and everything is new to him. He is feeling insecure and nervous because he doesn't have any friends yet. His new school has a good reputation, and he is looking forward to making friends and getting involved in school activities. His old school had very limited activities, so Spencer is not sure what he is good at or where he will fit in.

Jeremy, a peer leader from the Health Education Club, met him the first day of school and introduced him to each of his teachers, took him from class to class, invited him to sit with his friends at lunch, and made sure he got on the right bus to go home. What a relief!

The next day, Jeremy introduced him to all the club advisors, and they gave him a copy of the yearbook and information about each of the clubs. Spencer is very excited! He would like to become a peer leader because Jeremy was so helpful to him, and he now has the confidence to join the robotics and the afterschool workout clubs.

Spencer feels so much better and looks forward to going to school each day. He had no idea he would be interested in becoming a peer leader, but he is learning and loving it. He has a new student tomorrow morning, and he is looking forward to showing him around just as Jeremy had done for him. He is meeting lots of other students in robotics and the workout club. He is feeling very good about his new school and about himself.

Oh, he is also doing fine in his academics. He knows where to go and what to do if he gets stuck. Spencer loves his new school!

5. To help the students understand accurate self-perception and recognize strengths, ask the questions shown in **Table 3.19**.
6. Ask the students to put away his or her materials then ask review questions.
   a. Why is it important to identify strengths and interests? (1.8.1)
   b. How does the school affect personal health practices and behaviors *by helping students identify and connect their interests and strengths with academics, school clubs, and activities?* (2.8.4)
   c. How does knowing your interests and strengths affect how you perceive yourself? (SEL-Accurate self-perception)

Table 3.19 Relationship between Identifying Interests/Strengths and Personal Health, Influence of the School to Help Students Identify Interests and Strengths, and Changes in Self-Perception

Question	Answer
What are two relationships *Spencer discovered* between healthy behaviors *such as identifying interests and strengths,* and personal health? (1.8.1)	When Spencer first moved to his new home, he didn't know anyone and didn't know much about his new school except it had a good reputation. He felt insecure and nervous. After Jeremy introduced him to staff, students, and different activities, Spencer became very excited about his new school and his confidence increased.
What are two ways Spencer's school affects personal health practices and behaviors *by helping students identify and connect their interests and strengths with academics, school clubs, and activities*? (2.8.4)	Jeremy took Spencer from class to class and introduced him to his teachers, invited him to lunch, introduced him to the club advisors so he could see all the activities the school offered, and made sure he got on the right bus after school. As a result, Spencer became interested in peer leadership, robotics, and the afterschool workout club. Spencer likes his academic classes and where to go and what to do if he needs help.
Self-Awareness: Accurate self-perception, recognizing strengths How did Spencer's self-perception change in different situations? How Spencer recognized a personal strength he didn't know he had?	Spencer was first feeling insecure and nervous and unsure of himself before school started. Once he got to know his teachers, other students, and all the activities available, he gained confidence. Spencer didn't know anything about peer leadership until he went to his new school. He is now a peer leader and enjoys helping other new students.

   d. What is one way to help recognize your strengths? (SEL-Recognizing strengths)

7. Exit ticket

   How does recognizing your strengths help you have an accurate self-perception? (Self-Awareness: accurate self-perception, recognizing strengths)

Grades 9–12: Self-Awareness: Accurate Self-Perception/ Recognizing Strengths

Lesson Overview: Sexually Transmitted Infections (STIs). Students learn the hazards of participating in unprotected sexual intercourse and how alcohol consumption contributes to unprotected sex.

- 27.4% of high school students report being sexually active. (Center for Disease Control and Prevention, 2020)

- 45.7% of high school students report not using a condom during their last intercourse. (Centers for Disease Control and Prevention, 2020)
- Half of all STIs occur in young people aged 15–24 years.
- One in four new STI cases occurs in teenagers.
- Young people aged 15–24 account for 70% of all gonorrhea infections and 63% of chlamydia infections.
- Young people aged 13–24 account for approximately one in every four new HIV infections in the United States. (American Sexual Health Association, 2020)

Materials needed:

- **Worksheet 3.9 Consequences of STI Infection**

   Table 3.20 provides an overview of the lesson objectives, assessment, and instruction for this lesson.

Table 3.20 Lesson Objectives, Assessment, and Instruction

Step 1 – Lesson Objectives	Step 2 – Assessment
The verb of the *infused* performance indicator and the SEL competency generate the assessment and instruction.	Design the assessment based on the objectives. Ask yourself the question, "What can my students do to show me they have met the standard?"
1.12.9 <u>Analyze</u> the potential severity of injury or illness if engaging in unhealthy behaviors *such as having intercourse without using a condom.* (Joint Committee on National Health Education Standards, 2007, p. 25)	1.12.9 <u>Analyze</u> the potential severity of injury or illness *of one STI* if engaging in unhealthy behaviors *such as having intercourse without using a condom.*

2.12.9 <u>Analyze</u> how some health-risk behaviors, *such as drinking alcohol*, influences the likelihood of engaging in unhealthy behaviors *such as having intercourse without using a condom.* [Joint Committee on National Health Education Standards, 2007, p. 27]	2.12.9 <u>Analyze</u> how some health-risk behaviors, *such as drinking alcohol*, influences the likelihood of engaging in unhealthy behaviors *such as having intercourse without using a condom.*
Self-Awareness: Accurate self-perception, recognizing strengths	Students explain how self-perception changes in different situations. Students explain how a peer recognizes a personal strength he didn't know he had.

Step 3 – Instruction

Design the instruction so that students learn the content, skill, and competency to be successful on the assessment. Ask the question, "What do I need to teach so that the students will be successful when assessed?"

Step 3 – Instruction

1. Define
   a. Analyze: To scrutinize something or someone in order to understand how it or they work(s).
   b. Self-perception: The complete understanding that a person has of who they are as a whole (physically, emotionally, mentally, and psychologically).
2. 1.12.9 <u>Analyze</u> the potential severity of injury or illness if engaging in unhealthy behaviors *such as having intercourse without using a condom.*
   a. Use **Worksheet 3.9 Consequences of STI Infection** to help students analyze the cause, effects, and treatment of STIs. (1.12.9)
3. 2.12.9 <u>Analyze</u> how some health-risk behaviors, *such as drinking alcohol*, influences the likelihood of engaging in unhealthy behaviors *such as having intercourse without using a condom.*

   Students complete the True/False to learn about the effects of Sexual Risk Behaviors. (Centers for Disease Control and Prevention, 2020) Design a game (Kahoot.com) or a True/False sort or a verbal True/False using a white board or red, yellow, and green circles. (2.12.9)
   a. T F Teen substance use is associated with sexual risk behaviors that put teens at risk for STIs. (T)
   b. T F The more a teen abuses substances, the likelihood of having sex decreases but the number of partners increases. (F-the likelihood of having sex increases and the number of partners increases.
   c. T F Sexual risk behaviors are the highest with teens who drink alcohol. (F-the risk is the highest with teens who use marijuana, cocaine, prescription drugs, and other illicit drugs.)
   d. T F Adolescents who report no drug use are the least likely to engage in sexual risk taking. (T)
   e. T F According to Youth Online, CDC, of the students who are currently sexually active (29%), 19% drank alcohol or used drugs before the last sexual intercourse. (T)
   f. T F Association with drug-using peers is not a risk factor for sexual risk behaviors. (F. A common risk factor for substance use and sexual risk behaviors include association with substance-using peers.)
   g. T F When the teen's school environment is supportive and parents are engaged with their lives, teens are less likely to use alcohol and engage in sexual behaviors that put them at risk for HIV, STIs, or pregnancy. (T)
4. Read the practice prompt. Students answer the reflection questions and discuss.

Practice Prompt: Alicia and Danne

Alicia and Danne have been friends since middle school. Lately, Alicia is worried about Danne because she is behaving strangely. Danne always needs to go to the bathroom and can't seem to sit still. She often goes to the nurse with pain in her abdomen. When Alicia asks Danne what is wrong, Danne doesn't answer.

On Friday night, they were going to Natty's house for pizza and a movie. Alicia is a little shy in a group

(continues)

Practice Prompt: Alicia and Danne *(continued)*

but was looking forward to going. When they got to the house, Henry was there. He said, "Hi" but Danne didn't answer. She pulled Alicia away from him and told her not to get friendly with him. "He was bad news," she said. Natty's older brother was home and he took out some beers and passed them around. Danne grabbed one and drank it right down. Alicia was getting worried about her.

When Alicia found Danne sick in the bathroom, she asked her what was going on. Danne told her she was with Henry last weekend and they got drunk and had sex. Henry said he would use a condom, but he didn't. A few days later, Danne had a terrible itch in her crotch and some white smelly substance on her underwear. Alicia knew right away Danne had an STI but she didn't know which one.

The next day, Alicia took Danne to the health clinic to be tested. Alicia never thought she could do

something like that, but she knew if the STI wasn't treated, Danne could get very sick. She also knew from health class that teens can be tested and treated for an STI without their parents knowing. Otherwise, Danne wouldn't go.

Danne tested positive for gonorrhea. The doctor prescribed an antibiotic and told her she would be fine in several days but to use a condom every time she had sex because some STIs don't have symptoms and make you very sick.

Danne thanked Alicia for being such a good friend. She is not sure she would have the strength to go to the clinic on her own. Alicia felt good that she helped her friend. She was surprised she was so determined to help Danne because she considered herself shy and not one to take control of a situation. Not this time!

5. To help the students understand accurate self-perception and recognizing strengths, ask the questions shown in **Table 3.21**.
6. Ask the students to put away their materials then ask review questions.
   a. Select an STI and explain the severity of illness if not treated. (1.12.9)
   b. What is a sexual risk behavior? (2.12.9)
   c. What is the relationship between drinking alcohol and sexual risk taking? (2.12.9)
   d. Explain how accurate self-perception changes with different situations. (SEL-Accurate self-perception)
   e. What is one way to help recognize your strengths? (SEL-Recognizing strengths)
7. Exit ticket

   How does recognizing your strengths help you have an accurate perception of yourself? (**Self-Awareness**: Accurate self-perception, recognizing strengths)

Table 3.21 Injury or Illness Related to Sexually Transmitted Infections, How One Risk Factor Contributes to Another, and Changes in Self-Perception

Question	Answer
What was the potential severity of injury or illness *of gonorrhea* if engaging in unhealthy behaviors *such as having intercourse without using a condom*? (1.12.9)	Danne contracted gonorrhea and experienced abdominal pain, itchy crotch, and smelly discharge because she had intercourse without using a condom.
How do some health-risk behaviors, *such as drinking alcohol,* influence the likelihood of engaging in unhealthy behaviors *such as having intercourse without using a condom*? (2.12.9)	Danne got drunk with Henry and had intercourse without a condom.
Self-Awareness: Accurate self-perception, Recognizing strengths How did Alicia's self-perception change in different situations?	Alicia always considered herself shy, but that perception changed when she looked back and realized how she took control of the situation and got Danne the help she needed.
How did Alicia recognize a personal strength she didn't know she had?	Alicia didn't realize she had the personal strength to take charge of the situation and get Danne the help she needed.

Self-Confidence/Recognizing Strengths

"Students need to believe in themselves if they are to truly engage in learning. Teachers, in turn, need to help students develop self-confidence."

(Frey, Fisher, & Smith, 2019, p. 26)

For students to develop self-confidence, they need to believe in themselves and their abilities. This conviction is accomplished over time by discovering talents, learning content, and demonstrating skills and SEL competencies.

Adults with self-confidence are not compelled to discuss their successes admit when they have made a mistake and use the mistake to improve themselves. They acknowledge compliments, recognition from others, and the resources that have helped them achieve. Our goal is for children to develop their self-confidence and be able to demonstrate these characteristics.

In the classroom, effective feedback helps students develop self-confidence. (Frey, Fisher, & Smith, 2019, pp. 27-28) When observing students practicing during a lesson or preparing for their authentic assessment, compare the student evidence to the performance indicators and SEL competencies in the lesson or challenge.

Rather than saying, "Very good!" which may result in the students feeling good about what they are doing but not knowing why, say, "Your work demonstrates that you are using the performance indicators and SEL competency to design your role play. That connection shows me that you understand how to demonstrate the content, skill, and competency!"

To help students stay focused on the performance indicators and SEL content, design a self-check of all the requirements of the practice or authentic assessment. Using the self-check is an excellent formative assessment for the teacher. It paces student work and enhances student self-confidence to complete a demonstration of lesson objectives or the authentic assessment.

In skills-based health/SEL education, students gain self-confidence and recognize their strengths by learning a skill in progressive steps and demonstrating their competence in response to a prompt.

- Step 1: Explain why it is important to learn the skill, the relevance to a student's life, and how the skill connects to other skills.
- Step 2: Explain the steps of the skill.
- Step 3: Model the skill.
- Step 4: Provide student practice time. Design age-appropriate and relevant practice prompts that challenge the students to practice and demonstrate the skill.
- Step 5: Formatively assess student skill practice and provide effective feedback. (Joint Committee on National Health Education Standards, 2007, p. 14)

PreK–2 Lesson: Self-Awareness: Self-Confidence/Recognizing Strengths

Lesson Overview: Preventing the Spread of Communicable Disease. In this lesson, students learn the connection between school health education instruction and personal health by identifying that the skills of handwashing, covering the mouth when sneezing or coughing, support personal health practices and behaviors.

As a result of this content knowledge and skill, self-confidence is increased and students recognize that they have the personal strength to discipline themselves to keep a social distance, sneeze in the sleeve, cough into their shirts, and use the steps of handwashing to keep their hands clean.

Note:

- Because of the length of the health class and the age of the children, the content of the lesson may be taught over several lessons.
- Normally, coughing and sneezing into the sleeve and handwashing are found in Standard 7, practicing health behaviors. However, 2.2.2 Identify what the school does to support personal health practices and behaviors (Joint Committee on National Health Education Standards, 2007, p. 26) also aligns well when we include the role of the health education teacher as part of what the school does to support personal health practices and behaviors.

Materials needed:

- "Glo Germ" powder or a similar product to demonstrate the importance of proper handwashing to rid the hands of germs.

Table 3.22 provides an overview of the lesson objectives, assessment, and instruction for this lesson.

Table 3.22 Lesson Objectives, Assessment, and Instruction

Step 1 – Lesson Objectives	Step 2 – Assessment
The verb of the *infused* performance indicator and the SEL competency generate the assessment and instruction.	Design the assessment based on the objectives. Ask yourself the question, "What can my students do to show me they have met the standard?"
1.2.1 <u>Identify</u> that healthy behaviors, *such as preventing being infected,* affect personal health. (Joint Committee on National Health Education Standards, 2007, p. 24)	1.2.1 Students <u>identify</u> *the difference between a bacterial and a virus* and healthy behaviors *to prevent being infected.*
2.2.2 <u>Identify</u> what the school does to support personal health practices and behaviors *in addition to teaching about preventing communicable infections.* (Joint Committee on National Health Education Standards, 2007, p. 26)	2.2.2 Students <u>identify</u> *three ways* the school protects their health and *demonstrate* the skills taught by the health educator *such as social distancing, sneezing in the sleeve, covering the mouth when coughing, and the proper steps of handwashing* that support personal health practices and behaviors.
Self-Awareness: Self-confidence, recognizing strengths	Students explain why social distancing, sneezing into the sleeve, or covering the mouth when coughing increases self-confidence not to spread germs or to become infected. Students explain why using the steps of handwashing increases self-confidence not to get sick or to sicken others. Students explain why having the discipline to wash hands is a personal strength.

Step 3 – Instruction
Design the instruction so that students learn the content, skill, and competency to be successful on the assessment. Ask yourself the question, "What do I need to teach so that the students will be successful when assessed?"

Step 3 – Instruction

1. Define
   a. Describe: To use words that help others envision the physical attributes of a person, place, or thing.
   b. Demonstrate: To show how something is accomplished.
   c. Self-confidence: The ability to depend on one's own strength, talent, and ability.
2. 1.2.1 <u>Identify</u> that healthy behaviors, *such as preventing being infected,* affect personal health.
   a. Explain the difference between a virus and bacteria **Table 3.23**.
   b. Demonstrate (model) how to cough and sneeze into the sleeve. (KidsHealth from Nemours, 2020) to prevent being infected.
      i. Bend your arm at the elbow and sneeze into the bend.
      ii. Students practice sneezing into the sleeve and covering the mouth when coughing.
      iii. Formatively assess
         a) Explain that germs are spread through the air or from person to person when someone coughs or sneezes.

b) Use "Glo Germ" to demonstrate how "germs" are spread from one person to another by touch.
   c. Demonstrate (model) the steps for handwashing to prevent being infected. After the demonstration, students who have the "Glo Germs" on their hands practice handwashing while the teacher formatively assesses and provides effective feedback.
      i. **Wet** the hands with clean, running water; turn off the tap; and apply soap.
      ii. **Lather** the hands by rubbing them together with the soap. Lather the back of the hands, between the fingers, and under the fingernails.
      iii. **Scrub** the hands for at least 20 seconds. To check the time, sing Happy Birthday twice.
      iv. **Rinse** the hands well under clean, running water.
      v. **Dry** the hands using a clean towel or air dry. (Center for Disease Control and Prevention, 2020)
3. 2.2.2 <u>Identify</u> what the school does to support personal health practices and behaviors *in*

Table 3.23 **The Difference between a Virus and a Bacteria**

Bacteria	One-celled plant that gets nutrients from the environment to live, including the human body. They can grow in or outside the body. There are good bacteria that keep our digestive system healthy and others that make us sick. Examples of the bacteria that make us sick are those that cause ear infections, strep throat, tonsillitis, cavities, and pneumonia. An antibiotic kills the bacteria.
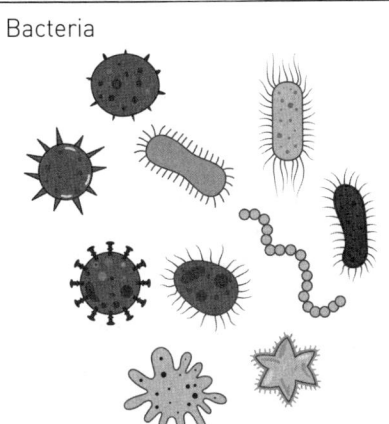	
Virus	Viruses must be inside the body to grow. They cause chicken pox, cold, flu, measles, and other illnesses. Our body's immune system kills the virus.
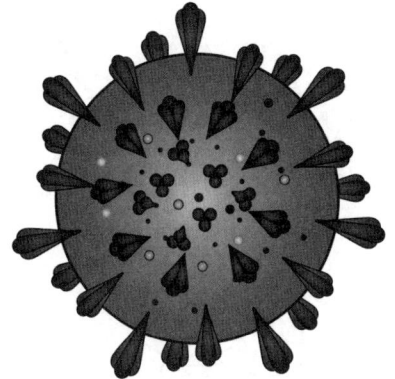	

Data from KidsHealth from Nemours. (2020, January 20). What are Germs? Retrieved from KidsHealth from Nemours: KidsHealth.org/en/kids/germs.html

addition to teaching about preventing communicable infections.

a. Ask the children, "What does the school do to help protect us from getting or spreading germs?"
   i. Soap in the lavatories.
   ii. Hand dryers in the lavatories.
   iii. Hand sanitizers
   iv. School nurse
   v. Health education
4. Read the practice prompt. Students answer the reflections questions and discuss.

Practice Prompt: Tanzena

Tanzena is looking forward to a family trip to Disney World during the February vacation. Last year, she remembers that many of her classmates got sick with the flu just before vacation and eventually, so did she. Tanzena is worried she will get sick again and her vacation will be ruined!

This year, Mrs. Applegate, the elementary health teacher, taught the class how cold and flu germs are passed from one person to another by shaking hands, touching something that has germs on it then touching eyes, mouth, or nose, and breathing in air that has germs from a cough or sneeze.

She showed the class pictures of bacteria and virus and how they make us sick. She demonstrated how to protect oneself and others from the germs by fist or elbow "bumping" to greet another person, sneezing and coughing into the sleeve, social distancing, and the effective way to use hand sanitizer and wash hands.

After Mrs. Applegate explained how germs are spread, showed the germ pictures, and demonstrated the skills, she gave the students time to practice. Around the room, there were different stations.

■ Station 1. The children sorted pictures of bacteria and viruses. Tanzena checked the answer key

(continues)

Practice Prompt: Tanzena   *(continued)*

and found she sorted most of the pictures correctly.

- Station 2. The children looked at pictures then practiced fist and elbow "bumping," the proper way to use hand sanitizer, and standing 6 feet away from a person who may be sick.
- Station 3. This station was fun! The children washed their hands while singing "Happy birthday" twice, the amount of time Mrs. Applegate told them would wash off the germs.
- Station 4. The children practiced coughing and sneezing in their sleeve or pulling up their shirts and sneezing into it.

Mrs. Applegate also told the children that the school works hard to prevent the spread of germs by providing soap, hand dryers, hand sanitizers, having a nurse in the building, and health education classes.

Tanzena thinks differently now about getting sick and knows she can get sick even if she cannot see the germs. However, she feels more confident because she knows how to prevent the spread of germs, how to get rid of germs on her hands, and how the school is helping her stay healthy.

5. Guide the students through the assessment questions in **Table 3.24**.
6. Ask the students to put away their materials then ask review questions.
    a. How does a virus spread? (1.2.1)
    b. How does a bacterium spread? (1.2.1)
    c. How should you greet others when they may have an infection? (1.2.1)
    d. What is the proper way to sneeze into the sleeve? (2.2.2)
    e. What is the proper way to cover the mouth when coughing? (2.2.2)
    f. What are the proper steps of handwashing? (2.2.2)

    g. How does knowing how germs are spread and the skills to keep germs from spreading give us confidence? (SEL-Self-Awareness: Self-confidence)
7. Exit ticket (Self-Awareness: Self-confidence, recognizing strengths)

    You just saw your friend rinse his hands before eating! He didn't use soap! What would you do? What would you say?

    Alternate: Sing "Cough, Cough, Cough, and Sneeze to the tune of "Row, Row, Row Your Boat."

    Cough, cough, cough and sneeze, but not into your hand,

Table 3.24 **The Difference between a Virus and Bacteria, How the School Protects the Health of Students, and Change in Self-Confidence**

Question	Answer
How did Tanzena identify *the difference between a bacteria and a virus* and healthy behaviors *to prevent being infected*? (1.2.1)	Tanzena sorted pictures, identifying bacteria and viruses. Tanzena learned about strategies to protect herself from people who may be infected.
What are *three ways* the school protects their health and *demonstrate* the skills taught by the health educator *such as social distancing, sneezing in the sleeve, covering the mouth when coughing, and the proper steps of handwashing* that support personal health practices and behaviors? (2.2.2)	Tanzena learned that the school protects her health by having soap and hand dryers in the lavatories, hand sanitizer, a school nurse, and a health educator. Tanzena practiced fist or elbow "bumping" instead of shaking hands; using hand sanitizer frequently; and standing 6 feet away from someone who may be sick. Tanzena practiced washing her hands, coughing and sneezing in her sleeve or shirt.
Self-Awareness: Self-confidence, recognizing strengths How did Tanzena's self-confidence change after she learned about how to protect herself against getting sick?	Tanzena's self-confidence increased after she learned how to protect herself.

Use a tissue or an elbow, that's the law of the land.

Wash, wash, wash your hands, wash them every day.

After you go and before you eat, keeps yucky germs away!

Keep, keep, keep your hands, out of your eyes, mouth, nose.

Stay away from colds and flu, so you can stay on your toes! (KidsHealth in the Classroom, 2020)

Grades 3–5: Self-Awareness: Self-Confidence/Recognizing Strengths

Lesson Overview: Responding to Emergency. In this lesson, students gain self-confidence when they learn when and how to react to an emergency and call 911. By practicing this skill and gaining confidence in being able to recognize a dangerous situation and how to respond, they recognize their own **personal strengths**.

Note: There are many safety situations to use in this lesson. Choose the situation that best relates to your students.

Materials needed:

- Cell phones or a facsimile
- Pictures of dangerous and not dangerous situations
- **Worksheet 3.10 When to Tell**

Table 3.25 provides an overview of the lesson objectives, assessment, and instruction for this lesson.

Step 3 – Instruction

1. Define
   a. Demonstrate: To show how something is accomplished.
   b. Destructive: To cause something or someone to be harmed or broken.
   c. Disturbing: Behavior that results in others feeling worried, anxious, nervous, and alarmed.
   d. Emergency: A situation that calls for quick action to find a solution.
   e. Self-confidence: The ability to depend on one's own strength, talent, and ability.
   f. Personal strengths: A talent or positive quality of a person.
2. 1.5.1 <u>Describe</u> the relationship between healthy behaviors, *such as knowing what to do in an emergency,* and personal health
   a. Ask students
      i. When should a person call 911? (Emergency)
      ii. What is an example of an emergency that requires a call to 911?
   b. Show pictures of different situations that are/are not destructive, dangerous, and disturbing

Table 3.25 Lesson Objectives, Assessment, and Instruction

Step 1 – Lesson Objectives	Step 2 – Assessment
The verb of the *infused* performance indicator and the SEL competency generate the assessment and instruction.	Design the assessment based on the objectives. Ask yourself the question, "What can my students do to show me they have met the standard?"
1.5.1 <u>Describe</u> the relationship between healthy behaviors, *such as knowing what to do in an emergency,* and personal health. (Joint Committee on National Health Education Standards, 2007, p. 24)	1.5.1 <u>Describe</u> *one* relationship between healthy behaviors, *such as knowing what to do in an emergency,* and personal health.
2.5.1 <u>Describe</u> how the family influences personal health practices and behaviors *such as how to respond to emergencies.* (Joint Committee on National Health Education Standards, 2007, p. 26)	2.5.1 <u>Describe</u> *one way* the family influences a child's personal health practices and behaviors *such as knowing how to respond to emergencies.*
Self-Awareness: Self-confidence, Recognizing strengths	▪ Explain how learning what to do in an emergency increases self-confidence. ▪ Explain how learning what to do in an emergency helps to recognize the personal strength to act.

Step 3 – Instruction
Design the instruction so that students learn the content, skill, and competency to be successful on the assessment. Ask the question, "What do I need to teach so that the students will be successful when assessed?"

and ask them to identify in which situations it would be appropriate to call 911.

  c. Explain that knowing what to do in an emergency increases self-confidence.

3. 2.5.1 <u>Describe</u> how the family influences personal health practices and behaviors *such as how to respond to emergencies*

  a. Parents teach the children what to do in an emergency.

  b. Families practice how to respond in emergencies.

4. Read the practice prompt. Students answer the reflection questions and discuss.

Practice Prompt: Lyda

Someone in Lyda's family always seems to be sick, having an accident, or being in the middle of an emergency. Lyda's mom and dad decided they needed to teach their children what to do in an emergency.

Lyda was scared when her mom started talking about what to do in an emergency but after a while she felt better knowing what to do.

Her dad is a fire fighter and described situations when she should dial 911; then they practiced. She didn't think she would ever have to call 911 but now she had the inner strength and confidence to do it!

One day, she went to Lyndon's house after school. He was hungry so he asked Lyda if she would like some popcorn. Lyda thought he was going to use the microwave, but he poured oil in a pan and told her when it got hot, he would pour the popcorn into the pot. They started playing a video game and forgot about the oil. All of a sudden, they both smelled smoke and ran to the stove. It was on

---

fire! Lyda didn't hesitate, she grabbed the phone and called 911. She told the policewoman there was a fire. She gave her name, Lyndon's address, and his phone number. The policewoman told them to go outside and that the firefighters were on their way.

Lyndon couldn't move so Lyda pulled him outside and called her parents. She told Lyndon to call his parents also. They were going to be really mad because he was not supposed to use the stove when home alone.

The firefighters put out the fire and told the children they did the right thing to call 911. Both parents arrived shortly afterward. Lyndon was right; his parents were mad but very glad he was safe. Lyda's parents were very proud of her for knowing what to do in the emergency, but she will not be going to a friend's house anymore, unless a parent is home!

Lyda was proud of herself for knowing what to do and doing it.

---

5. Guide the students through the assessment questions in **Table 3.26**.

6. Ask the students to put away their materials then ask review questions.

  a. What is an example of a destructive situation that would require calling 911?

  b. What is an example of a dangerous situation that would require calling 911?

  c. What is an example of a disturbing situation that would require calling 911?

  d. How did Lyda feel after she safely responded to the fire emergency? (1.5.1) (SEL-Self-Awareness: Self-confidence, recognizing strengths)

Table 3.26 Describing What to Do in an Emergency, How the Family Influences a Child to Know What to Do in an Emergency, and Self-Confidence

Question	Answer
What is *one* relationship between healthy behaviors, *such as knowing what to do in an emergency*, and personal health? (1.5.1)	Because Lyda knew what to do in an emergency, she had the self-confidence to act when the oil in the pan caught on fire.
What is *one way* the family influences a child's personal health practices and behaviors, *such as knowing how to respond to emergencies?* (2.5.1)	Lyda's family taught her to call 911 and practiced with her. Now, when there is an emergency, she has the confidence to know what to do.
Self-Awareness: Self-confidence, recognizing strengths How did learning what to do in an emergency increase Lyda's self-confidence? How did learning what to do in an emergency help Lyda recognize she had the personal strength to act?	Lyda learned to call 911 and get away from danger. Knowing how to react gave her the confidence to act. Knowing what to do in an emergency gave Lyda the strength to react to the emergency.

e. How did Lyda's family influence her personal strength and self-confidence so that she knew what to do in an emergency? (2.5.1)

7. Exit ticket (Self-Awareness: Self-confidence, recognizing strengths)

You saw someone fall off the curb. She can't move and is screaming in pain. What should you do? How does having self-confidence help you cope with an emergency?

Use **Worksheet 3.10 When To Tell** to reinforce the content, skill, and SEL competency.

Grades 6–8: Self-Awareness: Self-confidence/Recognizing Strengths

Lesson Overview: Reducing Screen Time When with Friends. In this lesson, students become aware of the benefits and barriers to reducing screen use and how social media affects time with friends.

In 2015, 10% of tweens used social media every day compared with 13% in 2019. (Rideout, 2019, p. 20)

Note: A sample lesson plan for this grade span is found at the end of the chapter.

Materials needed:

- **Worksheet 3.11 Benefits and Barriers to Limiting Screen Time When out with Friends.**

- **Worksheet 3.12 How Using Social Media Affects Teenagers**

Table 3.27 provides an overview of the lesson objectives, assessment, and instruction for this lesson.

Step 3 – Instruction

1. Define
   a. Demonstrate: To show how something is accomplished.
   b. Describe: To use words that help others envision the physical attributes of a person, place, or thing.
   c. Analyze: To scrutinize something or someone in order to understand how it or they work(s).
   d. Self-confidence: The ability to depend on one's own strength, talent, and ability.
   e. Personal strengths: A talent or positive quality of a person.

2. 1.8.7 <u>Describe</u> the benefits of and barriers to practicing healthy behaviors *such as cutting down on social media when out with friends*
   a. Model the problem: Model being preoccupied with social media on the cell phone. Express concern over what you are reading; comment on having to respond; all of a sudden, bring your attention back to the class.
   b. Ask the students
      i. "What was your reaction to being ignored?"

Table 3.27 Lesson Objectives, Assessment, and Instruction

Step 1 – Lesson Objectives	Step 2 – Assessment
The verb of the *infused* performance indicator and the SEL competency generate the assessment and instruction.	Design the assessment based on the objectives. Ask yourself the question, "What can my students do to show me they have met the standard?"
1.8.7 <u>Describe</u> the benefits of and barriers to practicing healthy behaviors *such as cutting down on social media when out with friends.* (Joint Committee on National Health Education Standards, 2007, p. 25)	1.8.7 <u>Describe</u> the *three* benefits of and *three* barriers to practicing healthy behaviors *such as cutting down on social media when out with friends.*
2.8.6 <u>Analyze</u> the influence of technology *(social media)* on personal and family *relationships.* (Joint Committee on National Health Education Standards, 2007, p. 27)	2.8.6 <u>Analyze</u> *three* influences *social media* has on personal *relationships.*
Self-Awareness: Self-confidence, recognizing strengths	Demonstrate self-confidence when encouraging friends to decrease social media use when out socializing.
	Demonstrate the personal strength to speak up when encouraging friends to decrease social media use when out socializing.

Step 3 – Instruction
Design the instruction so that students learn the content, skill, and competency to be successful on the assessment. Ask yourself the question, "What do I need to teach so that the students will be successful when assessed?"

ii. "Have you ever experienced being out with friends and everyone was on their phones rather than talking to each other? How does it make you feel?"

iii. Use the **Worksheet 3.11 Benefits and Barriers to Limiting Screen Time When out with Friends** to brainstorm the benefits and barriers to limiting screen time when with friends. Discuss. (Self-Awareness: Self-confidence/Recognizing strengths.)

3. 2.8.6 <u>Analyze</u> the influence of technology (*social media*) on personal and family *relationships*.

   a. **Use Worksheet 3.12 How Using Social Media Affects Teenagers** to read about how screen time affects relationships. Discuss.

   b. How screen time affects relationships
      1) Depression
      2) Anxiety
      3) Loneliness
      4) Lack of development of social and interpersonal skills
      5) Saying things in texts that would not be said in person
      6) Choose to be on screen than interact in real time.

4. Read the practice prompt. Students answer the reflection questions and discuss

Practice Prompt: Harrison

Harrison and Ian were hanging out after school waiting for their ride home. Both were on their phones checking their messages. They look forward to being able to use their phones after school to catch up on what everyone is doing. Teachers won't let them use their phones for texting or using other social media apps. Althea joined them. The boys said "Hi" but didn't look up from their screens. Althea was very upset and was hoping that the boys would pay attention and listen to her. She needed her friends.

After school, Althea got a terrible text from two of her friends. They were making fun of her for who she sat with at lunch. Althea felt badly for a girl who was sitting alone so she sat with her. Her friends were at a nearby table and were being rude, laughing at her, pointing at her, and making comments. After lunch, her friends wouldn't talk to her. She tried texting them but they ghosted her.

When she saw Harrison and Ian, she wanted to tell them what happened, but they wouldn't talk to her either. She thought they were friends! She couldn't sleep all night and had a head and

belly ache in the morning. She didn't want to go to school.

Harrison and Ian found out what happened the next day and wondered why Althea didn't come to them for help. She told them she did, but they didn't pay any attention to her when she approached them yesterday afternoon. The boys had no clue! It made them think. Maybe when friends are together, they could keep their phones away and just talk to each other. They all want to be good friends, so they are going to give it a try.

Because of that experience, Althea gained more confidence to be assertive when she is with others who stay on their phones rather than socialize in real time. She challenges her friends to put away their phones when they are together and wait to check them when their time together is over. Some of her friends don't agree but have decreased the screen time when they are together.

She no longer cares what her old girl friends think. Her new friends care about her and they spend time together socializing and having fun.

5. Guide the students through the assessment questions in **Table 3.28**.

6. Ask the students to put away their materials then ask review questions.

   a. What is one benefit of limiting screen time when with friends? (1.8.7)

   b. What is one barrier to limiting screen time when with friends? (1.8.7)

   c. What is one influence social media has on healthy personal relationships? (2.8.6)

7. Exit ticket (Self-Awareness: Self-confidence, recognizing strengths)

   Give an example of how coping with a challenging social experience can give you the strength and confidence to better deal with a similar situation another time.

Grades 9–12: Self-Awareness: Self-confidence/Recognizing Strengths

Lesson Overview: Body Image. In this lesson, students analyze how the perception of norms that surround body image influence unhealthy behaviors and propose ways to prevent health problems related to body image.

Learning about the impact of media on body image and the effects of eating disorders empowers teens to eat healthy and exercise to look good.

The National Eating Disorders Association reports that one in every 3.8 television commercials portrays an "Attractiveness Message." The message is that

Table 3.28 Benefits of and Barriers to Cutting down Social Media Use, Influence of Social Media on Relationships, and Self-Confidence

Question	Answer
What are the *three* benefits of and *three* barriers to practicing healthy behaviors *such as cutting down on social media when out with friends*? (1.8.7)	Benefits of cutting down on social media when with friends ■ Spend more time socializing ■ Practice communication skills ■ Develop friendship skills Barriers to cutting down on social media when with friends ■ Teens like their phones and don't want to limit their use. ■ Would rather communicate by text than in person. ■ Want to keep up with what everyone is saying and doing. They don't want to miss out on anything.
What are three influences *social media* has on personal *relationships*. (2.8.6)	■ Depression ■ Anxiety ■ Loneliness ■ Lack of development of social and interpersonal skills ■ Saying things in texts that would not be said in person ■ Choose to be on screen rather than interact in real time.
Self-Awareness: Self-confidence, recognizing strengths How did Althea demonstrate self-confidence when encouraging friends to decrease social media use when out socializing? How did Althea demonstrate the personal strength to speak up when encouraging friends to decrease social media use when out socializing?	When her friends agreed that they will try putting their phones away when they were together, Althea gained confidence to be assertive when she is with others who stay on their phones rather than socialize in real time. Before this incident, Althea would never have had the personal strength to ask her friends to give up their phones. Now, she has the strength to be assertive because she knows what happens when friends are distracted and don't care about each other.

extreme thinness is much more attractive than normal, healthy weight. Young men who read fitness magazines are more dissatisfied with their body. A popular teen magazine for girls encourages them to exercise to be more attractive, not to be healthy. (Mirror Mirror Eating Disorder Help, 2020)

Materials needed:

- **Worksheet 3.13 Tips for Feeling Your Best About Your Body Image**

  Table 3.29 provides an overview of the lesson objectives, assessment, and instruction for this lesson.

Table 3.29 Lesson Objectives, Assessment, and Instruction

Step 1 – Lesson Objectives	Step 2 – Assessment
The verb of the infused performance indicator and the SEL competency generate the assessment and instruction.	Design the assessment based on the objectives. Ask yourself the question, "What can my students do to show me they have met the standard?"
1.12.5 <u>Propose</u> ways to reduce or prevent injuries and health problems *related to body image*. (Joint Committee on National Health Education Standards, 2007, p. 25)	1.12.5 <u>Propose</u> *three* ways to reduce or prevent injuries and health problems *related to body image*.
2.12.5 <u>Evaluate</u> the effect of media on personal *(body image)* and family health. (Joint Committee on National Health Education Standards, 2007, p. 27)	2.12.5 <u>Evaluate</u> *two* effects of media on personal *(body image)* and family health.
Self-Awareness: Self-confidence, recognizing strengths	Demonstrate self-confidence and personal strength when they demonstrate three ways to reduce or prevent injuries and health problems *related to body image*.

(continues)

Table 3.29 Lesson Objectives, Assessment, and Instruction *(continued)*

Step 3 – Instruction

Design the instruction so that students learn the content, skill, and competency to be successful on the assessment. Ask the question, "What do I need to teach so that the students will be successful when assessed?"

Step 3 – Instruction

1. Define
   a. Propose: To present a new idea for serious consideration and discussion by other people.
   b. Evaluate: To judge a person or thing after methodically examining the situation.
   c. Body image: The beliefs and feelings a person has about their body.
   d. Self-confidence: The ability to depend on one's own strength, talent, and ability.
   e. Personal strengths: A talent or positive quality of a person.
2. 1.12.5 <u>Propose ways</u> to reduce or prevent injuries and health problems *related to body image.*
   a. Use **Worksheet 3.13 Tips for Feeling Your Best about your Body Image** to make a poster that proposes ways to reduce health problems associated with body image.
3. 3. 2.12.5 <u>Evaluate</u> the effect of media on personal *(body image)* and family health

   Formative assessment: The influence of media on body image assessment (Use red, yellow, green circles for False, Not Sure, and True; Kahoot and Quizlet are also fun and easy formative assessment tools) (2.12.5)
   a. T F By the time a girl is 17, she has seen 250,00 commercials that emphasize the importance of beauty and physical attractiveness. (T)
   b. T F Women in typical ads are typical, normal, healthy women. (F) The women are not typical, normal, healthy women.
   c. T F Fashion models weigh the same as the average woman. (F) They weigh substantially less than the average woman.

   d. T F The average American woman has the assets to become a fashion model. (F) Only 1% of young women have the potential to be a supermodel.
   e. T F Advertisers deliberately try to normalize unrealistically thin bodies in ads to drive product purchase and consumption. (T) (Randy M. Page., 2015, pp. 167-168)
   f. T F Young men who see the idealized male muscular body and know that they will never achieve, sometimes experience body dissatisfaction and eating disorders. (T)
   g. T F Boys have more body dissatisfaction than girls. (F) More girls have body dissatisfaction.
   h. T F Boys and girls (9–14 years old) who make an effort to look like the figures in the media were less likely than their peers to develop weight concerns and become constant dieters. (F) More likely than their peers to develop weight concerns and become constant dieters.
   i. T F Exposure to unrealistic and often unhealthy body images can influence young people's perception of their own body shape and size as well as their own sense of body satisfaction. (T)
   j. T F The effect of media does not lead to harmful weight loss behaviors. (F) The effect of media does lead to harmful weight loss behaviors. (Anne M. Morris & Debra K. Katzman, 2003)
4. Read the practice prompts. Students answer the reflection questions and discuss.

Practice Prompt: Sofia

Sofia grew up watching television, reading fashion magazines, and of course, using social media. Sophia thinks the advertisements in the magazines make thin women seem to be normal and she wonders if she should ask her mom to buy some of the diet products advertised. She has friends who try to look like the models, and they diet constantly. Sophia doesn't want to do that.

As a child, Sophia was a little overweight. Her mom is an excellent cook, and Sofia loved to eat everything she cooked. Sometimes she ate too much, but it tasted so good. Now that she is in high school, she is very aware of her weight and how thin the other girls are and how thin all the models and TV/movie actresses look. She is starting to put herself down because she has tried to diet but she can't lose weight. She has tried not eating breakfast but that only gives her a headache and she can't concentrate, making her feel even worse. Her friends tell her she looks fine. In fact, her body isn't much different from her friends.

One day the health teacher taught a lesson on body image and how the media effects how teens think about themselves. The light went on! It was as if the teacher was talking about her! She decided there were some things she could change and others she couldn't. She stopped putting herself down and immediately

felt better. She found out the right weight for her and learned how to balance her foods and eat the right portion. She even enjoys physical education now and joined the afterschool wellness club where she does Yoga and works the machines. She likes to look in the mirror and watch her body make the different poses. She didn't think she could ever do that! She is even encouraging her friends to join her. With the exercise and healthy eating, her body is looking much better, and Sophia is feeling much better.

Practice Prompt: Maruis

Maruis grew up watching television, reading muscle magazines, and of course, using social media. The magazines always showed men with bulging muscles. He knew he would never look that way, but also wasn't very happy with how he did look. He has friends who try to look like the men in the magazine, and they diet constantly. Maruis doesn't want to do that.

As a child, he was a little overweight. His mom is an excellent cook and Maruis loved to eat everything she cooked. Sometimes he ate too much but it tasted so good. Now that he is in high school, he is very aware of his weight and how better built the other boys are. Everyone looks better than he does. He is starting to put himself down because he has tried to diet but he can't lose weight. He has tried not eating breakfast but that only gives him a headache and he can't concentrate which makes him feel even worse.

His friends tell him he looks fine. In fact, his body isn't much different from his friends.

One day, the health teacher taught a lesson on body image and how the media affects how teens think about themselves. The light went on! It was if the teacher was talking about him! He decided there were some things he could change and others he couldn't. He stopped putting himself down and immediately felt better. He found out the right weight for him and learned how to balance his foods and eat the right portion. He even enjoys physical education now and joined the afterschool wellness club where he works the machines and lifts the free weights. He likes to look in the mirror and watch his body while he is working out. He didn't think he could ever do that! He is even encouraging his friends to join him. With the exercise and healthy eating, his body is looking much better and Maruis is feeling much better.

5. Guide the students through the assessment questions in **Table 3.30**.
6. Ask the students to put away their materials then ask review questions.
    a. What is one tip to feel good about your body image? (1.12.5)
    b. How does the media influence our body image? (2.12.5)
    c. How did the characters in the story develop the strength and self-confidence to change their behavior? (Self-Awareness: Self-confidence, recognizing strengths)

Table 3.30 Ways to Prevent Injuries and Health Problems Related to Body Image, Effects of Media on Body Image, and Self-confidence

Question	Answer
What are *three* ways for *Sophia and Maruis* to reduce or prevent injuries and health problems *related to body image?* (1.12.5)	<ul><li>Stop putting themselves down.</li><li>Realize there were some things they could change and others they couldn't.</li><li>Find their healthy weight, balance their foods, and eat the right portion.</li><li>Enjoy physical education.</li><li>Join the afterschool wellness club.</li><li>Take steps to manage their weight and body image, they feel better about themselves.</li></ul>

(continues)

Table 3.30 Ways to Prevent Injuries and Health Problems Related to Body Image, Effects of Media on Body Image, and Self-confidence *(continued)*

Question	Answer
What are *two* effects of media on personal (*body image*) and family health? (2.12.5)	Sophia thinks the advertisements in the magazines make thin women seem to be normal and she wonders if she should ask her mom to buy some of the diet products advertised.
	The men's magazines always showed men with bulging muscles. He knew he would never look like that, but he wasn't very happy with how he did look.
	Sophia and Maruis have friends who try to look like the models in the magazines and they are always dieting.
Self-Awareness: Self-confidence, recognizing strengths How did Sophia and Maruis gain the self-confidence and personal strength to demonstrate three ways to reduce or prevent injuries and health problems *related to body image*.	After their health class, Sophia and Maruis had the personal strength and self-confidence to change their behavior. They realized there were some things they could not change about themselves but there were some things they could change. Knowing this, they both started eating healthier and exercising. Their bodies began to look better with good nutrition and muscle toning from exercising.

7. Exit ticket (Self-Awareness: Self-confidence, recognizing strengths)

   Give an example of how recognizing a personal strength and having self-confidence helps to cope with the influence of media.

Self-Efficacy

What is the difference between self-esteem and self-efficacy?

Self-esteem is how much we value, respect, and feel confident about ourselves. It develops when we receive praise or are successful at mastering a challenge. (Mary H. Bronson, 2009) Students with good self-esteem feel good about themselves, feel liked and accepted, are proud of what they accomplish, and believe in themselves. (TeensHealth from Nemours, 2020) In skills-based health education, self-esteem develops when students succeed in demonstrating functional health knowledge, a skill, and a SEL competency.

A person who demonstrates self-efficacy has confidence in their ability to perform a health behavior or reach a goal. (Randy M. Page., 2015, p. 39) Students with high self-efficacy demonstrate confidence in their ability to exert control over their motivation, behavior, and environment. They become advocates for themselves and have fewer negative emotional reactions when confronted with difficulties. (Transforming Education, 2020) In skills-based health education, self-efficacy develops when students are challenged with

a performance assessment and believe that they can figure out how to successfully complete the challenge and show proficiency in functional health knowledge, a skill, and a SEL competency.

There are four ways a teacher can help a student develop self-efficacy.

- *Mastery experiences:* The teacher coaches the child through a series small steps of content/skill/SEL competency to develop their self-confidence. When the student successfully completes the small steps, he or she has the confidence to pursue a more complicated task. Success increases self-efficacy whereas failures challenge self-efficacy.
- *Vicarious experiences:* Provide experiences where the student sees another peer succeeding at a behavior. By observing the peer, he or she may gain the confidence in his ability to perform.
  - Play a video of another student performing in a role play. After watching, the student may gain the confidence to role play, also.
  - Show step-by-step pictures of students completing a skill, such as the steps for handwashing, fitting a bicycle helmet, CPR, first aid, the Heimlich maneuver, etc. (Standard 7-Practicing Healthy Behaviors) The pictures make clear how to successfully complete a task and with effective feedback from the teacher and practice, the child develops the confidence to try the new skill.

- Read a children's book that provides examples of how students resolved conflict (Standard 4: Interpersonal Communication; SEL Healthy Relationships: Communication). (Frey, Fisher, & Smith, 2019, pp. 29-30) Once the child sees how to use the conflict resolution skill, he or she may have the confidence to use it him- or herself.
- *Verbal persuasion:* To encourage the student and provide guidance and feedback as the student is trying a new skill or behavior.
- *Positive emotional state:* To encourage the development of self-efficacy, be enthusiastic about teaching functional health knowledge, a skill, and a SEL competency. The teacher's enthusiasm and support decreases student stress and anxiety about performing. (Frey, Fisher, & Smith, 2019, p. 39)

PreK–2: Self-Awareness: Self-Efficacy

Lesson Overview: Dental Health. In this lesson, children learn to identify trusted adults, such as the school nurse, when seeking help for a dental health issue. They also learn why it is important to see a dentist every six months. Learning this content and skill results in increased self-confidence and a sense of self-efficacy.

About one of five (20%) children aged five to 11 have at least one untreated decayed tooth.

Children aged five to 19 from low-income families are twice as likely (25%) to have cavities, compared with children from higher-income households. (11%) (Center for Disease Control and Prevention, 2020)

Materials needed:

- Pictures of a dentist
- Pictures of the different types of teeth
- Picture of a tooth with a cavity.

Table 3.31 provides an overview of the lesson objectives, assessment, and instruction for this lesson.

Step 3 – Instruction

1. Define
   a. Describe: To use words that help others envision the physical attributes of a person, place, or thing.
   b. Identify: To recognize a particular person or an object.
   c. Self-awareness: An accurate understanding of a person's own values, emotions, and wants and needs.
   d. Self-efficacy: The ability to take action, complete a task, and attain goals. (Frey, Fisher, & Smith, 2019)

Table 3.31 Lesson Objectives, Assessment, and Instruction

Step 1 – Lesson Objectives	Step 2 – Assessment
The verb of the *infused* performance indicator and the SEL competency generate the assessment and instruction.	Design the assessment based on the objectives. Ask yourself the question, "What can my students do to show me they have met the standard?"
1.2.5 <u>Describe</u> why it is important to seek health care *when you have a toothache.* (Joint Committee on National Health Education Standards, 2007, p. 24)	1.2.5 Students <u>describe</u> why it is important to seek health care *when you have a toothache.*
3.2.1 <u>Identify</u> trusted adults and professionals who help promote *dental* health. (Joint Committee on National Health Education Standards, 2007, p. 28)	3.2.1 Students <u>identify</u> *one* trusted adult in the school and *one trusted adult in the* community who help promote *dental* health.
Self-Awareness: Self-efficacy	Explain two ways to increase self-efficacy when faced with a health issue.

Step 3 – Instruction	
Design the instruction so that students learn the content, skill, and competency to be successful on the assessment. Ask the question, "What do I need to teach so that the students will be successful when assessed?"	

2. 1.2.5 <u>Describe</u> why it is important to seek health care *when you have a toothache*
   a. Ask the children why it is important to see the dentist when they have a toothache.
      i. If not treated, the tooth may have to be pulled.
      ii. A cavity in a tooth may be cleaned and filled, resulting in stopping the pain.
3. 3.2.1 Identify trusted adults and professionals who help promote *dental* health.
   a. What kind of health care does a dentist give?
   b. Why is it important to have a family dentist?
   c. Why it is important to go the dentist every six months?
4. Read the practice prompt. Students answer the reflection questions and discuss.

Practice Prompt: Nina

Nina has a toothache. She has never been to a dentist. She also has a headache and cannot concentrate on her work. She wants to cry. Her teacher noticed that she didn't look well and sent her to the nurse. The nurse told Nina that she thinks she may have a problem with a tooth and recommended that her parents take her to the dentist.

The nurse explained that the toothache was only going to get worse and may lead to other problems. She gave Nina the name of several dentists in the community.

When Nina went home, her mom saw that she was pale and not feeling well. Nina told her she went to the nurse and she thinks Nina has a problem with a tooth. Nina gave her mother the list of local dentists, but her mom told her the pain would go away with a good night's sleep. Nina told her mom that she needs to see a dentist right away because the toothache is only going to get worse and may lead to other problems.

Nina's mom listened to her, called the dentist, and got an appointment that afternoon. Sure enough, Nina had a cavity. The dentist explained that it was good that she came today because although the cavity was deep, he could fill it. If she waited longer, he might have had to pull the tooth. Now that Nina has a dentist, she is scheduled for a cleaning and regular check-up in six months.

To help Nina keep her teeth healthy, the dental hygienist showed Nina how to brush and floss her teeth.

Nina is grateful to her teacher and the nurse for helping her. She feels confident now that she has knowledge to keep her teeth healthy, the skills to brush and floss, and has set a goal to practice

good dental hygiene every day. She plans to share that information with family and friends. Not only did her self-confidence increase but so did her self-efficacy.

5. Guide the students through the assessment questions in **Table 3.32**.
6. Ask the students to put away their materials then ask review questions.
   a. Why is it important to seek health care when you have a toothache? (1.2.5)
   b. Who is a trusted adult in school and professional in the community who help promote *dental* health? (3.2.1)
   c. How can a child increase his or her self-efficacy? (SEL-Self-Awareness: Self-efficacy)
7. Exit ticket (Self-Awareness: Self-Efficacy)
   a. Neva was nervous about going to gym because she is not good at physical activity. The teacher taught simple skills that she was able to do then the teacher put two skills together and Neva was able to do them, also. Now, Neva looks forward to going to gym. She has gained self-_____.
   b. Benjamin doesn't get discouraged when he is working on a hard assignment. He keeps trying and doesn't get upset. He knows to ask the teacher if he needs help. Benjamin shows self-_____.

Grades 3–5: Self-Awareness: Self-Efficacy

Lesson Overview: Transition to Middle School. Transitioning from the elementary school to the middle school is a big change for students. In this lesson, the student examines how he or she feels about moving to the middle school before experiencing "Move up" day and after. The lesson could be adjusted to help students cope with any new experience.

Resources:

- Moving up to Middle School—https://media .centervention.com/pdf/Middle-school-transition -worksheet.pdf

Materials needed:

- **Worksheet 3.14 Graphic Organizers to Monitor Feelings Before and After Move-Up Day**
- **Worksheet 3.15 Self-efficacy Exit Ticket**
- Combination locks

Table 3.32 Why It Is Important to Seek Help for a Toothache, Identification of Dental Health Resources, and Self-Efficacy

Question	Answer
Why was it important for Nina to seek health care *when having a toothache?* (1.2.5)	The dentist told Nina that it was good that she came in for treatment because the cavity was deep, but he could fill it. If she had waited, he might have had to pull the tooth.
Who is *one* trusted adult in the school and *one trusted adult in the* community who Nina contacted to promote *dental* health? (3.2.1)	The teacher and the school nurse are the trusted adults Nina identified in school. The dentist is the trusted adult Nina identified in the community.
Self-Awareness: Self-efficacy How did Nina's self-efficacy develop as a result of facing a health issue?	Nina's self-efficacy developed because she now has the confidence to keep her teeth healthy and knows what to do and where to go if she has a toothache. She plans to share that information with family and friends.

Table 3.33 provides an overview of the lesson objectives, assessment, and instruction for this lesson.

Step 3 – Instruction

1. Define
   a. Describe: To use words that help others envision the physical attributes of a person, place, or thing.
   b. Identify: To recognize a particular person or an object.
   c. Self-esteem: A feeling about the worth of the self.
   d. Self-efficacy: The ability to take action, complete a task, and attain goals. (Frey, Fisher, & Smith, 2019)
2. 1.5.2 Identify examples of emotional, intellectual, physical, and social health *when moving up to a new school.*
   a. Ask the children to write down their biggest fear on a sticky note about moving up to the middle school and splash it on the board. Be prepared for:
      i. Getting lost
      ii. Making friends
      iii. Lunch

Table 3.33 Lesson Objectives, Assessment, and Instruction

Step 1 – Lesson Objectives	Step 2 – Assessment
The verb of the *infused* performance indicator and the SEL competency generate the assessment and instruction.	Design the assessment based on the objectives. Ask yourself the question, "What can my students do to show me they have met the standard?"
1.5.2 Identify examples of emotional, intellectual, physical, and social health *when moving up to a new school.* (Joint Committee on National Health Education Standards, 2007, p. 24)	1.5.2 On a graphic organizer, students identify *two* feelings for each component before and after Move Up Day. Reflect on the effect of Move Up Day on self-esteem.
2.5.4 Describe how the school and community supports personal health practices and behaviors *for new students to the middle school building.* (Joint Committee on National Health Education Standards, 2007, p. 28)	2.5.4 Students describe *two* things that a school does to welcome new students and give them the confidence that they need to succeed in the new setting. (self-efficacy)
Self-Awareness: Self-efficacy	Explain how to develop self-efficacy when moving to a new school.

Step 3 – Instruction
Design the instruction so that students learn the content, skill, and competency to be successful on the assessment. Ask the question, "What do I need to teach so that the students will be successful when assessed?"

      iv. Bathrooms
      v.   Opening lockers
      vi. Late to class
      vii. Teachers too hard
      viii.Classes too hard

   b. Discuss the responses and how they affect self-esteem. Fill out **Worksheet 3.14 Graphic Organizers to Monitor Feelings Before and After Move-Up Day** to help students identify how they feel today (physical, emotionally, intellectually, and socially) about moving to the middle school.

3. 2.5.4 <u>Describe</u> how the school and community support personal health practices and behaviors *for new students to the middle school building.*

   a. Explain the Move Up program. It is designed to increase your self-efficacy during transition.

      a. Each elementary school visits the middle school on different days (*Self-efficacy-Mastery experiences*)

      b. During the visit, you will meet the principal, the teachers, and peer leaders. (*Self-efficacy: Verbal persuasion*)

      c. A student tour guide will walk us through the school, lavatories, cafeteria, and gym. (*Self-efficacy: Vicarious experiences*)

      d. Tomorrow, peer leaders come to talk to our students, in small groups, to answers your questions (*Self-efficacy: Positive emotional state, vicarious experiences*)

      e. After the visit by the peer leaders, students filled out the second graphic organizer: Vicarious experiences) to identify how they felt (physically, emotionally, intellectually, and socially), after the Move Up Day and the visit from the peer leader.

4. Read the practice prompt. Students answer the reflection questions and discuss.

Practice Prompt: Tracie

Tracie is nervous about going to middle school. She has heard so many horrible stories about getting lost, being bullied in the lavatory, the cafeteria having bad food, and the teachers being mean. She gets a headache and stomach ache just thinking about it. Tracie is a good student, but she wonders if the middle school courses are going to be too hard for her. She knows how to study and feels good about her accomplishments in elementary school, but middle school may be too hard.

She has friends at her school but students from two other elementary schools will also be at the middle school. She is afraid she will lose her current friends and won't be able to make new friends. She is a mess!

On Move Up day, Tracie's school visited the middle school. It wasn't at all what she thought. She felt much better right away. The middle school guides were really nice and showed them all around the building. They were very friendly and made her feel welcome. Terry, her guide, is the older brother of one of her friends. He told her not to worry because he will watch out for her next year. The lunch in the cafeteria was really good and the lavatories were clean. There was plenty of soap and tissues, and a noisy hand dryer that dried her hands really fast!

Best of all, during the assembly, she learned about all of the afterschool clubs and supports available. She made good friends in the afterschool clubs at her school and believes she can do the same in the new school.

Rather than being afraid, Tracie now feels good about the move and looks forward to meeting her new teachers, being challenged by new subjects, and making new friends. She hasn't had a headache or stomach ache since Move Up day!

5. Guide the students through the assessment questions in **Table 3.34**.
6. Ask the students to put away their materials then ask review questions.

   a. How would you feel before a Move Up Day and after a Move Up Day? (1.5.2)

   b. What are two ways the school supports the student's development of self-efficacy during the transition from elementary to middle school? (2.5.1)

   c. What is one example of how a child can increase his or her self-efficacy when moving to a new school? (SEL-Self-Awareness: Self-Efficacy)

7. Exit ticket (Self-Awareness: Self-Efficacy) **Worksheet 3.15 Self-Efficacy Exit Ticket** Circle one way we learned to increase self-efficacy then explain how it would help you develop self-efficacy.

Grades 6–8: Self-Awareness: Self-Efficacy

Lesson Overview: Influence of Advertising on Vaping. Students learn how to influence a peer, not to Juul, and to analyze eCigarette

Table 3.34 Effects of Move Up Day on Components of Health, the School's Role in Move Up Day, and Self-Efficacy

Question	Answer
How did Move Up Day affect Tracie's health? (1.5.2) Emotional → Intellectual → Physical → Social (cycle)	Emotional ■ Felt more confident ■ Everyone was nice and made her feel welcome Intellectual ■ Knows there is after-school support for subjects ■ Looks forward to being challenged Physical ■ No headache ■ No stomach ache Social ■ Looking forward to making new friends in her classes and afterschool clubs. Self-esteem ■ Feels good about going to the middle school.
What were two things that the school did to welcome new students and give them the confidence they need to believe they will succeed in the new setting? (2.5.4)	The school organized a Move Up Day so the students would be more comfortable entering the school in the fall. The middle school has a peer leader program and a member of the club visited the elementary school to talk to the children about life in the middle school.
Self-Awareness: Self-efficacy How can a student develop self-efficacy when moving to a new school?	Visit the school so you know your way around (mastery experiences, vicarious experiences) Talk to your teacher about the move and get to know the middle school teachers before school starts (verbal persuasion) Practice opening your locker Be prepared (positive emotional state)

advertisements to understand how they influence people to vape.

In a Population Assessment of Tobacco and Health, 41% of youth aged 12 to 13 years, as well as half of older adolescents who had never used tobacco, were receptive to at least one tobacco advertisement. Across each age group, 28%–33% were most receptive to eCigarette advertisements. (Pierce JP, 2017)

3.7%-15.7% of middle school students report currently using an electronic vapor product. In the territories, 20%-32.4% report current use. (Center for Disease Control and Prevention, 2020)

Presenting in front of peers is challenging. This lesson helps students build confidence to present their authentic assessment about vaping to the class. Student self-esteem is enhanced by receiving targeted feedback about the content and skill preparation of the assessment. In small steps the students will gain confidence until they believe (self-efficacy) they can successfully present in front of the class.

Resources:

- Interactive resources about the effects of vaping http://www.scholastic.com/youthvapingrisks/interactive/ (Scholastic, 2020)
- Teens and eCigarettes https://www.drugabuse.gov/drug-topics/trends-statistics/infographics/teens-e-cigarettes https://www.cdc.gov/tobacco/basic_information/e-cigarettes/Quick-Facts-on-the-Risks-of-E-cigarettes-for-Kids-Teens-and-Young-Adults.html
https://pediatrics.aappublications.org/content/139/6/e20163353

Materials needed:

- **Worksheet 3.16 Effects of eCigarettes on the Body**
- **Worksheet 3.17 Sorting Advertising Strategies**

Table 3.35 provides an overview of the lesson objectives, assessment, and instruction for this lesson.

Table 3.35 Lesson Objectives, Assessment, and Instruction

Step 1 – Lesson Objectives	Step 2 – Assessment
The verb of the *infused* performance indicator and the SEL competency generate the assessment and instruction.	Design the assessment based on the objectives. Ask yourself the question, "What can my students do to show me they have met the standard?"
1.8.9 <u>Examine</u> the potential seriousness of injury or illness if engaging in unhealthy behaviors *such as vaping.* (Joint Committee on National Health Education Standards, 2007, p. 25)	1.8.9 Role play influencing a peer, not to Juul because of the seriousness of injury or illness associated with eCigarettes on the body.
2.5.6. <u>Describe</u> ways that technology influences personal health *such as advertisements for vaping products.* (Joint Committee on National Health Education Standards, 2007, p. 26)	2.5.6 <u>Analyze</u> the eCigarette ads and sort under the advertising strategy. Describe how the ad influences teens to vape. Students present their findings and share their rationale.
Self-Awareness: Self-efficacy	To build efficacy, allow the students to practice at their seats then standing up but away from the whole group but close enough so they can observe others practicing. Formatively assess and provide support. (mastery experience, vicarious experience, verbal persuasion, positive emotional state)

Step 3 – Instruction
Design the instruction so that students learn the content, skill, and competency to be successful on the assessment. Ask the question, "What do I need to teach so that the students will be successful when assessed?"

Step 3 – Instruction

1. Define
   a. Describe: To use words that help others envision the physical attributes of a person, place, or thing.
   b. Examine: Look carefully at someone or something to determine the condition.
   c. Self-esteem: A feeling about the worth of the self.
   d. Self-efficacy: The ability to take action, complete a task, and attain goals. (Frey, Fisher, & Smith, 2019)
2. 1.8.9 <u>Examine</u> the potential seriousness of injury or illness if engaging in unhealthy behaviors *such as vaping.*
   a. Using **Worksheet 3.16 Effects of eCigarettes on the Body,** provide time for students to prepare a role play where they influence a peer, not to Juul because of the harmful effects of eCigarettes on the body.
   b. To build efficacy, or the belief in the ability to complete the role play, allow the students to practice at their seats, then standing up but away from the whole group but close enough so they can observe others practicing. Formatively assess and provide support. (mastery experience, vicarious experience, verbal persuasion, positive emotional state)
3. 2.5.6. <u>Describe</u> ways that technology influences personal health *such as advertisements for vaping products*
   a. Use **Worksheet 3.17 Sorting Advertising Strategies** to sort eCigarette ads under advertising strategies **Table 3.36**.
   b. Students present their findings and share their rationale.
   c. To build efficacy, allow the students to practice at their seats then standing up but away from the whole group but close enough so they can observe others practicing. Formatively assess and provide support. (mastery experience, vicarious experience, verbal persuasion, positive emotional state)
4. Read the practice prompt. Students answer the reflection questions and discuss.

Table 3.36 Advertising Strategies

Technique	Example	Hidden Message
Bandwagon	Group of people using the eCigarette.	Everyone is using it and you should too.
Rich and Famous	The eCigarette is shown in an expensive setting.	The eCigarette will make you feel rich and famous.
Free Gifts	The vendor offers redeemable coupons or discounts for the purchase of e-cigarettes.	It is a deal that is too good to be true.
Great Outdoors	The advertisement shows a person using an eCigarette outdoors.	If the eCigarette is associated with nature, it must be healthy.
Good Times	People smoking eCigarettes are shown as smiling, laughing, and having a good time.	The eCigarette will add fun to your life.
Testimonial	People who have used eCigarettes to quit smoking or smoke an eCigarette instead of a tobacco cigarette to feel healthy.	The eCigarette worked for them and it can work for you, too.

Data from Mary H. Bronson, P. (2009). Glencoe Health. Woodland Hills, CA: McGraw Hill, pg. 47

Practice Prompt: Jonas

Jonas and his group were assigned an in-class project to examine the effects of Juuling on the body and the influence of advertising on middle school students. The evidence he collected proved how dangerous eCigarettes are to the body and how advertisements are geared toward youth.

He wanted the 5th graders to know that most Juuls contain the addictive drug nicotine. In fact, one Juul pod contains the same amount of nicotine as 20 cigarettes. Because brains grow new memories the more we do something, Juuling over and over creates strong connections and makes it more difficult to quit. He also wants the younger students to understand that teens first use a Juul because they are curious about the different flavors.

The team wrote a prompt about a girl named Althea. Jonas enjoyed gathering examples of eCigarette advertisements, creating a graphic organizer about the effects of smoking on the teenage body, and writing the prompt. However, he does not want to present in front of the class. In fact, he is petrified. He had a bad experience last year and he is now afraid of public speaking.

Here is the prompt:

Althea likes the look of Juul. They have colorful caps and they are sleek and easy to put into a pocket undetected. The advertisements make Juuling look like fun. The older women look sophisticated and the younger girls all look like they are popular.

She thinks smoking cigarettes is disgusting and dirty but Juuling seems really cool. Her older sister Juuls and Althea knows where she hides the stick and the pods. She sneaks a few puffs when she can. She likes the taste of the different flavors and that teachers and her parents cannot smell smoke on her clothes.

Lately, the more she smokes, the more she wants to smoke. She is wondering if there is nicotine in the Juul. She noticed that she is developing a cough and gets winded when running. Her sister is trying to cut down because she has some high school friends who started smoking cigarettes after they had been Juuling for a while. She doesn't want to get addicted and she doesn't want to smoke cigarettes; she is just curious and likes the way she looks when she is smoking.

Jonas's friends convinced him he could present. First, they practiced their presentation at their seats. Jonas did the research on how eCigarettes affect the body so that was his part. He was confident that he knew the facts but was still scared to present. After they practiced at their seats, they went to the back of the room to practice. The other groups were also practicing in the room so Jonas could see how the other groups were practicing. It gave him more confidence to see the other students struggling, also. Mrs. Page came by to watch, make suggestions, and gave encouragement.

After much practice and increased self-confidence, he believes he can present in front of the class. He knows this is an important topic and he wants to help his peers stop vaping.

Table 3.37 Effects of Juuling on the Body, the Influence of Juuling Advertisements, and Self-efficacy

Question	Answer
Using the information in the prompt, what were *three effects of Juuling on Althea's body* that may lead to injury or illness? (1.8.9)	■ The more Althea Juuls, the more she wants to Juul. ■ Althea fears becoming addicted. ■ Althea developed a cough and gets winded when running.
Using the information in the prompt, which advertising strategy most influenced Althea to try Juuling? (2.5.6)	■ Ads with older women made them look wealthy and sophisticated. (Rich and famous) ■ Ads with younger women made them look like they were popular and having fun. (Good times)
Self-Awareness: Self-efficacy How did Jonas develop the self-efficacy to present his project to the class?	■ The group first practiced at their seats. ■ The group then practiced standing up but away from the whole group. ■ Jonas observed the other students struggling and practicing. ■ Mrs. Page formatively assessed the group and provided support and encouragement. ■ After much practice and increased self-confidence, he believed he could present in front of the class. He knows this is an important topic and he wants to help his peers stop vaping. (mastery experience, vicarious experience, verbal persuasion, positive emotional state) (Self-Awareness: Self-efficacy)

5. Guide the students through the assessment questions in **Table 3.37**.
6. Ask the students to put away their materials then ask review questions.
   a. What are two effects of eCigarettes on the teen body? (1.5.9)
   b. How did Juul advertisements influence the character in the prompt? (2.5.6)
   c. How can a teen increase his or her self-efficacy to present in front of the class? (SEL-Self-Awareness: Self-efficacy)
7. Exit ticket (Self-Awareness: Self-efficacy)
   Give an example of how a teen builds self-efficacy to do something.

Grades 9–12: Self-Awareness: Self-Efficacy

Lesson Overview: CPR. Students learn that knowing how to give CPR affects their components of health and how the school health program that taught the course gave them confidence.

Approximately 90% of people who suffer out-of-hospital cardiac arrests die. CPR, especially if performed immediately, can double or triple a person's change of survival. (American Heart Association, 2020)

Note: This lesson, although about CPR, does not teach the steps of CPR. Because it is a self-awareness lesson with an emphasis on self-efficacy and aligned with Standard 2, analyzing influences, it addresses motivation and how a school empowers a student to act.

Materials needed:

• **Worksheet 3.18 How Giving CPR Effects Emotional, Intellectual, Physical, and Social Health**

Table 3.38 provides an overview of the lesson objectives, assessment, and instruction for this lesson.

Table 3.38 Lesson Objectives, Assessment, and Instruction

Step 1 – Lesson Objectives	Step 2 – Assessment
The verb of the *infused* performance indicator and the SEL competency generate the assessment and instruction.	Design the assessment based on the objectives. Ask the question, "What can my students do to show me they have met the standard?"
1.12.2 <u>Describe</u> the interrelationships of emotional, intellectual, physical, and social health *when able to give CPR.* (Joint Committee on National Health Education Standards, 2007, p. 25)	1.12.2 Students <u>describe</u> two feelings experience in each component of wellness when they successfully give CPR.

2.12.4. <u>Evaluate</u> how the school and community affects personal health practices and behavior *by learning CPR*. (Joint Committee on National Health Education Standards, 2007, p. 27)	2.12.4 Student <u>evaluates</u> how the school CPR program gave the confidence to perform CPR on a family member.
Self-Awareness: Self-efficacy	Student writes a letter to the principal explaining how the school gave him or her the confidence and belief that he or she could administer CPR. (mastery experience, vicarious experience, verbal persuasion, positive emotional state)

Step 3 – Instruction

Design the instruction so that students learn the content, skill, and competency to be successful on the assessment. Ask the question, "What do I need to teach so that the students will be successful when assessed?

Step 3 – Instruction

1. Define
   a. Describe: To use words that help others envision the physical attributes of a person, place, or thing.
   b. Evaluate: To judge a person or thing after methodically examining the situation.
   c. Self-efficacy: The ability to take action, complete a task, and attain goals. (Frey, Fisher, & Smith, 2019)
2. 1.12.2 <u>Describe</u> the interrelationships of emotional, intellectual, physical, and social health *when able to give CPR*.
   a. Use **Worksheet 3.18, How Giving CPR Affects Emotional, Intellectual, Physical, and Social Health** to read Jacob's story and then describe two of the feelings he felt for each component as a result of saving his grandfather's life by giving CPR.
3. 2.12.4. <u>Evaluate</u> how the school and community affects personal health practices and behavior *by learning CPR*.
   a. Examine the school mission and explain how it supports the teaching of CPR and first aid.
   b. To practice the skill, instruct the students to write a letter as Jacob's grandmother to Jacob's principal, Mrs. Nambia. Explain that the whole family has been affected by Jacob knowing how to react in an emergency and give CPR. Express gratitude to the school for supporting health education and providing the resources for the health teachers to include CPR in their program.
4. Read the practice prompt. Students answer the reflection questions and discuss.

Practice Prompt: Demetry

Demetry attends Lakeview High School. The school's mission is to provide a safe and healthy school environment where students learn the content and skills needed to meet life's challenges.

Demetry knew the CPR unit was taught in the spring and he was dreading it. The piles of mannequins, tucked away in the corner would soon be on the floor, challenging students to give rescue breaths and compressions. Yuck!

The day arrived. Mrs. Connolly was standing outside the classroom with a baby mannequin in her arms! In the classroom, tables were grouped, and each had a baby, disinfecting wipes, face shields, and a self-check with step-by-step directions. Everyone made comments about the babies but it was because they were anxious. The babies look real!

Demetry babysits his younger siblings so he knows he should learn CPR. His grandmother lives with the family, and she has a weak heart. "Change your attitude," he told himself.

The school has automated external defibrillators (AEDs) in several places around the school and the health teacher has been teaching first aid and CPR for a long time. Several students have been awarded the Valor Award for using their first aid and CPR skills in school and in the community.

(continues)

Practice Prompt: Demetry *(continued)*

Mrs. Connolly taught the students about the circulatory and respiratory systems in order to understand why first aid and CPR works. Today, she demonstrated what to do when you find an unresponsive infant. She gently shook the baby saying, "Are you OK?" The students laughed but Mrs. Connolly explained that the rescuer is trying to see if the baby responds to a voice. The baby didn't respond so she checked for breathing and pulse. She found none so she gave CPR. After a minute, she made baby crying noises and lifted the baby to her shoulders. The students laughed but were also relieved.

After Demetry saw the demonstration and knew he could look at the pictures and steps, he felt better. He watched his classmates for a while. When it was his turn, it took him a few times to get it right but with Mrs. Connolly coaching him, he did it! It wasn't so bad! In a few days, they moved on to the child then the adult. By that time, he was over his nervousness and he just got to work give rescue breaths and compressions. He was proud of himself

and believed if he needed to give first aid or CPR, he could do it.

A few months later, he was helping his grandmother cook. All of a sudden, she called Demetry's name and collapsed. He knew just what to do. He checked for responsiveness but found none. He called to his mother and told her to call 911. He began CPR. The paramedics came a few minutes later and told Demetry that his quick response saved his grandmother's life. Demetry was exhausted and felt a little nauseous but was very relieved.

Demetry's mother called the health teacher and principal and told them she was so glad they teach CPR because her son saved her mother's life by knowing just what to do and to have the confidence to do it. During the spring awards ceremony, Demetry received the Valor Award from the Superintendent. His grandmother was called to the stage to give Demetry the award. His classmates all stood up and clapped. Demetry was very proud of himself and grateful to the school for teaching him CPR.

5. Guide the students through the assessment questions in **Table 3.39**.
6. Ask the students to put away their materials then ask review questions.
   a. What is one feeling from each of the wellness components that Demetry felt after giving CPR? (1.12.2)
   b. How can a school evaluate if a CPR program is successful? (2.12.4)
   c. How can a teen increase his or her self-efficacy to present in front of the class? (SEL-Self-Awareness: self-efficacy)
7. Exit ticket (Self-Awareness: Self-efficacy)

   Give an example of how a teen builds self-efficacy by learning and giving CPR.

Growth Mindset

The skill of the teacher is evident when a frustrated student says that he/she cannot demonstrate a skill or competency and the teacher says, "You mean you cannot demonstrate the skill, yet!" (Frey, Fisher, & Smith, 2019, pp. 29-30)

How we think about our intelligence affects how hard we try, or engage with others, our motivation, achievement on tests, and our grades in school. We have a fixed or growth mindset or a combination of both depending on the situation. (Transforming Education, 2020)

A person with a fixed mindset believes his/her basic qualities of intelligence and talent are static and do not change. He believes that effort is irrelevant because personal talent is the key to success, not how hard a person tries. A person with this mindset is concerned if people think he is smart, gets upset when he makes a mistake, and gives up on more difficult tasks. (Transforming Education, 2020) He second guesses himself and may give up when challenged rather than trying a different approach. However, the good news is that a person with a fixed mindset can progress to a growth mindset and a person with a fixed mindset in one area may have a growth mindset in another area. For example, a child may have a fixed mindset about speaking in public and advocating for a health issue (Standard 8) but may have a growth mindset when researching valid and reliable sources of information (Standard 3).

One strategy to help high risk or impoverished students move from a fixed to a growth mindset is to help them interact with others through writing and discussions. (Frey, Fisher, & Smith, 2019, p. 33) In the skills-based health/SEL classroom, this development occurs when students work in groups to write prompts, act them out through role play, then discuss how the presenters demonstrated the content, skill, and SEL competency. This strategy demonstrates that students are able to embrace a challenge, keep trying

Table 3.39 Effects on Components of Health When Students are able to give CPR, How the School Affects Personal Health, and Self-Confidence

Question	Answer
What are two feelings Demetry experienced in each component of wellness after successfully giving CPR? (1.12.2)	Emotional health ■ Anxious ■ Relieved ■ Practice, coaching, and the self-check gave him confidence to learn CPR ■ Felt great that he saved his grandmother's life. Intellectual health ■ He knew the CPR steps ■ He understood why CPR works Social health ■ He felt proud receiving the Valor Award ■ His family was very proud of him Physical health ■ Exhausted ■ Nauseous
How did the school and community affect personal health practices and behavior *by teaching CPR*? (2.12.4.)	
■ What is the mission of Lakeview High School?	The school's mission is to provide a safe and healthy school environment where students learn the content and skills needed to meet life's challenges.
■ Is the school meeting the mission? Provide the evidence.	Yes. Demetry learned CPR and used it to save his grandmother's life.
■ Two positive effects of the school teaching CPR on student health practices and behaviors.	Demetry learned CPR; Demetry gained self-efficacy to perform CPR.
■ Negative effects of the school teaching CPR on student health practices and behaviors.	Increased student anxiety prior to the beginning of CPR.
■ Other evaluation comments	Demetry was recognized by the school by being given the Valor Award for saving his grandmother's life.
Self-Awareness: Self-efficacy How did the school give Demetry the confidence and belief that he could administer CPR? (mastery experience, vicarious experience, verbal persuasion, positive emotional state)	The health teacher modeled the CPR skills (mastery experience); students practiced in front of everyone else (vicarious experience); the teacher accurately assessed the students as they practiced and provided effective and targeted feedback (verbal persuasion); the teacher was enthusiastic as she greeted the students with the baby mannequin and modeled the skills (positive emotional state)

even when an adjustment in the work is needed, learn from the formative assessment given by the teacher, and gain confidence by watching peers successfully complete the same challenge. (Frey, Fisher, & Smith, 2019, p. 32)

A person with a growth mindset believes that mistakes are a way to learn. He believes he achieves through effort and perseverance. If failure occurs, this person figures out a way to cope with it and does not blame himself. A person with a growth mindset stays with a difficult task until completion. Having a growth mindset is important because it affects all parts of our lives and gives us the confidence to develop the skills necessary to meet life's challenges. (Frey, Fisher, & Smith, 2019, pp. 32, 33)

Importance of Feedback in Helping Students Develop a Growth Mindset

Using feedback to help children become self-aware and develop a growth mindset enhances teaching and learning and the acquisition of the sub-competencies. Feedback should always refer to the performance indicators and competencies and provide guidance on how to achieve them. Saying, "Well done" may cause the child to feel good but ask the question, "What did I do that was well done?" In contrast, if the feedback is, "Mary, your tracing of the map from your classroom to the nurse's office really showed me that you can (3.2.2) identify ways to locate school health helpers!" (Joint Committee on National Health Education Standards, 2007, p. 28) Now, Mary knows why the teacher is complimenting her. (self-awareness)

Another classroom strategy includes giving children a practice prompt and challenge that provides the opportunity for them to demonstrate content, skill, and SEL competency. As the students practice meeting the challenge, the teacher provides effective feedback, fundamental to assessment and instruction. Giving effective feedback is fundamental to assessment and instruction. Research by Carol Dweck in 2007 documented how different types of feedback impacted student motivation.

As students worked on a puzzle, the researcher complimented the first group on their strategy of building the puzzle from the outside edges in. Students with this growth mindset believed that mistakes were a part of learning and that being smart is a result of hard work and persistence, not innate ability.

The second group received feedback complimenting them about their innate ability to do puzzles. Because of the feedback, the first group outperformed the second. The second group developed a fixed mindset meaning that they believed that their puzzle abilities were innate or predetermined. These students believed they did not have to work so hard and viewed mistakes as negative. (Posey, 2019)

What Is the Relationship between Self-Confidence, Self-Efficacy, and Growth Mindset?

When a student is self-confident, he has a sense of his own self-worth based on his accomplishments. When a student is efficacious, he believes he has what it takes to achieve a goal or a task. A student with a growth mindset believes that his abilities may change over time due to how hard he tries, his ability to stay with a difficult task, and his willingness to practice until he achieves his goal.

A student with high self-efficacy and a growth mindset is self-confident. He believes he can persevere through challenges and meet his goal if he tries hard and learns new coping skills. (Transforming Education, 2020)

In skills-based health education instruction, self-confidence, self-efficacy, and developing a growth mindset are inherent in our practice. We teach students skills and competencies, one step at a time, and provide time to practice and acquire them. We formatively assess and provide effective feedback to help the student gain confidence and succeed.

There are several pedagogical strategies to encourage a growth mindset in the classroom.

- *Praising effort and process rather than just the results.* (Transforming Education, 2020) For example, "You did an excellent job on that presentation! Your role play demonstrated that you tried very hard to follow the rubric and that you understand the content and skill learned in class."
- *Nurturing a classroom culture that accepts risk taking.* (Transforming Education, 2020) For example, "Remember we worked together to design our classroom norms and that we all agreed that we value the challenge of a difficult task rather than choosing easier tasks?"
- *Emphasizing process and perseverance.* (Transforming Education, 2020) For example, "Look at the sample content posters and the role plays of previous students. On this wall, is the rough draft of the project. After giving feedback to the students about showing proficiency in the performance indicators and SEL competencies, look at how the projects improved! Let's work together, I am here to help you succeed."
- *Thinking of the brain as something that develops over time.* (Transforming Education, 2020) For example, "Let's grow our brain today! We are going to learn something new and practice. By practicing and trying hard to achieve, we strengthen our brain."
- *Encouraging students to help each other by offering tips to success.* (Transforming Education, 2020) After the completion of an authentic assessment, (role play, video, comic strip, or drawing, etc.) take time for the students to write a "Tips for Success" for the next group of students assigned to the same task.
- *Framing mistakes as part of learning.* (Transforming Education, 2020) Show a video clip of a professional performer (actor, performer, musician, orator, etc.). Ask the students to reflect on how much practice it took to be so proficient. Ask the students their opinion about the mistakes the person may have made on the way to achieving his/her status. Ask about the value of making mistakes and staying with the practice if they want to succeed.

- *Specifically rewarding effort or process in addition to outcomes.* (Transforming Education, 2020) As part of the nonstandards portion of the analytical rubric, provide credit for effort.
- *Communicating high expectations.* (Transforming Education, 2020) Introduce the performance indicators and SEL competency at the beginning of the unit and each lesson. Define the verbs and competency so the students understand them. Model the steps to the skill and provide student practice time and effective, targeted feedback. This pedagogical practice sets high expectations for the students.

PreK–2: Self-Awareness: Growth Mindset

Lesson Overview: Working in a Group.

Students may believe they do not work well in a group. By examining the health benefits of working in a group as well as expressing needs, wants, and feelings, the students may move from the fixed to a growth mindset.

Note:

- The skill performance indicator is from the grade span 3–5. However, it is adjusted to be age-appropriate.
- This resource may be appropriate for a PreK–2 mindset overview https://ideas.classdojo.com/i /growth-mindset-1

Materials needed:

- **Worksheet 3.19 Moving from a Fixed to Growth Mindset**

Table 3.40 provides an overview of the lesson objectives, assessment, and instruction for this lesson.

Step 3 – Instruction

1. Define
   a. Identify: To recognize a particular person or an object.
   b. Demonstrate: To show how something is accomplished.
   c. Self-awareness: An accurate understanding of a person's own values, emotions, and wants and needs.
   d. Fixed mindset: A person believes his/her basic qualities including intelligence and talent, are unchanging and unchangeable traits. (Frey, Fisher, & Smith, 2019, pp. 30-31)
   e. Growth mindset: A person believes their basic abilities can be developed through focused efforts, dedication, and hard work. (Frey, Fisher, & Smith, 2019, p. 31)
2. 1.2.1 <u>Identify</u> that healthy behaviors *such as participating in a group* affect personal health.
   a. Ask the children to raise their hand if they like to
      1) Work in a group. Ask the children to explain why.

Table 3.40 Lesson Objectives, Assessment, and Instruction

Step 1 – Lesson Objectives	Step 2 – Assessment
The verb of the *infused* performance indicator and the SEL competency generate the assessment and instruction.	Design the assessment based on the objectives. Ask yourself the question, "What can my students do to show me they have met the standard?"
1.2.1 <u>Identify</u> that healthy behaviors *such as participating in a group* affect personal health. (Joint Committee on National Health Education Standards, 2007, p. 24)	1.2.1 Students <u>identify</u> *one way participating in a group* affects their personal health.
2.5.3 Identify how peers influence healthy and unhealthy behaviors *when working in a group.* (Joint Committee on National Health Education Standards, 2007, p. 26)	2.5.3 Students <u>identify</u> two ways peers influence healthy and unhealthy behaviors *when working in a group.*
Self-Awareness: Growth mindset	Give an example of how a person changes his or her mindset from fixed to growth.
Step 3 – Instruction	
Design the instruction so that students learn the content, skill, and competency to be successful on the assessment. Ask the question, "What do I need to teach so that the students will be successful when assessed?"	

2) Work alone. Ask the children to explain why.

  b. Ask the children if they can change their feelings about working in a group.

    i. Explain that when a person believes that he or she cannot do something well because that is the way they are, that is a fixed mindset.

    ii. Explain that when a person believes that if he or she tries hard and stay with a difficult task, he or she can succeed, that is a growth mindset.

    iii. Explain that with practice and perseverance, a person is able to change his or her attitude about liking or not liking working in a group. (Moving from fixed to growth mindset)

  c. Use **Worksheet 3.19 Moving from a Fixed to Growth Mindset** to show how attitudes can change with good rules and coaching. (Self-Awareness: Self-Efficacy)

3. 2.5.3 Identify how peers influence healthy and unhealthy behaviors *when working in a group.*

  a. Ask the students to brainstorm how peers influence healthy and unhealthy behaviors when working in a group. Use the lists below to guide the discussion.

  b. Peers influencing healthy behaviors

    1) Group success depends on the hard work of each person.

    2) Individual members are accountable for learning content, skill, SEL competency.

    3) Group members

      a) Encourage and help one another.

      b) Set a goal and everyone works to meet the goal.

      c) Listen to one another.

      d) Are respectful of one another.

  c. Peers influencing unhealthy behaviors

    a. Some group members ignore or belittle group members who they perceive as low achievers.

    b. Some group members socialize while others work.

    c. Some group members dominate and tell others what to do rather than deciding as a group. (Slavin, 2014)

1. Read the practice prompt. Students answer the reflection questions and discuss.

Practice Prompt: Natalie

In health class, Mrs. Sorrento always places students in groups to do a variety of activities. Natalie is a quiet girl and does not like to work in a group or role play in class. She tried to be a good group member but was always worried that the group didn't think she was smart. When she made mistakes in the group, they got frustrated with her and started telling her what to do. Other members of the group didn't do any work. They just talked all the time. After a while, the group ignored her. Natalie got very upset with herself and she found it was easier to give up and let someone else do the work.

She doesn't have many friends as a result, but she is used to that. Until now, teachers would let her do whatever she was most comfortable doing, as long as she participated and completed her work. Mrs. Sorrento was different.

She wanted to help Natalie gain confidence to work in a group. Mrs. Sorrento encouraged Natalie to first sit with the group then slowly take on a role in the group activities. When Natalie found the other students were kind to her, accepted and encouraged her, she felt different about being in a group. She began to look forward to health class to be with her new friends.

Natalie has always liked to write. If she makes mistakes in her writing, she doesn't get upset. She just makes the changes and keeps writing. Mrs. Sorrento challenged the group to write a prompt then act it out. Natalie took a chance and volunteered to write the prompt and her group loved it! Natalie was pleased but told the group, "I don't want to role play so can I write the prompts instead of acting them out?"

One day, one of her group mates, who had a speaking role in a class presentation, was absent. Her group asked Natalie to act in the role play. She said, "I can't speak in front of the class. I never speak in front of the class!" Her teammates encouraged her by explaining she would only be saying the words she already wrote. It would be easy. She didn't want to but didn't want to let her group mates down.

The group had time to practice and encouraged and supported Natalie. They told her that the role play doesn't have to be perfect—she just had to try her best! She practiced and practiced and listened to the suggestions of her group to make the role play better.

On the day of the presentation, with her nerves on edge, she participated in the role play. She felt good! She felt great! She was smiling and enjoyed watching the faces of her peers as she acted out the words she wrote!

After class, Natalie told Mrs. Sorrento that she enjoyed her new role and looks forward to acting again.

Table 3.41 How Participating in a Group Affects Personal Health, Influence of Peers, and Growth Mindset

Question	Answer
What is *one way participating in a group* affected Natalie's personal health? (1.2.1)	In Mrs. Sorrento's class, Natalie became less shy, more social, and more confident in her writing and speaking ability.

<u>What are</u> two ways Natalie's peers influenced healthy and unhealthy behaviors *when working in a group*? (2.5.3)	Healthy behaviors in Mrs. Sorrento's group
	■ The members were kind to Natalie.
	■ The group accepted and encouraged Natalie.
	■ Natalie took a chance and volunteered to write a prompt.
	■ The group encouraged Natalie to participate in the role play and take the place of a person who was absent. She did and now believes she can not only write the role plays but also act in them.
	Unhealthy behaviors of a previous group
	■ When Natalie made a mistake, the members got frustrated with her and started telling her what to do.
	■ Some members of the group didn't do any work. They just talked all the time.
	■ The group ignored Natalie.
	■ Because of the reaction of the group,
	  • Natalie got very upset with herself and found it was easier just to give up and let someone else do the work.
	  • Natalie doesn't have many friends.

Self-Awareness: Self-Confidence, recognizing strengths How did Natalie change her mindset from fixed to growth?	Natalie's fixed mindset of not participating in a group and not being comfortable working in a group was changed to a growth mindset when her group supported her and gave her the confidence to speak the words she had written.

5. Guide the students through the assessment questions in **Table 3.41**.
6. Ask the students to put away their materials then ask review questions.
   a. What is one positive result of working in a group? (1.2.1)
   b. What is one way peers influence healthy behaviors? (2.5.2)
   c. What is one way peers influence unhealthy behaviors? (2.5.2)
   d. If someone believes if they work hard, they can improve or achieve, do they have a fixed or growth mindset?
7. Exit ticket (Self-Awareness: growth mindset) What is one thing you can do to influence healthy behaviors in a group?

Grades 3–5: Self-Awareness: Growth Mindset

Lesson Overview: Making Friends.
Students describe how having a growth mindset enhances their health and ways the peers influence healthy and unhealthy behaviors.

Navigating social challenges is enhanced when children understand that a person who has not been friendly or respectful is able to change his or her behavior, rather than believing that if a peer is mean, he or she will always be mean. A student who believes that behavior can change exhibits a growth mindset.

This lesson introduces the growth mindset and ways to use it to cope with the influence of peers.

Resources:
- Mindset of a Champion: Carson Byblow/TEDx Youth@AASSofia (6:48 minutes)
- www.mindsetworks.com
- Developing a Growth Mindset! Dr. Nagler's Laboratory: You Tube
- To introduce the concept of "Growth mindset," watch the five minute video from https://ideas.classdojo.com/i/growth-mindset-1
- My Mindset Matters: https://media.centervention.com/pdf/growth-mindset-worksheet.pdf
- Explain the neuroscience from the Mindset Kit https://www.mindsetkit.org/topics/teaching-growth-mindset/explain-the-neuroscience
- Stanford University, PERTS: https://www.perts.net/

Table 3.42 Lesson Objectives, Assessment, and Instruction

Step 1 – Lesson Objectives	Step 2 – Assessment
The verb of the *infused* performance indicator and the SEL competency generate the assessment and instruction.	Design the assessment based on the objectives. Ask yourself the question, "What can my students do to show me they have met the standard?"
1.5.1 <u>Describe</u> the relationship between healthy behaviors *such as having a growth mindset* and personal health. (Joint Committee on National Health Education Standards, 2007, p. 24)	1.5.1 Students <u>describe</u> *three ways* having a growth mindset enhances personal health.
2.5.3 <u>Identify</u> how peers influence healthy behaviors (*growth mindset*) and unhealthy behaviors (*fixed mindset*). (Joint Committee on National Health Education Standards, 2007, p. 26)	2.5.3 Students <u>identify</u> *three ways* peers influence healthy behaviors (*growth mindset*) and unhealthy behaviors (*fixed mindset*).
Self-Awareness: Growth mindset	Students list three reasons why it is healthier to have a growth mindset than a fixed mindset.

Step 3 – Instruction
Design the instruction so that students learn the content, skill, and competency to be successful on the assessment. Ask the question, "What do I need to teach so that the students will be successful when assessed?"

Materials needed:

- **Worksheet 3.20 Influencing Peers to Move from a Fixed to Growth Mindset**

Table 3.42 provides an overview of the lesson objectives, assessment, and instruction for this lesson.

Step 3 – Instruction

1. Define
   a. Identify: To recognize a particular person or an object.
   b. Describe: To use words that help others envision the physical attributes of a person, place, or thing.
   c. Self-awareness: An accurate understanding of a person's own values, emotions, and wants and needs.
   d. Influence: The ability to bring about a change by using persuasion.
   e. Fixed mindset: A person believes his/her basic qualities including intelligence and talent, are unchanging and unchangeable traits. (Frey, Fisher, & Smith, 2019, pp. 30-31)
   f. Growth mindset: A person believes his/her basic abilities can be developed through focused efforts, dedication, and hard work. (Frey, Fisher, & Smith, 2019, p. 31)
2. 1.5.1 <u>Describe</u> the relationship between healthy behaviors *such as having a growth mindset* and personal health.
   a. View the YouTube video, "Mindset of a Champion." This video is a Ted Talk for kids. Carson

Byblow is a 5th grade student who describes fixed and growth mindsets that include his own struggle with reading to the stories of athletic and media stars.
   b. Place a fixed mindset sign on one side of the class and a growth mindset sign on the other side. After viewing the video, read characteristics of a fixed growth mindset and ask the children to move to the sign that fits the description (**Figure 3.6**).
      1) Characteristics of a fixed mindset.
         a) I was born with a certain amount of intelligence and it cannot be changed.
         b) If I show a lot of effort, that means I do not have much ability.
         c) I am focused on looking smart rather than learning.
         d) I avoid asking questions when I don't understand something.
         e) If I have to try hard, I am not smart.

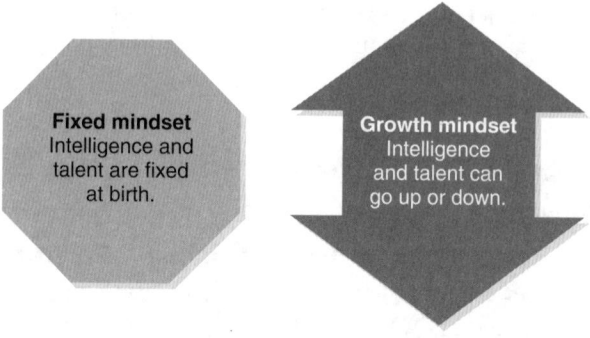

Figure 3.6 Fixed Mindset vs. Growth Mindset.

f) I give up when faced with a challenge or setback because I believe it means I am not smart.

2) Characteristics of a growth mindset
   a) I believe that intelligence grows over time by challenging myself.
   b) When I challenge myself and try, I can get smarter.
   c) My main goal is to learn.
   d) I ask questions when I do not understand something because I know that is how to learn.
   e) I like challenges.
   f) I try hard. (Blackwell, 2007)

b. Ask the children
   1) How does having a growth mindset affect your health? (gain confidence, develop self-esteem, develop self-efficacy, positive mental health because of accomplishing something difficult and reaching goals.)
   2) How does having a fixed mindset affect your health? (decrease confidence, self-esteem, and self-efficacy, decrease in mental health because of a lack of trying and working hard and giving up. (Self-Awareness: Growth mindset)

3. 2.5.3 Identify how peers influence behaviors (*Growth mindset*) and unhealthy behaviors.
   a. Activity.
      1) Use **Worksheet 3.20 Influencing Peers to Move from a Fixed to a Growth Mindset** to identify influences on behaviors.
      2) Review

4. Read the practice prompt. Students answer the reflection questions and discuss.

Practice Prompt: Marinda

Marinda is a shy 5th grade student who has trouble making friends. She thought she made friends with Amalia and her group but when Marinda checked her social media, the group told her she couldn't hang around with them. She was devastated. She didn't want to get hurt anymore, so she stopped trying to make friends. She thought other children just didn't like her for some reason. She thought about asking her classmates why Amalia doesn't want to be friends, but she didn't. She is very lonely.

Donato noticed that Marinda was always by herself, so he sat with her at lunch and asked how she was doing. Marinda almost started crying but she told him nothing was wrong. He asked her if she would like to move to his table and eat with his

friends. Marinda said, "No, thank you." She was afraid once they got to know her, they would reject her.

Donato ate lunch with Marinda and told her how much he enjoyed her story in health class about trying new things. Marinda laughed and told him she can write about being adventuresome, but she can't do it in real life. He asked her if she would help him with his health project. He had to write a part for the role play. She said, "OK."

For the next few days, Marinda and Donato worked together in the library on the role play. It was a challenge, but they did it and it felt good! They talked and laughed and had a good time. Donato introduced Marinda to his friends. and they made her feel very welcome. Maybe there was nothing wrong with her and she could make friends. Marinda was starting to feel confident, speaking more in class, and asking questions when she didn't understand something. She offered to help her friends who had trouble writing. She was happy.

5. Guide the students through the assessment questions in **Table 3.43**.
6. Ask the students to put away their materials and then ask review questions.
   a. What is a benefit of having a growth mindset? (1.5.1)
   b. What is one characteristic of a person with a fixed mindset?
   c. How can someone change from a fixed to a growth mindset?
   d. How do peers influence others to have a fixed or growth mindset? (2.5.3)
7. Exit ticket (Self-Awareness: fixed/growth mindset) Give an example of something you have a fixed mindset about and how you can change it to a growth mindset.

Grades 6–8: Self-Awareness: Growth Mindset

Lesson Overview: Using a Growth Mindset to Quit Marijuana. In this lesson, students learn the likelihood of injury or illness when smoking marijuana along with how smoking marijuana may lead to other harmful behaviors.

In 2019, 11.8% of 8th graders reported using marijuana in the past year and 6.6% in the past month. (National Institute of Drug Abuse, 2020)

Resources:

- The YouTube video, Growing Your Brain, provides a good introduction to the concept of fixed and growth mindsets. https://www.youtube.com/watch?v=WtKJrB5rOKs&feature=youtu.be

Table 3.43 How a Growth Mindset Enhances Health, Is Influenced by Peers, and Advantages of a Growth Mindset

Question	Answer
What are *three ways* having a growth mindset enhanced Marinda's personal health? (1.5.1)	Although writing the role play was difficult, Marinda did it and it felt good. Making new friends gave Marinda confidence. Marinda started speaking more in class and asking questions when she didn't understand something.
What were *three ways* Marinda's peers influenced healthy behaviors (growth mindset) and unhealthy behaviors (fixed mindset)? (2.5.3)	Peers influenced unhealthy behaviors when ■ They told Miranda through social media that she couldn't hang around with them. ■ Marinda stopped trying to make friends because she thought others just didn't like her. ■ Marinda lost confidence in reaching out to other peers. Peers influenced healthy behaviors when Donato ■ Sat with Marinda at lunch ■ Complimented her on her writing and about trying new things. ■ Asked her to help him write the role play. ■ Introduced her to his friends and they made her feel very welcome.
Self-Awareness: Growth mindset List *three reasons* why it is healthier to have a growth mindset than a fixed mindset.	Develop ■ Confidence ■ Self-esteem ■ Self-efficacy ■ Mental health because of accomplishing something difficult and reaching goals

Material needed:

- Worksheet 3.21 Grades 6–8 Mindset Self-Quiz
- Worksheet 3.22 Growth Mindset and Marijuana
- Worksheet 3.23 Changing Fixed Mindset Language to Growth Mindset Language

Table 3.44 provides an overview of the lesson objectives, assessment, and instruction for this lesson.

Table 3.44 Lesson Objectives, Assessment, and Instruction

Step 1 – Lesson Objectives	Step 2 – Assessment
The verb of the *infused* performance indicator and the SEL competency generate the assessment and instruction.	Design the assessment based on the objectives. Ask yourself the question, "What can my students do to show me they have met the standard?"
1.8.8 Examine the likelihood of injury or illness if engaging in unhealthy behaviors *such as using marijuana.* (Joint Committee on National Health Education Standards, 2007, p. 25)	1.8.8 Students examine *three examples* of injury or illness associated with using marijuana.
2.8.9 Describe how some health risk behaviors, *such as smoking marijuana,* influence the likelihood of engaging in unhealthy behaviors (Joint Committee on National Health Education Standards, 2007, p. 27)	2.8.9 Students describe *three* additional unhealthy behaviors that may result from using marijuana.
Self-Awareness: Growth mindset	Students explain how having a growth mindset helps a teen make a healthy decision about using marijuana.

Step 3 – Instruction

Design the instruction so that students learn the content, skill, and competency to be successful on the assessment. Ask the question, "What do I need to teach so that the students will be successful when assessed?".

Step 3 – Instruction

1. Define
   a. Examine: Look carefully at someone or something to determine the condition.
   b. Describe: To use words that help others envision the physical attributes of a person, place, or thing.
   c. Fixed mindset: A person believes their basic qualities including intelligence and talent, are unchanging and unchangeable traits. (Frey, Fisher, & Smith, 2019, pp. 30-31)
   d. Growth mindset: A person believes their basic abilities can be developed through focused efforts, dedication, and hard work. (Frey, Fisher, & Smith, 2019, p. 31)

2. Background information about fixed and growth mindset
   a. View the YouTube video, Growing Your Brain to learn the difference between fixed and growth mindset.
   b. Follow the viewing of the video with **Worksheet 3.21 Grades 6–8 Mindset Self-Quiz**
      i. Fixed mindset: Questions 1, 2, 3, 5
      ii. Growth mindset: Questions 4, 6, 7
   c. Characteristics of a fixed mindset.
      i. I was born with a certain amount of intelligence and it cannot be changed.
      ii. If I show a lot of effort, it means I do not have much ability.
      iii. I am focused on looking smart rather than learning.
      iv. I avoid asking questions when I don't understand something.
      v. If I have to try hard, I am not smart. I give up when faced with a challenge or setback because I believe it means I am not smart.
   d. Characteristics of a growth mindset.
      i. I believe that intelligence grows over time by challenging myself.
      ii. When I challenge myself and try, I can get smarter.
      iii. My main goal is to learn.
      iv. I ask questions when I do not understand something because I know that is how to learn.
      v. I like challenges.
      vi. I try hard. (Blackwell, 2007)

3. 1.8.8 <u>Examine</u> the likelihood of injury or illness if engaging in unhealthy behaviors *such as using marijuana.*
   a. Read the information on **Worksheet 3.22 Growth Mindset and Marijuana**
      1) On the back of the paper, use the first graphic organizer to write down the short- and long-term effects of using marijuana.

4. 2.8.9 <u>Describe</u> how some health risk behaviors, *such as smoking marijuana,* influence the likelihood of engaging in unhealthy behaviors.
   a. Read the information on **Worksheet 3.22 Growth Mindset and Marijuana**
      1) Use the second graphic organizer to analyze how using marijuana may lead to other unhealthy behaviors. (Self-Awareness: Growth mindset)

5. Read the practice prompt. Students answer the reflection questions and discuss.

Practice Prompt: Lamonte and Tyrone

Lamonte and Tyrone have been friends for a long time. Lamonte finds school difficult and doesn't think he is very smart. Consequently, he gives up easily and doesn't try. He is embarrassed to ask questions because he doesn't want to look stupid in front of the class. At the beginning of the school year, Lamonte started smoking weed and hanging out with a different group of friends. He has changed a lot. Before smoking weed, he would always exercise, and worry about school; now he doesn't seem to care about either. He gets moody, is putting on weight, and can't seem to think problems through. He quit cross country because he got too winded to run long distance. Lamonte is nervous because his heart pounds when he is not even running.

The new user friends smoke weed but also experiment with other drugs and do other things

(continues)

Practice Prompt: Lamonte and Tyrone (continued)

Lamonte is not comfortable with but finds interesting and exciting. One Friday night, Lavoy, one of Lamonte's new friends, had a party. His parents were away for the weekend. Teens were vaping and smoking marijuana. After a while, Lamonte went into the liquor cabinet and took out some rum. He mixed it with orange juice and told everyone it was a healthy drink. Everyone laughed. Some of the girls were taking pills that made them silly. He noticed the boys and girls pairing off and going into the bedrooms. Lamonte got a little nervous when he saw what was going on, but he stayed at the party anyway. After all, these kids were his friends. When one of his friends came back after being with a girl, Lamonte asked what was going on. His friend said, "Come on, getting together is more fun when you are high!" Lamonte asked if he used a condom. The friend looked at him, laughed, and said, "I don't need a condom." Lavoy's older brother, who had been drinking, drove everyone home. Lamonte was glad he got home safely.

Although Lamonte and Ty loved playing sports, lately, they don't get together anymore to throw the ball. Ty is an optimistic boy who likes a challenge and is not afraid to fail a few times until he finally figures things out. He knows if he asks for help and keeps trying, he will succeed.

Ty is worried about Lamonte and wants to help him. After school last week, they walked home from school together. Ty asked Lamonte about quitting weed. Lamonte said he knew weed was getting in the way of school and sports, but he didn't think he could quit. He quit once before but then went right back to it. He told Ty that maybe, if he were smarter, he would have the willpower to quit but he knows he is not as smart as many of his peers.

Ty asked if he could help. After a little encouragement, Lamonte said, "Yes." First, they agreed they would hang out together and Lamonte would not hang out with his user friends. Right away, Lamonte felt better. They started hitting balls at the playground and throwing the football. These activities helped Lamonte believe he could change. His head started to clear, and he was less moody. Ty helped him with homework and that helped a lot. It showed him he could learn some of the hard things being taught and gave him the confidence to ask the teacher some questions. Lamonte knew the schoolwork was not going to be easy but if he tried and asked for help, he might be able to figure things out.

The boys are good friends again. Ty has stopped smoking weed. Both boys feel really good about themselves and about each other!

6. Guide the students through the assessment questions in **Table 3.45**.
7. Ask the students to put away their materials then ask review questions.

a. What is one short-term effect of smoking marijuana? (1.8.8)
b. What is one long-term effect of smoking marijuana? (1.8.8)

Table 3.45 Injuries/illnesses Related to Marijuana Use, Risky Behaviors Associated with Marijuana Use, and the Advantage of Having a Growth Mindset

Question	Answer
What are *three examples* of injury or illness that Lamonte experienced when using marijuana? (1.8.8)	Lamonte ■ Was moody ■ Became winded when running ■ Felt his heart pounding ■ Couldn't think through problems
What were *three* additional risky behaviors that Lamonte experienced as a result of using marijuana? (2.8.9)	Additional risky behaviors ■ Was friendly with peers who experimented with other drugs. ■ Became friendly with peers who were sexually active and not using a condom. ■ Stayed at a party where peers were using drugs. ■ Drove with someone who had been drinking.
Self-Awareness: Growth mindset How did having a growth mindset help Lamonte quit using marijuana?	A growth mindset helped Lamonte quit smoking by giving him confidence and showing him that he can succeed if he tries hard and doesn't give up. Supplemental: **Worksheet 3.23 Changing Fixed Mindset Language to Growth Mindset Language.**

c. How does marijuana influence the likelihood of engaging in other unhealthy behaviors? (2.8.9)

d. How may a fixed mindset contribute to drug use?

e. How may a growth mindset help keep a teen drug free? (Wang, 2019)

8. Exit ticket (Self-Awareness: fixed/growth mindset) Give an example of something you have a fixed mindset about and how you can change it to a growth mindset.

Grades 9–12: Self-Awareness: Growth Mindset

Lesson Overview: Mindset. Students describe the relationships between a growth mindset and the components of health and the perception that the mindset is fixed.

Resources:

- Fixed vs. Growth Mindset - https://www.youtube.com/watch?v=x0Y4QhdqUMA
- Mindset Assessment - http://blog.mindsetworks.com/what-s-my-mindset
- PERTS A Mindset for 9th Graders is an online "Growth mindset" program specifically for grade 9 students. https://neptune.perts.net/static/programs/hg17/information_packet.pdf
- Quizlet is a formative assessment tool to check content knowledge. The product is accessed through subscription but this sample is available at https://quizlet.com/107610977/growth-mindset-vs-fixed-mindset-self-test-flash-cards/
- Implicit theories of intelligence predict achievement across an adolescent transition: A longitudinal study and intervention (Yeager, 2016)

Materials needed:

- **Worksheet 3.24 Grades 9–12 Mindset Self-Quiz**
- **Worksheet 3.25 Famous Person Growth Mindset Sort**
- **Worksheet 3.26 Challenging the Mindset Voice**

Table 3.46 provides an overview of the lesson objectives, assessment, and instruction for this lesson.

Step 3 – Instruction

1. Define
   a. Describe: To use words that help others envision the physical attributes of a person, place, or thing.
   b. Analyze: To scrutinize something or someone in order to understand how it or they work(s).
   c. Fixed mindset: A person believes their basic qualities including intelligence and talent, are unchanging and unchangeable traits. (Frey, Fisher, & Smith, 2019, pp. 30-31)
   d. Growth mindset: A person believes their basic abilities can be developed through focused

Table 3.46 Lesson Objectives, Assessment, and Instruction

Step 1 – Lesson Objectives	Step 2 – Assessment
The verb of the *infused* performance indicator and the SEL competency generate the assessment and instruction.	Design the assessment based on the objectives. Ask yourself the question, "What can my students do to show me they have met the standard?"
1.12.2 Describe the interrelationships of emotional, intellectual, physical, and social health *when developing a growth mindset.* (Joint Committee on National Health Education Standards, 2007, p. 25)	1.12.2 Students describe *three* interrelationships between having a growth mindset and emotional, intellectual, physical, and social health. Students choose either a famous person or another example of their choice.
2.12.7 Analyze how the perception of norms, *regarding mindset*, influence health and unhealthy behaviors. (Joint Committee on National Health Education Standards, 2007, p. 27)	2.12.7 Write a short paragraph to analyze the perception that a mindset is fixed vs. the ability to have a mindset that allows for growth.
Self-Awareness: Growth mindset	Students explain how having a growth mindset helps a teen decrease stress.

Step 3 – Instruction
Design the instruction so that students learn the content, skill, and competency to be successful on the assessment. Ask the question, "What do I need to teach so that the students will be successful when assessed?"

efforts, dedication, and hard work. (Frey, Fisher, & Smith, 2019, p. 31)

2. Background information about fixed and growth mindsets
   a. View the YouTube video, Growing Your Brain to learn the difference between fixed and growth mindset. (see resource above)
   b. If online access is available, students take the Mindset Assessment: http://blog.mind-setworks.com/what-s-my-mindset; If online access is not available, use **Worksheet 3.24 Grades 9–12 Mindset Self-Quiz** to determine mindset.
   c. Additional information from the article, Implicit theories of intelligence predict achievement across an adolescent transition: A longitudinal study and intervention, provides a list of fixed and growth mindset characteristics.
   d. Characteristics of a fixed mindset.
      1) I am born with a certain amount of intelligence and it cannot be changed.
      2) If I show a lot of effort, it means I do not have much ability.
      3) I am focused on looking smart rather than learning.
      4) I avoid asking questions when I don't understand something.
      5) If I have to try hard, I am not smart.
      6) I give up when faced with a challenge or setback because I believe it means I am not smart.
   e. Characteristics of a growth mindset
      1) I believe that intelligence grows over time by challenging myself.
      2) When I challenge myself and try, I can get smarter.
      3) My main goal is to learn.
      4) I ask questions when I do not understand something because I know that is how to learn.
      5) I like challenges.
      6) I try hard. (Blackwell, 2007)

3. 1.12.2 Describe the interrelationships of emotional, intellectual, physical, and social health *and a growth mindset.*
   a. Using the **Worksheet 3.25 Famous Person Growth Mindset Sort** (**Table 3.47**), cut the paper into strips, then cut the name from the story. Students match the name to the story. When complete, discuss the possible effects of a famous person's growth mindset story on their emotional, intellectual, physical, and social health.
   b. For further study, research each person and map their characteristics to the growth mindset characteristics. Discuss.

4. 2.12.7 Analyze how the perception of norms, *regarding mindset,* influence health and unhealthy behaviors.
   a. The norm for some teens may be the fixed mindset. To challenge the fixed mindset voice, complete **Worksheet 3.26 Challenging the Mindset Voice**

5. Read the practice prompt. Students answer the reflection questions, and discuss.

Table 3.47 The Mindset Story of Famous People

Famous Person	Growth Mindset Story
Walt Disney	Fired from the Kansas City Star because his editor felt he lacked imagination and had no good ideas.
Oprah Winfrey	Publicly fired from her first television as an anchor in Baltimore for getting too emotionally invested in her stories.
Steven Spielberg	Was rejected by the University of Southern California School of Cinematic Arts multiple times.
R. H. Macy	Had a series of failed retail ventures throughout his early career.
Soichiro Honda	His unique vision got him ostracized by the Japanese business community.
Colonel Harland David Sanders	Fired from dozens of jobs before founding a fried chicken empire.
Sir Isaac Newton	His mother pulled him out of school as a boy so he could run the family farm. He failed miserably.

Thomas Edison	Teachers told him he was too stupid to learn anything.
Sidney Poitier	When he first auditioned for the American Negro Theatre, he flubbed his lines and spoke in a heavy Caribbean accent. The director stopped the audition and told him to get a job as a dishwasher.
Albert Einstein	As a child, he had some difficulty communicating and learning in a traditional manner.

Data from Business Insider. (2020, March 19). 29 incredibly successful people who failed at first. Retrieved from Business Insider: https://www.businessinsider.in/29-incredibly-successful-people-who-failed-at-first/articleshow/48010383.cms

Practice Prompt: Melia

Melia enjoys hearing her peers talk about the "Future Health Teacher Club." She likes her high school but doesn't think she is smart enough to even think about being a teacher. Her mother and father graduated high school, are very smart, and both work in the service industry. It is expected that she will do the same. Some of her peers think Melia is smart, which she likes, so when she doesn't understand something, she pretends she does. She won't do something new unless she knows she will succeed with little effort. If things get too hard, she quits.

One day, a member of the "Future Health Teacher Club" spoke to her health class. He explained that they work together with their advisor to plan events and lessons to teach to the elementary and middle school students. As a little girl, Melia played teacher with her younger sister and she enjoyed it. She found that she had to really know what she was teaching, or her sister would get bored. Because her student was her sister, Melia met the challenge, and they both had a lot of fun. This club appealed to her.

Her friend, Marissa, decided to apply and convinced Melia to join her. The girls went to a few meetings and saw that the club members supported each other. Melia had butterflies in her stomach, but she was interested. The advisor provided great suggestions for events and lessons. They were accepted!

Melia first volunteered to help at the COVID-19 informational night for parents. She didn't speak but was nervous and excited at the same time. She helped with the planning, set up, and clean up. It was challenging to work with so many different people, but she knew what to do and did it well. She was very proud of herself. Her parents were in the audience and they were very proud of her also.

During the second year of the club, she volunteered to teach a lesson on handwashing, sneezing, social distancing, and coughing in the sleeve to prevent the spread of germs. She practiced with her little sister to make sure she could explain all the facts, demonstrate the skills, and gain some confidence. The lesson went very well. The teachers from the school were very pleased to see her and complimented Melia on how she demonstrated the personal hygiene skills and how she engaged the students to practice. It seems like all the hard work was paying off. She could actually teach!

As time went on, she got more involved, worked harder, and accomplished more. Eventually, Melia believed she could fully participate in the club activities. She was learning a lot, making new friends, and she liked it! She feels that she is really growing socially, emotionally, and intellectually.

Melia is beginning to think she may succeed in college and believes she has what it takes to be a skills-based health teacher, if she puts her mind to it.

6. Guide the students through the assessment questions in **Table 3.48**.
7. Ask the students to put away their materials then ask review questions.
   a. How does a fixed mindset affect emotional, intellectual, physical, and social health and interfere with a teen reaching his/her potential? (1.12.2)
   b. How may a growth mindset affect emotional, intellectual, physical, and social health and interfere with a teen reaching his/her potential? (1.12.2)
   c. How would a teen change the norm that if he or she has a fixed mindset, it will always be fixed. (2.12.7)
8. Exit ticket (Self-Awareness: fixed/growth mindset) Give an example of something you have a fixed mindset about and how you can change it to a growth mindset.

Table 3.48 **Relationship between a Growth Mindset and the Components of Health, Influence of Beliefs About Mindset, and Advantage of Having a Growth Mindset**

Question	Answer
What were *three* interrelationships between having a growth mindset and emotional, intellectual, physical, and social health that Melia experienced? (1.12.2)	Growth mindset and emotional health. ■ Melia likes knowing her peers think she is smart. ■ Feels more confident ■ When Melia was a child, she enjoyed teaching her sister. ■ Melia was proud of herself when she helped during the parent COVID-19 presentation. ■ Melia's parents were proud of her when she helped during the parent COVID-19 presentation. Growth mindset and intellectual health. ■ She practiced with her little sister to make sure she could explain all delete the facts, demonstrate the skills, and gain some confidence. ■ Was challenged to do different things Growth mindset and physical health. ■ Melia had butterflies in her stomach, but she was interested. ■ During the COVID-19 presentation, she didn't speak but was nervous and excited at the same time. Growth mindset and social health. ■ Melia's peers think she is smart. ■ Marissa encouraged Melia to join peer leaders. ■ Made new friends ■ As Melia gained confidence, she got more involved, worked harder, and accomplished more. Eventually, Melia believed she could fully participate in the club activities. She was learning a lot, making new friends, and she liked it!
Write a short paragraph to <u>analyze</u> the perception that Melia had about a fixed mindset vs. the ability to have a mindset that allows for growth. (2.12.7)	At first, Melia was accepting of her fixed mindset but was intrigued when she heard about the "Future Health Teacher Club." As a member of the club, she accepted that she could meet difficult challenges and succeed if she tried hard. She realized she was learning a lot and liked that feeling. Eventually she began to believe she could be a skills-based health teacher if she put her mind to it.
Self-Awareness: Growth mindset How did Melia's growth mindset help her decrease stress?	With a growth mindset, a teen becomes comfortable with working hard and being challenged because he or she knows that it results in learning and feeling good about the accomplishment. The teen learns to ask questions when he or she doesn't understand something and to accept targeted feedback as a way of improving performance, not as a criticism.

Sample Lesson Plan for Analyzing Influences/Self-Awareness

Unit: *State the unit of the lesson.*	Analyzing influences
Topic: *State the topic of the lesson.*	Reducing Screen Time When with Friends *Self-Awareness: Self-confidence/Recognizing strengths*
Grade level: *State the grade level of the lesson.*	Grades 6–8
Time allotment: *State the time allotted for the lesson.*	45 minutes
Lesson summary: *Provide a summary of the lesson.*	Students become aware of the benefits of and barriers to reducing screen use and how social media affects time with friends.
Risk behavior data: *Provide time rationale for this lesson by accessing the risk behavior the lesson reduces.*	In 2015, 10% of tweens used social media every day as compared to 13% in 2019. (Rideout, 2019, p. 20)
Standards and SEL competency to reduce the risk factor(s): *List the standard 1 and skills standards and the SEL competency/sub-competency.*	1.8.7 <u>Describe</u> the benefits of and barriers to practicing healthy behaviors. 2.8.6 <u>Analyze</u> the influence of technology on personal and family health. Self-Awareness: Self-confidence, Recognizing strengths
Objectives: *The objectives are the infused performance indicators and SEL competency.*	1.8.7 <u>Describe</u> the benefits of and barriers to practicing healthy behaviors *such as cutting down on social media when out with friends.* 2.8.6 <u>Analyze</u> the influence of technology *(social media)* on personal and family *relationships.* Self-Awareness: Self-confidence, Recognizing strengths
Lesson assessment: *Design an assessment for each infused performance indicator and SEL competency.*	1.8.7 <u>Describe</u> the *three* benefits of and *three* barriers to practicing healthy behaviors *such as cutting down on social media when out with friends.* 2.8.6 <u>Analyze</u> *three* influences *social media* has on personal *relationships.* Demonstrate self-confidence when encouraging friends to decrease social media use when out socializing. Demonstrate the personal strength to speak up when encouraging friends to decrease social media use when out socializing.

Lesson instruction: *Provide a detailed description of how content, skill, and SEL competency are taught, "bell to bell."*	Review/Preview
	■ How many tweens use social media every day? (13% in 2019 compared to 10% in 2015)
	■ Think about you and your friends: Is there any benefit to cutting down on social media use? Are there any barriers to cutting down on use?
	Lesson Objectives
	    Explain each of the infused performance indicators and SEL competency/sub competency and how the students will demonstrate proficiency.
	Lesson
	■ Model the problem: Model being preoccupied with social media on the cell phone. Express concern over what you are reading; comment on having to respond; bring your attention back to the class.
	    ● Ask the students
	        1) "What was your reaction to being ignored?"
	        2) "Have you ever experienced being out with friends and everyone was on their phones rather than talking to each other? How does it make you feel?"

- Use the **Worksheet 3.11 Benefits and Barriers to Limiting Screen Time When out with Friends**, to brainstorm the benefits and barriers to limiting screen time when with friends. Discuss.

- Use **Worksheet 3.12 How Using Social Media Affects Teenagers** to read about how screen time affects relationships.
  - Use the content below to discuss how screen time affects relationships
    1) Depression
    2) Anxiety
    3) Loneliness
    4) Lack of development of social and interpersonal skills
    5) Saying things in texts that would not be said in person
    6) Choose to be on screen rather than interact in real time.

- Read the practice prompt then ask the students the re-enforcement questions.

Practice Prompt: Harrison and Ian

Harrison and Ian were hanging out after school waiting for their ride home. Both were on their phones checking their messages. They look forward to being able to use their phones after school to catch up on what everyone is doing. Teachers won't let them use their phones for texting or using other social media apps. Althea joined them. The boys said "Hi" but didn't look up from their screens. Althea was very upset and was hoping that the boys would pay attention and listen to her. She needed her friends.

After school, Althea got a terrible text from two of her friends. They were making fun of her for who she sat with at lunch. Althea felt badly for a girl who was sitting alone so she sat with her. Her friends were at a nearby table and were being rude, laughing at her, pointing at her, and making comments. After lunch, her friends wouldn't talk to her. She tried texting them but they ghosted her.

When she saw Harrison and Ian, she wanted to tell them what happened, but they wouldn't talk to her either. She thought they were friends! She couldn't sleep all night and had a head and belly ache in the morning. She didn't want to go to school.

Harrison and Ian found out what happened the next day and wondered why Althea didn't come to them for help. She told them she did, but they didn't pay any attention to her when she approached them yesterday afternoon. The boys had no clue! It made them think. Maybe when friends are together, they could keep their phones away and just talk to each other. They all want to be good friends, so they are going to give it a try.

Because of that experience, Althea gained more confidence to be assertive when she is with others who stay on their phones rather than socializing in real time. She challenges her friends to put away their phones when they are together and wait to check them when their time together is over. Some of her friends don't agree but have decreased the screen time when they are together.

She no longer cares what her old girl friends think. Her new friends care about her and they spend time together socializing and having fun.

- Reinforcement questions

What are the *three* benefits of and *three* barriers to practicing healthy behaviors *such as cutting down on social media when out with friends?* (1.8.7)	The benefits of cutting down on social media when with friends ■ Spend more time socializing ■ Practice communication skills ■ Develop friendship skills The barriers to cutting down on social media when with friends ■ Teens like their phones and don't want to limit their use.

		<ul><li>Would rather communicate by text than in person.</li><li>Want to keep up with what everyone is saying and doing. They don't want to miss out on anything.</li></ul>
	What are three influences *social media* has on personal *relationships?* (2.8.6)	<ul><li>Depression</li><li>Anxiety</li><li>Loneliness</li><li>Lack of development of social and interpersonal skills</li><li>Saying things in texts that would not be said in person</li><li>Choose to be on screen rather than interact in real time</li></ul>
	Self-Awareness: Self-confidence, recognizing strengths How did Althea demonstrate self-confidence when encouraging friends to decrease social media use when out socializing? How did Althea demonstrate the personal strength to speak up when encouraging friends to decrease social media use when out socializing?	When her friends agreed that they will try putting their phones away when they were together, Althea gained confidence to be assertive when she is with others who stay on their phones rather than socialize in real time. Before this incident, Althea would never have had the personal strength to ask her friends to give up their phones. Now she has the strength to be assertive because she knows what happens when friends are distracted and don't care for each other.

	<ul><li>End of class review: Ask the students to put away their materials then ask review questions.<ul><li>What is one benefit of limiting screen time when with friends? (1.8.7)</li><li>What is one barrier to limiting screen time when with friends? (1.8.7)</li><li>What is one influence social media has on healthy personal relationships? (2.8.6)</li></ul></li><li>Exit ticket (Self-Awareness: Self-confidence, recognizing strengths) Give an example of how coping with a challenging social experience can give you the strength and confidence to better deal with a similar situation another time.</li></ul>
Materials: *List the materials used to plan and implement the lesson, including formative assessments.*	<ul><li>Worksheet 3.11 Benefits and Barriers to Limiting Screen Time When out with Friends.</li><li>Worksheet 3.12 How Using Social Media Affects Teenagers</li></ul>
Resources: *What resources were used to plan and implement the lesson?*	N/A
Differentiated instruction: *What modifications are being made for students with disabilities and English learners?*	Students work in groups, specifically designed to support students with disabilities or English Learners.
Sample student products: *Provide exemplars of how other students successfully complete this assignment.*	Show previously completed worksheets.

Collaboration: *Are the students completing the activity individually, in pairs, in groups, etc.?*	Students work in groups of four to pair up or work as a group.
Teacher reflection: *What can I do to improve this lesson next time it is taught?*	Will vary.

References

Tucci, A. (2020). *3 Easy ways to get your teenager to eat breakfast*. Retrieved from Super Kids Nutrition https://www.superkidsnutrition.com/3-easy-ways-to-get-your-teenager-to-eat-breakfast/

American Academy of Dermatology. (2020). *What kids should know about what causes a sunburn*. Retrieved from American Academy of Dermatology https://www.aad.org/public/parents-kids/healthy-habits/parents/kids/sunburn-cause

American Heart Association. (2020). *Next Generation of Life Savers*. Retrieved from American Heart Association, CPR & First Aid, Emergency Cardiovascular Care: https://cpr.heart.org/en/training-programs/community-programs/generation-of-heartsavers

American Sexual Health Association. (2020, February 24). *STIs and young people*. Retrieved from American Sexual Health Association https://www.ashasexualhealth.org/teachers/stis-and-young-people/

Armstrong, T. (2019). *Mindfulness in the Classroom*. Alexandria: ASCD.

Blackwell, L. T., Trzesniewski, K. H., Dweck, C. S. (2007). Implicit theories of intelligence predict achievement across an adolescent transition: A longitudinal study and an intervention. *Child Development, 78*(1), 246–263.

Business Insider. (2020, March 19). *29 incredibly successful people who failed at first*. Retrieved from Business Insider https://www.businessinsider.in/29-incredibly-successful-people-who-failed-at-first/articleshow/48010383.cms

CASEL. (2019, September 21). *What is SEL?* Retrieved from CASEL: https://casel.org/what-is-sel/

Centers for Disease Control and Prevention. (2020, March 3). *Children's oral health: Overview*. Retrieved from Center for Disease Control and Prevention https://www.cdc.gov/oralhealth/basics/childrens-oral-health/index.html

Center for Disease Control and Prevention. (2020, September 4). *High School YRBS, 2019 Results, Overweight*. Retrieved from Center for Disease Control and Prevention: https://nccd.cdc.gov/youthonline/App/Results.aspx?TT=B&OUT=0&SID=HS&QID=H67&LID=LL&YID=RY&LID2=&YID2=&COL=&ROW1=&ROW2=&HT=&LCT=&FS=&FR=&FG=&FA=&FI=&FP=&FSL=&FRL=&FGL=&FAL=&FIL=&FPL=&PV=&TST=&C1=&C2=&QP=&DP=&VA=CI&CS=Y&SYID=&EYID=&SC=&SO=

Centers for Disease Control and Prevention. (2020, January 13). *When and How to Wash Your Hands*. Retrieved from Handwashing: Clean Hands Save Lives https://www.cdc.gov/handwashing/when-how-handwashing.html

Centers for Disease Control and Prevention. (2020, February 24). *High School YRBS, 2017 Results, Did not wear a condom*. Retrieved from Centers for Disease Control and Prevention: https://nccd.cdc.gov/youthonline/App/Results.aspx?TT=B&OUT=0&SID=HS&QID=H64&LID=LL&YID=RY&LID2=&YID2=&COL=&ROW1=&ROW2=&HT=&LCT=&FS=&FR=&FG=&FA=&FI=&FP=&FSL=&FRL=&FGL=&FAL=&FIL=&FPL=&PV=&TST=&C1=&C2=&QP=&DP=&VA=CI&CS=Y&SYID=&EYID=&SC=&SO=

Centers for Disease Control and Prevention. (2020). *Substance Use and Sexual Risk Behaviors Among Youth*. Retrieved from the Centers for Disease Control and Prevention https://www.cdc.gov/healthyyouth/substance-use/pdf/dash-substance-use-fact-sheet.pdf

Cha, S., Masho, S. W., Mezuk, B. (2016). Age of sexual debut and cannabis use in the United States. *Substance Use and Misuse, 51*(4), 439–448.

Choose MyPlate, US Department of Agriculture. (2020). *Eat Healthy, Fruits*. Retrieved from Choose MyPlate, US Department of Agriculture https://www.choosemyplate.gov/eathealthy/fruits

Collaborative for Academic and Social Emotional Learning. (2020). *CASEL Competencies*. Retrieved from CASEL https://casel.org/wp-content/uploads/2020/12/CASEL-SEL-Framework-11.2020.pdf

Collaborative for Academic Social Emotional Learning. (2020). Retrieved from CASEL.org: https://casel.org/wp-content/uploads/2017/08/Sample-Teaching-Activities-to-Support-Core-Competencies-8-20-17.pdf

Connolly, M. (2018). *Skills-based health education*. Burlington: Jones and Bartlett.

Frey, N., Fisher, D., & Smith, D. (2019). *All learning is social and emotional; helping students develop essential skills for the classroom and beyond*. Alexandria: ASCD.

Joint Committee on National Health Education Standards. (2007). *National Health Education Standards*, (2nd ed.). American Cancer Society.

Jones, L. (2018). *If we're teaching social emotional skills, we need to assess them*. Retrieved from We Are Teachers https://www.weareteachers.com/assess-sel-skills/

KidsHealth from Nemours. (2020). *Are video games bad for me?* Retrieved from KidsHealth by Nemours: https://kidshealth.org/en/kids/video-gaming.html

KidsHealth in the Classroom. (2020). *Grades 3 to 5 • Personal Health Series Screen Time*. Retrieved from KidsHealth in the Classroom https://classroom.kidshealth.org/classroom/3to5/personal/fitness/screen_time.pdf

KidsHealth from Nemours. (2020, January 20). *Personal Health Series: Germs, washing my hands*. Retrieved from Nemours: https://classroom.kidshealth.org/classroom/prekto2/personal/hygiene/germs_handout2.pdf

KidsHealth from Nemours. (2020). *Sharing is great! But* don't *share germs*. Retrieved from KidsHealth: https://classroom.kidshealth.org/classroom/prekto2/personal/hygiene/dont_spread_germs_k5.pdf

KidsHealth from Nemours. (2020). *What are Germs?* Retrieved from KidsHealth from Nemours KidsHealth.org/en/kids/germs.html

KidsHealth in the Classroom. (2020). *Cough, Cough, Cough and Sneeze*. Retrieved from KidsHealth in the Classroom, Personal Health Series, Cold and Flu: https://classroom.kidshealth.org/classroom/prekto2/problems/conditions/colds_flu_handout1.pdf

Linda Meeks, P. H. (2011). *Comprehensive School Health Education*, (7th ed.). New York: McGraw Hill.

Mary H. Bronson, P. (2009). *Glencoe Health*. Woodland Hills, CA: McGraw Hill.

Mirror Mirror Eating Disorder Help. (2020). *Media Influence on Body Image*. Retrieved from Mirror Mirror Eating Disorder Help https://www.mirror-mirror.org/media-influence-on-body-image.htm

Morris, A. M., Katzman, D. K. (2003). The Impact of the media on eating disorders in children and adolescents. *Paediatrics & Child Health*, 287(5), 287–289.

National Academies of Sciences. (2016). *Preventing Bullying Through Science, Policy, and Practice*. Washington DC: The National Academies Press. doi: 10.17226/23482.

National Health, Lung, and Blood Institute. (2020). *Aim for a Healthy Weight, Body Mass Index*. Retrieved from National Health, Lung, and Blood Institute: https://www.nhlbi.nih.gov/health/educational/lose_wt/BMI/bmi_tbl.htm

National Highway Transportation Safety Association. (2012). *Fitting Your Bike Helmet*. Retrieved from National Highway Transportation Safety Association https://www.nhtsa.gov/sites/nhtsa.dot.gov/files/8019_fitting-a-helmet.pdf

National Institute of Drug Abuse. (2020). *What is the scope of marijuana use in the United States?* Retrieved from National Institute of Drug Abuse https://www.drugabuse.gov/research-reports/marijuana/what-scope-marijuana-use-in-united-states

PsicoPico. (2019). *The Wheel of Emotions, by Robert Plutchick*. Retrieved from PsicoPico https://psicopico.com/en/la-rueda-las-emociones-robert-plutchik/

Pierce, J. P., Sargent, J. D., White, M. M., Borek, N., Portnoy, D. B., Green, V. R., ...Messer, K. (2017). Receptivity to tobacco advertising and susceptibility to tobacco products. *Pediatrics*, 139(6), e20163353.

Posey, A. (2019). *Engage the Brain: How to Design for Learning That Taps into the Poeert of Emotion*. Alexandria: Association for Supervision and Curriculum Development.

Randy M., & Page., T. S. (2015). *Promoting Health and Emotional Well-Being in Your Classroom*. Burlington, MA: Jones and Bartlett.

Rideout, V. a. (2019). *The Common Sense census: Media use by tweens and teens, 2019*. San Francisco: Common Sense Media.

Scholastic. (2020). *What You Need to Know About Vaping-Interactive*. Retrieved from Scholastic http://www.scholastic.com/youthvapingrisks/interactive/

Six Seconds The Emotional Intelligence Network. (2020). *Plutchik's Wheel of Emotions – 2017 Update*. Retrieved from Six Seconds: http://www.uvm.edu/~mjk/013%20Intro%20to%20Wildlife%20Tracking/Plutchik's%20Wheel%20of%20Emotions%20-%202017%20Update%20_%20Six%20Seconds.pdf

Slavin, R. E. (2014). Making cooperative learning powerful. *Educational Leadership, 72*, pp. 22–26.

stopbullying.gov. (2020). *Bullying as an Adverse Childhood Experience (ACE)*. Retrieved from stopbullying.gov https://www.stopbullying.gov/resources/research-resources/bullying-as-an-ace

TeensHealth from Nemours. (2020). *5 Ways to Reach a Healthy Weight*. Retrieved from TeensHealth from Nemours https://teenshealth.org/en/teens/weight-tips.html?WT.ac=t-ra

TeensHealth from Nemours. (2020). *Dealing With Feelings When You're Overweight*. Retrieved from TeensHealth from Nemours https://teenshealth.org/en/teens/feelings-overweight.html

TeensHealth from Nemours. (2020). *What is Self-Esteem*. Retrieved from TeensHealth from Nemours: https://kidshealth.org/en/teens/self-esteem.html?ref=search

The Bronfenbrenner Center for Translational Research (BCTR). (2020). *Does screen time affect academic performance among youth?* Retrieved from Psychology Today: https://www.psychologytoday.com/us/blog/evidence-based-living/201910/does-screen-time-affect-academic-performance-among-youth

Transforming Education. (2020). *Introduction to Growth Mindset*. Retrieved from Transforming Education, https://www.transformingeducation.org/introduction-to-growth-mindset/

Transforming Education. (2020). *Introduction to Self-Efficacy*. Retrieved from Transforming Education, https://www.transformingeducation.org/introduction-to-self-efficacy/

USDA Choose MyPlate, US Department of Agriculture. (2020). *Eat Healthy, Vegetables*. Retrieved from USDA Choose MyPlate, US Department of Agriculture, https://www.choosemyplate.gov/eathealthy/vegetables

Wang, C. L., Luo, J., Niw, P., & Wang, D. (2019). Growth mindset can reduce the adverse effect of substance use on adolescent reasoning. *Frontiers in Psychology*, 10, 1852.

Washoe County School District: Social & Emotional Learning. (2019). *SEL Standards Language for Primary Grades*. Retrieved from https://www.washoeschools.net/cms/lib/NV01912265/Centricity/Domain/202/Social%20Emotional%20Learning/Resources%20for%20Staff/SEL%20Kid%20Friendly_Primary%20%20.pdf

Wheeler, S. (2016). Can a change in mindset help teens de-stress? *Mindful, Healthy Mind, Healthy Life*, https://www.mindful.org/can-change-mindset-help-teens-de-stress/.

Yeager, D. S., Lee, H. Y., & Jamieson, J. P. (2016). How to improve adolescent stress responses: Insights from integrating implicit theories of personality and biopsychosocial models. *Psychological Science*, 27(8), 1078–1091.

Yu, C. W. (2019). Is marijuana use significantly correlated with other risky behaviors such as binge drinking, cigarette smoking, and physical inactivity. *American Sociological Association*, 1–17.

Chapter 3—Appendix A
Self-Awareness: Scope, Sequence, Content, SEL–Competency/ Subcompetencies

<u>Note:</u> This page is organized by grade span, Standard 1, skill standards, the HECAT content areas, and SEL Competency/Subcompetencies.

The HECAT content areas include: AOD – Alcohol and Other Drugs; HE – Healthy Eating; MEH – Mental/ Emotional Health; PHW – Personal Health and Wellness; PA – Physical Activity; S – Safety; SH – Sexual Health; T – Tobacco; V – Violence Prevention

Accurately Recognizing One's Own Feelings and thoughts and their Influence on Behaviors				
Grade Span	Standard 1	Skill	HECAT Content Areas and Specific Content	SEL–Competency and Subcompetencies
PreK–2	1.2.2 <u>Recognize</u> that there are multiple dimensions of health *affected by the positive or negative effects of emotion.*	2.2.1 <u>Identify</u> how the family influences personal health practices and behaviors *of their children.*	Mental/Emotional Health: How the family influences emotions	SEL–Self-awareness: Identifying emotions, self-confidence
3–5	1.5.1 Describe the relationship between healthy behaviors *such as screen-free fun activities* and personal health.	2.5.6. <u>Describe</u> ways that technology, *especially screen time,* influences thoughts, feelings, and health behaviors.	Physical Activity: Reducing screen time when with friends	SEL–Self-awareness: Identifying emotions
6–8	1.8.2 <u>Describe</u> the interrelationships of emotional, intellectual, physical, and social health in adolescence *when being bullied.*	2.8.3 <u>Describe</u> how peers influence health and unhealthy behaviors *about bullying.* 2.8.10 <u>Explain</u> how the school and public health policies influence health promotion and disease prevention.	Violence prevention: Effects of bullying; role of peers and the school in prevention	SEL–Self-awareness: Identifying emotions
9–12	1.12.7 <u>Compare and contrast</u> the benefits of and barriers to practicing a variety of healthy behaviors *such as maintaining a healthy weight.*	2.12.8 <u>Analyze</u> the influence of personal values and belief on individual health practices and behaviors *such as maintaining a healthy weight.*	Personal Health and Wellness: Body image	SEL–Self-awareness: Identifying emotions
Accurately assessing one's interests, strengths and limitations, and possessing a well-grounded sense of self-efficacy and optimism and a "growth mindset."				
PreK–2	1.2.4 <u>List</u> ways to prevent common childhood injuries *to the head.*	2.2.1 <u>Identify</u> how the family influences personal health practices and behaviors *about bicycle safety.*	Safety: Bicycle safety; fitting a helmet	Self-awareness: Accurate self-perception, recognizing strength

3–5	1.5.1 <u>Describe</u> the relationship between healthy behaviors, *such as practicing sun safety*, and personal health.	2.5.3. <u>Identify</u> how peers influence healthy and unhealthy behaviors *about sun safety.*	Safety: Sun safety	Self-awareness: Accurate self-perception/ recognizing strengths
6–8	1.8.1 <u>Analyze</u> the relationship between healthy behaviors, *such as identifying interests and strengths*, and personal health.	2.8.4 <u>Analyze</u> how the school and community affect personal health practices and behaviors *by helping students identify and connect their interests and strengths with academics, school clubs, and activities.*	Mental/Emotional Health: Connecting interests and strengths to academics	Self-awareness: Accurate self-perception/ recognizing strengths
9–12	1.12.9 <u>Analyze</u> the potential severity of injury or illness if engaging in unhealthy behaviors *such as having intercourse without using a condom.*	2.12.9 <u>Analyze</u> how some health risk behaviors, *such as drinking alcohol,* influences the likelihood of engaging in unhealthy behaviors *such as having intercourse without using a condom.*	Sexual Health: STIs	Self-awareness: Accurate self-perception, recognizing strengths

Self-Confidence/Recognizing Strengths

PreK–2	1.2.1 Identify that healthy behaviors, *such as preventing being infected or infecting others*, affect personal health.	2.2.2 Identify what the school does to support personal health practices and behaviors *such as teaching about preventing communicable infections.*	Personal Health and Wellness: Preventing the spread of communicable diseases	Self-awareness: Self-confidence, recognizing strengths
3–5	1.5.1 <u>Describe</u> the relationship between healthy behaviors, *such as knowing what to do in an emergency*, and personal health.	2.5.1 <u>Describe</u> how the family influences personal health practices and behaviors *such as how to respond to emergencies.*	Safety: Responding to emergencies	Self-awareness: Self-confidence, recognizing strengths
6–8	1.8.7 <u>Describe</u> the benefits of and barriers to practicing healthy behaviors *such as cutting down on social media when out with friends.*	2.8.6 <u>Analyze</u> the influence of technology *(social media)* on personal and family *relationships.*	Mental/Emotional Health: Effects of social media	Self-awareness: Self-confidence, recognizing strengths
9–12	1.12.5 <u>Propose ways</u> to reduce or prevent injuries and health problems *related to body image.*	2.12.5 <u>Evaluate</u> the effect of media on personal *(body image)* and family health.	Mental/Emotional Health: Suicide prevention	Self-awareness: Self-confidence, recognizing strengths

Self-Efficacy

PreK–2	1.2.5 <u>Describe</u> why it is important to seek health care *when you have a tooth ache.*	3.2.1 <u>Identify</u> trusted adults and professionals who help promote *dental* health.	Personal Health and Wellness: Dental health	Self-awareness: Self-efficacy

(continues)

Accurately Recognizing One's Own Feelings and thoughts and their Influence on Behaviors *(continued)*

Grade Span	Standard 1	Skill	HECAT Content Areas and Specific Content	SEL–Competency and Subcompetencies
Self-Efficacy				
3–5	1.5.2 <u>Identify</u> examples of emotional, intellectual, physical, and social health *when moving up to a new school.*	2.5.4 <u>Describe</u> how the school and community supports personal health practices and behaviors *for new students to the middle school building.*	Mental/Emotional Health: Transition to middle school	Self-awareness: Self-efficacy
6–8	1.8.9 Examine the potential seriousness of injury or illness if engaging in unhealthy behaviors *such as vaping.*	2.5.6. Describe ways that technology influences personal health *such as advertisements for vaping products.*	Tobacco – Influence of advertisements on vaping	Self-awareness: Self-efficacy
9–12	1.12.2 Describe the interrelationships of emotional, intellectual, physical, and social health *when able to give CPR.*	2.12.4. Evaluate how the school and community affects personal health practices and behavior *by learning CPR.*	Safety: CPR	Self-awareness: Self-efficacy
Growth Mindset				
ProK–2	1.2.1 <u>Identify</u> that healthy behaviors *such as participating in a group* affect personal health.	2.5.3 Identify how peers influence healthy and unhealthy behaviors *when working in a group.*	Mental/Emotional Health: Participating in a group	Self-awareness: Self-confidence, recognizing strengths
3–5	1.5.1 <u>Describe</u> the relationship between healthy behaviors *such as having a growth mindset* and personal health.	2.5.3 <u>Identify</u> how peers influence behaviors *(Growth mindset)* and unhealthy behaviors *(Fixed mindset).*	Mental/Emotional Health: Making friends	Self-awareness: Growth mindset
6–8	1.8.8 <u>Examine</u> the likelihood of injury or illness if engaging in unhealthy behaviors *such as using marijuana.*	2.8.9 <u>Describe</u> how some health risk behaviors, *such as smoking marijuana,* influence the likelihood of engaging in unhealthy behaviors.	Alcohol and Other Drugs: Using a growth mindset to quit marijuana	Self-awareness: Growth mindset
9–12	1.12.2 Describe the interrelationships of emotional, intellectual, physical, and social health *when developing a growth mindset.*	2.12.7 Analyze how the perceptions of norms, *relating to mindset,* influence healthy and unhealthy behaviors.	Mental/Emotional Health: Developing a growth mindset	Self-awareness: Growth mindset

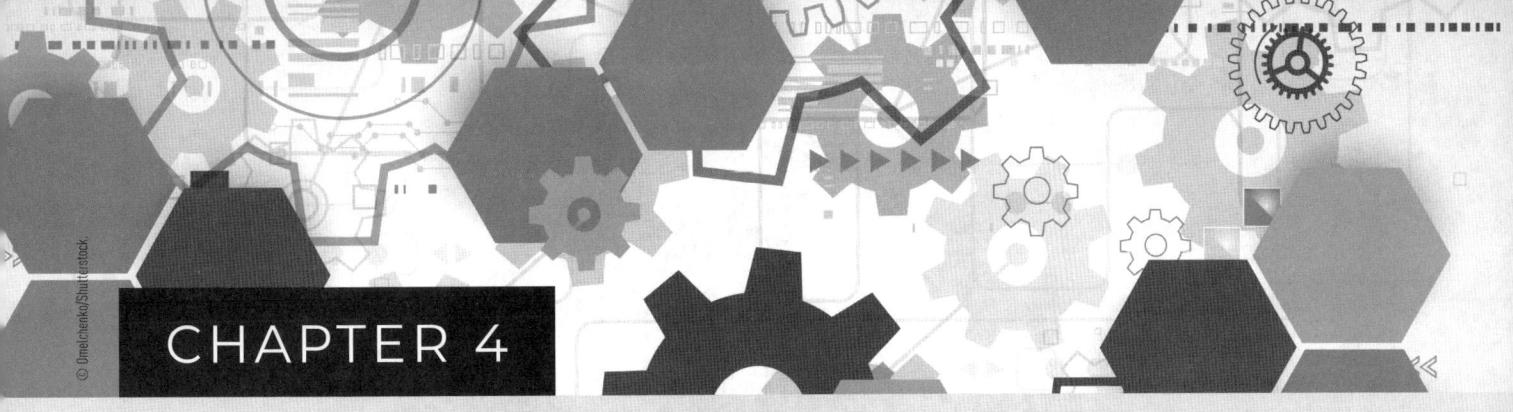

CHAPTER 4

Teaching Self-Management

LEARNING OBJECTIVES

Upon finishing this course, students will be able to:

- Plan skills-based health (SBH)/SEL lessons using backwards design and practice prompts.
- Incorporate the subcompetencies of self-management into assessment and instruction.

KEY TERMS

Goal setting   Organizational skills   Self-motivation
Impulse control   Self-discipline   Stress management

Social and Emotional Learning (SEL) Competencies*

- **SELF-MANAGEMENT Figure 4.1**
  - The ability to successfully regulate one's emotions, thoughts, and behaviors in different situations—effectively managing stress, controlling impulses, and motivating oneself. The ability to set and work toward personal and academic goals. (CASEL, 2019)

Introduction

Self-awareness and self-management are linked because they are skills that regulate an individual's emotions, thoughts, values, and behavior. They help us assess our strengths, set goals, manage, and motivate ourselves with a sense of confidence.

Students with self-management manage stress, delay gratification, motivate themselves, and set and work toward personal goals. They come to class prepared, pay attention in class, follow directions, allow others to speak without interrupting them, and work independently. (Transforming Education, 2020)

Self-management is unique in that it contains a classroom management component and an instructional component. Classroom management strategies are mentioned in **Table 4.1**. In planning a safe learning environment, teachers use a variety of self-management strategies that also enhance student **organizational skills**.

The most effective classroom self-management strategies are planned and provisioned well before they are needed. Break spots are set up away from the

*A scope and sequence document is included as an appendix at the end of this chapter.

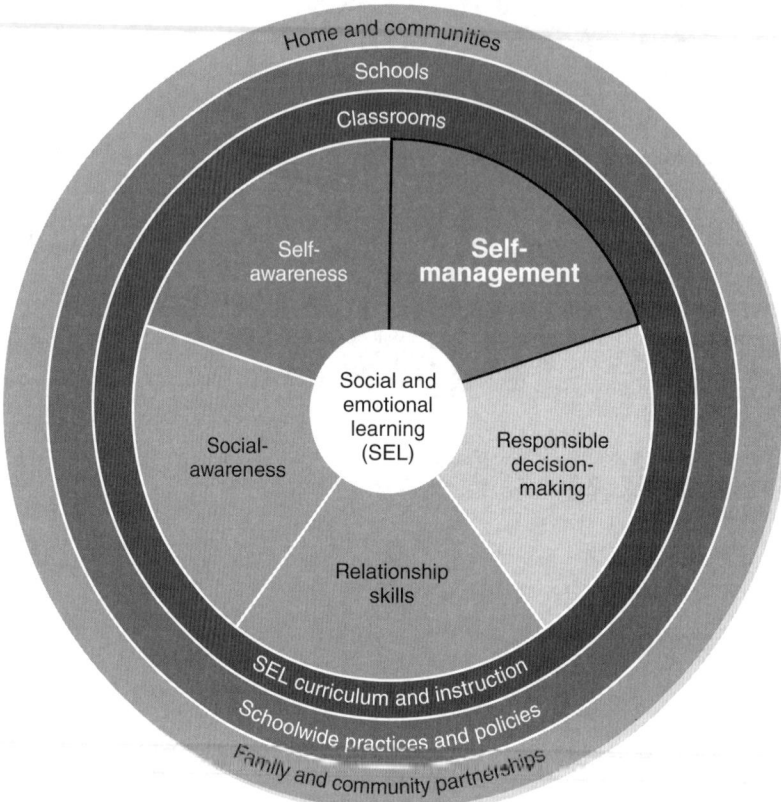

Figure 4.1 The CASEL Framework: Competency on Self-Management.

Table 4.1 Strategies to Support the Development of a Student's Self-management Skills

Strategy	Explanation
Class behavior agreement	Create a personalized classroom norms agreement with student input.
Are You Ready?	Students design a self-check and a tracking mechanism to assess their readiness to learn. For example: Do I have my pencil? Do I have everything I need for my group project?
Class expectations	Students design a behavior self-check to help them identify and track their classroom behavior. For example: ■ Am I practicing active listening? ■ Am I waiting for my peers to stop talking before I say something? ■ When I disagree, am I using appropriate language, tone; Am I raising my voice?
Being the best learner	Students determine, with the help of the teacher, the best way they learn and track progress. ■ What focusing strategy works best for me? ■ What gets in the way of being the best learner I can be? ■ What helps me be the best learner I can be?
The **WOOP** Method of Goal Setting	A positive thinking strategy to help students think positively. ■ **Wish:** Students think of a wish or goal they would like to have or accomplish. ■ **Outcome:** Students visualize what their life would be like if they got what they wished for or reached their goal. ■ **Obstacle:** Students identify a significant obstacle to their wish or goal. ■ **Plan:** Students identify a behavior that will help them overcome the obstacle and achieve their wish or goal. Brainstorm different obstacles and what can be done to overcome it.

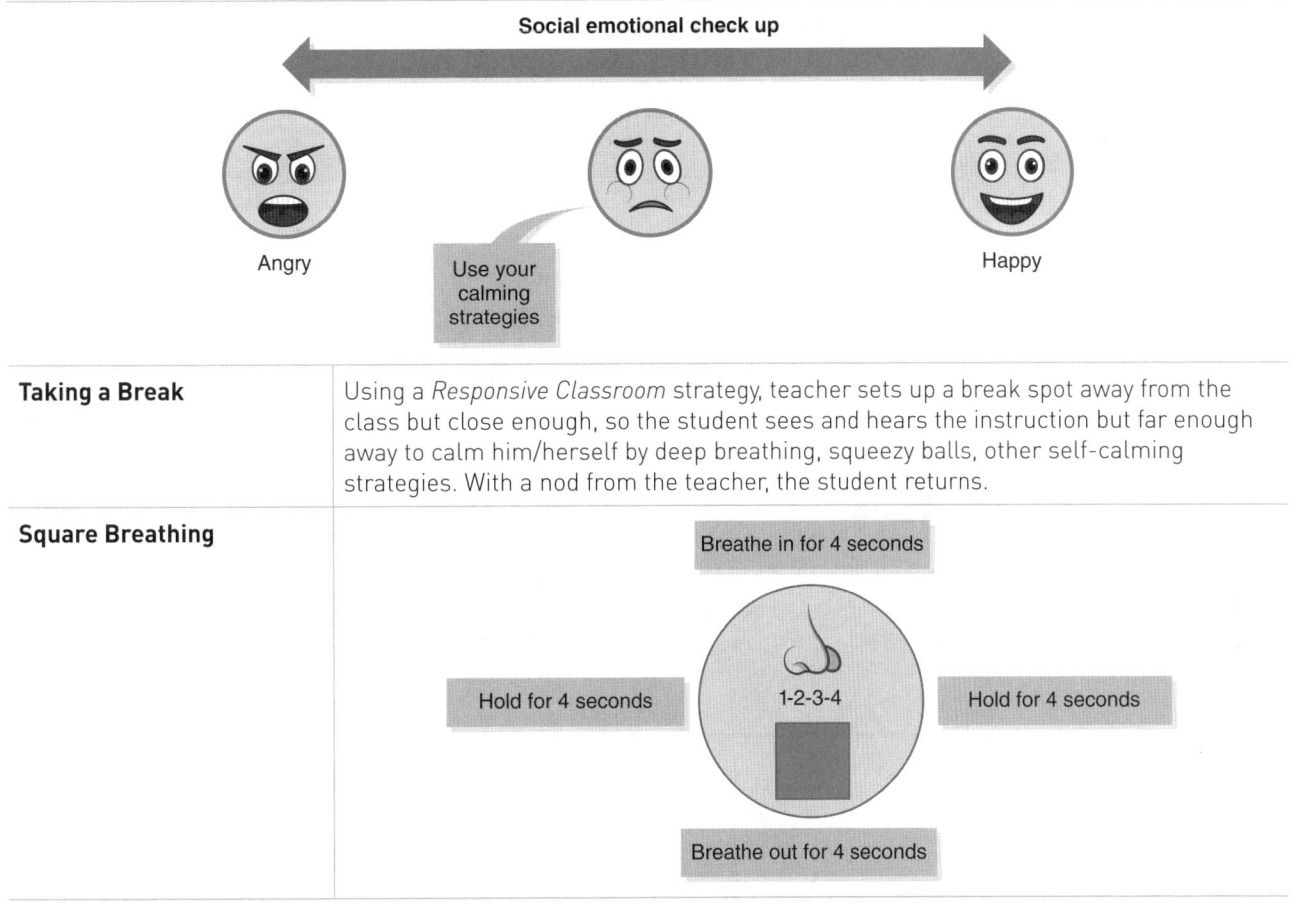

Taking a Break	Using a *Responsive Classroom* strategy, teacher sets up a break spot away from the class but close enough, so the student sees and hears the instruction but far enough away to calm him/herself by deep breathing, squeezy balls, other self-calming strategies. With a nod from the teacher, the student returns.
Square Breathing	

Data from Transforming Education. (2020, April 5). Self-Management, Sample Strategies. Retrieved from Transforming Education: https://www.transformingeducation.org/wp-content/uploads/2018/07/2018_Self-Management-Strategies_website.pdf

class but close enough, so the student still sees and listens to the instruction. Students understand that the break spot is temporary, and they are expected to use calming down strategies to resume self-control. The teacher and students model what that behavior looks like to set the expectations.

Other student strategies include encouraging a student to decide to spend time with peers that help them succeed in school; request a change of seat if the current table mates are distracting; use deep breathing when agitated, and walk away from trouble. To enhance organization skills, the students learn to write down assignments; set up a locker check list of items that need to be brought home at the end of the day; and plan a calendar and set deadlines to complete sections of a large project. (Transforming Education, 2020)

Self-management is an important skill/competency because higher self-management is associated with increased high school graduation rates and higher income levels. (Transforming Education, 2020) In adults, it is associated with being able to maintain a high level of motivation, control impulses, manage stress, set and achieve goals, meet responsibilities and

deadlines, and develop and maintain healthy habits. (My Learning Tools, 2020) Lower self-management is associated with chronic health problems, financial challenges, substance abuse, and criminal activity. (Transforming Education, 2020)

The CASEL self-management competency includes the National Health Education standard 6, **goal setting** and standard 7, practicing healthy behaviors.

Teachers help students self-manage through a variety of rituals, routines, collaborative rule setting, self-regulation activities to cope with **impulse control** and **self-discipline**, activities such as mindfulness, formative and summative assessments, and personal reflections.

When planning lessons, teachers use practice prompts as the daily vehicle to demonstrate and reinforce content, skill, and SEL competencies. During each lesson, the instructor teaches content, skill, and SEL competency and checks for understanding by distributing or reading a practice prompt and asking the students to answer follow up questions. Each of the questions refers to the infused performance

Table 4.2 Alignment of Self-Management to the National Health Education Standard 6 and Standard 7

Self-Management	The ability to successfully regulate emotions, thoughts, and behaviors in different situations such as managing stress, controlling impulses, and self-motivation. The ability to set and work toward personal and academic goals. (Collaborative for Academic and Social Emotional Learning, 2020)	▪ Impulse control ▪ Stress management ▪ Self-discipline ▪ Self-motivation ▪ Goal setting ▪ Organizational skills

The self-management competency is aligned with the National Health Education standard 6, students demonstrate the ability to use goal-setting skills to enhance health (Joint Committee on National Health Education Standards, 2007, p. 34) and standard 7, students demonstrate the ability to practice health-enhancon behaviors and avoid or reduce health risks. (Joint Committee on National Health Education Standards, 2007, p. 35)

Self-management: goal setting directly aligns to standard 6 of the National Health Education Standards. Consequently, when planning a unit, the assessment and instruction are already aligned, and no additional assessment or instruction is needed.

Self-management: **Stress management** directly aligns to standard 7 of the National Health Education Standards. When planning a stress management unit, the assessment and instruction are already aligned, and no additional assessment or instruction is needed.

Because of the increase in anxiety amongst youth (1 in 10 children in pre-school have suicidal thoughts; ⅓ of adolescents report feeling depressed or overwhelmed by stress; ¼ girls and ⅒ boys in high school try to harm themselves even when they are not attempting suicide, (Armstrong, 2019, p. 7). Stress management is a common component in comprehensive skills-based health programs.

indicators (lesson objective), assessment, content, and SEL competency.

Providing effective feedback to students as they practice helps guide and direct the student to proficiency of the performance indicator and SEL competency. Successful completion of a skill practice gives the student the self-confidence to learn other skills, develop self-efficacy, and ultimately a growth mindset. (Frey, Fisher, & Smith, 2019, p. 29)

Table 4.2 describes the alignment of self-management to the National Health Education standard 6 and standard 7.

Preview

Skills-Based Unit

In a skills-based/SEL unit, the planner accesses and analyzes data then selects a standard 1 and skills performance indicator to reduce the risk factor and infuses them with content. The SEL competency and sub-competency are aligned with the infused performance indicators. Once established, the instructor plans the assessment and instruction. When the content, skill, and competency are taught, the teacher distributes the performance task which consists of the unit prompt(s), the scoring rubric, back-up materials needed such as supplemental content, self-checks, and any other information the students need to show proficiency in the performance

indicators and SEL competency. Students organize and practice for a few days and present their work to the class. This summative assessment is scored with an analytical rubric.

Skills-Based Lessons

The sections that follow present infrastructure for a lesson, not a unit. Each begins with an overview, data (when available), and a list of resources. A table initiates backwards design. It consists of the infused performance indicators and SEL competencies as the lesson objectives. Assessments are designed for each of the performance indicators and competency. The prompt and the review questions engage the learner and help the teacher determine if the students met the lesson objectives. An exit question provides an opportunity for students to reflect on how to use what was taught.

When reading, let your imagination guide your planning. You may need more or fewer lessons to teach the material. You may like an idea and modify it to meet the needs of your students. You may find the worksheets valuable or may prefer to edit them.

When modifying, maintain the integrity of the backwards design. Teach content, skill, and SEL each day. If the lesson infrastructure contains too much material, plan an additional day(s) but maintain the integrity of aligning SEL and teaching content through the infused performance indicators. Refer to the sample lessons at the end of each

Table 4.3 Self-Management Sub Competencies

Impulse control	Self-motivation
Stress management	Goal setting
Self-discipline	Organizational skills

chapter to understand how to align SEL and teach content through the skill.

Organization

The learning activities for the core competency of self-management are divided into three sections:

- Regulating one's emotions, cognitions, and behaviors
- Setting and achieving personal and educational goals
- Persevering in addressing challenges

Each section below contains background information about the SEL subcompetency followed by lesson suggestions and resources.

The National Health Education Standards are grouped according to the grade spans PreK–2, grades 3–5, grades 6–8, and grades 9–12. The following examples follow that structure. The classroom examples may require the teacher to be creative and adjust instruction to accommodate the age and abilities of the students.

The heading of each section represents a self-management subcompetency (**Table 4.3**). The practice prompt is aligned with the competency and the infused performance indicators of the National Health Education Standards.

Section 1. Regulating One's Emotions, Cognitions, and Behaviors

(Collaborative for Academic Social Emotional Learning, 2020)

Impulse Control, Self-Discipline, Self-Motivation

PreK–2: Self-Management: Impulse Control, Self-Discipline, Self-Motivation

Lesson Overview: Effect of Impulse Control. In this lesson, students learn how impulse control affects the components of health. Also, students learn to manage their impulses by playing a variety of games that target each of the components of health.

The subcompetencies of impulse control, self-discipline, and **self-motivation** are combined in this lesson framework because a student needs to be motivated to exercise self-discipline over his/her impulses.

Resources:

- Cookie Monster-But Me Wait- https://www.yourtherapysource.com/blog1/2017/05/16/games-practice-self-regulation-skills/
  - Explanation of how to use bubbles to teach impulse control: https://momentousinstitute.org/blog/home-strategies-bubbles
  - Impulse control-Freeze Game-Ready-Set-Go! https://media.centervention.com/pdf/1002-Impulse-Control-Strategies-Ready-Set-Go.pdf
- Calming Activity-Deep breathing https://www.centervention.com/calming-activity-deep-breathing/?tx_post_tag=elementary
- Cool Down Corner– Retrieved from https://media.centervention.com/pdf/6002-Behavior-Strategies-Cool-Down-Corner.pdf
- Resource for parents https://www.centervention.com/5-ways-parents-can-help-children-develop-social-and-emotional-skills/

Materials needed:

- **Worksheet 4.1 PreK–2 What Do I Look Like When I Control My Impulses?**

Table 4.4 provides an overview of the lesson objectives, assessment, and instruction for this lesson.

Table 4.4 Lesson Objectives, Assessment, and Instruction

Step 1 – Lesson Objectives	Step 2 – Assessment
The verb of the *infused* performance indicator and the SEL competency generate the assessment and instruction.	Design the assessment based on the objectives. Ask yourself the question, "What can my students do to show me they have met the standard?"

(continues)

Table 4.4 Lesson Objectives, Assessment, and Instruction   *(continued)*

Step 1 – Lesson Objectives	Step 2 – Assessment
1.2.1 <u>Recognize</u> that *impulse control* affects multiple components of health. (Joint Committee on National Health Education Standards, 2007, p. 24)	1.2.1 Students <u>recognize</u> *one-way impulse control* affects emotional, intellectual, physical, and social health.
7.2.1 <u>Demonstrate</u> healthy practices and behaviors, *such as impulse control,* to maintain or improve personal health. (Joint Committee on National Health Education Standards, 2007, p. 26)	7.2.1 Students <u>demonstrate</u> *one-way* to control their impulses to maintain or improve their personal health.
Self-management: Impulse control Self-management: Self-discipline, Self-motivation	Students <u>recognize</u> *one-way impulse control* affects emotional, intellectual, physical, and social health. Students <u>demonstrate</u> self-discipline and self-motivation to control their impulses to maintain or improve their personal health.

Step 3 – Instruction
Design the instruction so that students learn the content, skill, and competency to be successful on the assessment. Ask yourself the question, "What do I need to teach so that the students will be successful when assessed?"

Step 3 – Instruction

1. Define
   a. Recognize: To identify a person or thing because there is a history of having seen or interacted with that person or thing in the past.
   b. Demonstrate: To show how something is accomplished.
   c. Impulse control: The ability to resist a strong, sudden urge.
   d. Self-discipline: A person's capacity to control his/her behavior.
   e. Self-motivation: The ability to encourage one's self to accomplish a task.
2. 1.2.2 <u>Recognize</u> that *impulse control* affects many different aspects of health. Because of limited time, select the activity from the list below that best meets the needs of your students.
   a. Impulse control affects emotional health. Students with impulse control are able to:
      1) Tolerate more frustration when problem solving.
      2) Feel better about themselves that they can control their impulses.
      3) **Play** Simon Says. <u>Note:</u> Make the game challenging to determine how well the students manage frustration and control their impulses.
         Children perform an action only when the leader says, "Simon says do...." For example, if the leader says,

"Simon says touch your head," students stay in the game if they touch their head. If Simon says, "Touch your nose," and the children touch their nose, they are out. (YTS Your Therapy Source, April)

<u>Reflection:</u> How does playing Simon says affect your ability to control your impulses? Comment on how student successfully/unsuccessfully exercised impulse control. Explain the benefits of being able to control impulses. What effect did playing the game have on your emotional health?

   b. Impulse control affects intellectual health. Students with impulse control are able to:
      1) Think before they act.
      2) Think about their answers before writing them down or answering a verbal question. (YTS Your Therapy Source, April)
      3) Achieve higher SAT scores in later grades.
      4) **Play** Body Part Mix Up.
         The leader calls out body parts and the children point to the part on their body. However, to make the game more challenging, create different rules each time the game is played. For example, each time the leader says, "head," the children touch their toes instead. This requires the children to stop and think before they react. If the leader calls

out "knees, head, elbow," the children should touch their knees, <u>toes,</u> and elbow. (YTS Your Therapy Source, April)

<u>Reflection:</u> How does playing Body Part Mix Up affect your ability to control your impulses? Comment on how student successfully/unsuccessfully exercised impulse control. Explain the benefits of being able to control impulses. What affect did playing the game have on your intellectual health?

<u>Note:</u> Self-control is twice as important as intelligence regarding academic achievement. (Amy Morin, 2020)

c. Impulse control affects physical health. Students with impulse control are able to:
1) Successfully stand in line.
2) Successfully wait their turn when playing a game.
3) **Play** Ready, Set, Wiggle. The purpose is to have the children wait to move until they hear a certain word.

The leader calls out Ready…Set…Wiggle and everyone wiggles their body. The leader calls out Ready…Set…Watermelon. The children should not move. The leader calls out Ready…Set…Wigs. The children should not move. The leader calls out Ready…Set…Wiggle. The children wiggle, again. The leader may change the wording used. (YTS Your Therapy Source, April)

<u>Reflection:</u> How does playing Ready, Set, Wiggle affect your ability to control your impulses. Comment on how students successfully/unsuccessfully exercised impulse control. Explain the benefits of being able to control impulses. What effect did playing the game have on your physical health?

d. Impulse control affects social health. Students with impulse control are able to:
1) Develop successful peer relationships.
2) Able to resist peer pressure.
3) Able to resolve conflict. (Amy Morin, 2020)
4) **Play** Mother May I? Before the game begins, discretely assign roles to the students.
   - Observe how the pairs successfully complete the game.
   - One pair of students pressures others to break the rules. Observe how students react.
   - One pair of students tries to start an argument with another pair. Observe how others react.

One child stands at the front of the room and is the leader (mother). The remaining students stand a distance from the leader. Children take turns asking, "Mother, may I take….. (a certain number of steps, hops, jumps, or leaps, to get to the leader. The leader approves or disapproves of the request by responding, "Yes, you may….or No, you may not."

When the game is over, discuss how well some pairs worked together; how pairs resisted/did not resist the pressure to break the rules; how the pairs resolved conflict.

<u>Reflection:</u> How does playing Mother, May I… affect your ability to control your impulses? Comment on how students successfully/unsuccessfully exercised impulse control. Explain the benefits of being able to control impulses. What effect did playing the game have on your social health?

3. 7.2.1 <u>Demonstrate</u> healthy practices and behaviors, *such as impulse control,* to maintain or improve personal health.
   a. What does impulse control look like? *Use pictures to illustrate each behavior.*
   1) Raising your hand to speak instead of calling out.
   2) Keeping your hands to yourself.
   3) Walking quietly in the hallway.
   4) Waiting your turn.
   5) Playing by the rules in class and during recess.
   6) Keeping your space, desk, and materials clean.
   7) Telling the truth.
   8) Trying your best. (Courtney Ward, 2020)
   b. Use **Worksheet 4.1 PreK–2 What Do I Look Like When I Control My Impulses?** to provide time for the students to reflect on how they control their impulses.
4. Read the practice prompt, students answer the reflection questions, and discuss.

Practice Prompt: Belinda

Belinda has always been fidgety. Sometimes she does something without thinking. Sometimes it doesn't matter and other times she gets in trouble or someone gets mad at her.

Now that she is in second grade, she wishes she was more in control of herself. The other day, she needed a pencil and instead of asking the teacher, Belinda took a pencil from another student when she wasn't looking. Her classmate was angry and told the teacher. Belinda doesn't know why she did it except she needed a pencil and she saw one not being used.

It makes her feel bad that she doesn't have better control. The teacher and her classmate were upset and Belinda felt bad. She couldn't concentrate on her work for the whole morning. She felt sick so she asked to go to the nurse. The nurse let her lie down and talked to her about why she is upset. After explaining, the nurse showed Belinda how to use the 4 Square to breathe deeply. Breath in for 4-3-2-1, hold for 4-3-2-1, breathe out 4-3-2-1, hold it 4-3-2-1.

The nurse told the teacher about Belinda and the teacher is going to set up a Break Space where Belinda can go to calm herself down. Belinda feels relieved that she can do something when she feels out of control.

The next day, Belinda brought several sharpened pencils to school. She apologized to her classmate and offered her a nice new pencil. The girls are friendly now and Belinda feels better because she knows she can go to the Break Space and get herself under control.

A few days later, Belinda became frustrated again because she raised her hand several times to answer a question, but the teacher didn't call on her! She was getting more and more agitated. She didn't want anyone to get mad at her again, so she caught the eye of the teacher and pointed to the Break Space. The teacher nodded and off she went. She practiced her 4 square breathing, squeezed the stress ball, drew a picture of why she was upset, practiced saying positive things to herself, and relaxed her body from head to toe. In a few minutes, she felt better and gestured to the teacher she would like to return to her seat. She got a nod and a smile.

Belinda still is impulsive but is feeling better because she is trying to control herself so she can get along better with others and concentrate on her schoolwork.

5. Use the review questions in **Table 4.5** to help the children understand how impulse control affects the components of health and how to control impulses.
6. End of class review. Ask the students to put away their materials then ask review questions.
   a. How does impulse control affect emotional health? (1.2.2)
   b. How does impulse control affect intellectual health? (1.2.2)
   c. How does impulse control affect physical health? (1.2.2)
   d. How does impulse control affect social health? (1.2.2)
   e. What is one way to show that you have control over your impulses? (7.2.1)
7. Exit ticket (Self-Awareness: Identifying emotions)

   Today, I started to.........without thinking but then I did............instead!

Table 4.5 How Impulse Control Affects the Components of Health and How to Control Impulses

Question	Answer
What is *one way impulse control* affected Belinda's components of health. (1.2.2)	
How did Belinda recognize that she did not demonstrate impulse control?	Belinda's Emotional Health ■ Wishes she had more impulse control. ■ Didn't feel good about herself when she took the pencil. Belinda's Physical Health ■ She felt sick after being caught taking the pencil Belinda's Social Health ■ The classmate was upset with her for taking the pencil and Belinda felt bad about that. Belinda's Intellectual Health ■ Belinda couldn't concentrate after the pencil incident.

How did Belinda recognize that she did demonstrate impulse control?	Belinda's Emotional Health ■ She tried to make amends by offering a new, sharp pencil to her classmate. ■ Belinda feels relieved to know that she will be able to use the Break Space when she gets fidgety. Belinda's Physical Health ■ She felt better after using the 4 square method to breathe. Belinda's Social Health ■ After apologizing and offering a new pencil, the girl was friendly toward Belinda. Belinda's Intellectual Health ■ Belinda learned a new skill, 4 square breathing, which helps her control her impulsiveness.
What was one way Belinda demonstrated control of her impulses to maintain or improve their personal health? (7.2.1)	When Belinda went to the Break Space, she practiced her 4 square breathing, squeezed the stress ball, drew a picture of why she was upset, practiced saying positive things to herself, and relaxed her body from head to toe.
SEL-Self-Management: Impulse control What is *one way impulse control* affects emotional, intellectual, physical, and social health. SEL-Self-Management: Self-discipline, self-motivation How did Belinda <u>demonstrate</u> self-discipline and self-motivation to control her impulses to maintain or improve her personal health?	Belinda learned to identify her impulses and wanted to control them so she could get along better with her classmates and improve her classwork. Belinda disciplined herself to ask permission to use the Break Space when she sensed she needed to calm down.

Grades 3–5: Self-Management: Impulse Control, Self-Discipline, and Self-Motivation

Lesson Overview: Impulse Control, Self-Discipline, and Self-Motivation. In this lesson, students learn how to practice impulse control and learn the importance of being motivated to use self-discipline to control their behavior.

The subcompetencies of impulse control, self-discipline, and self-motivation are combined in this lesson framework because a student needs to be motivated to exercise self-discipline over his/her impulses.

Note: A sample lesson plan for this grade span is found at the end of the chapter.

Resources:

- Emotion regulation activity: Calm Down tools. GRIN-Smart-Not-Smart-Calm-Down-Strategies .pdf (centervention.com)

Materials needed:

- **Worksheet 4.2 Effects of Controlling/Not Controlling Impulses on Personal Health**
- **Worksheet 4.3 Impulse Control Tools**

Table 4.6 provides an overview of the lesson objectives, assessment, and instruction for this lesson.

Table 4.6 Lesson Objectives, Assessment, and Instruction

Step 1 – Lesson Objectives	Step 2 – Assessment
The verb of the *infused* performance indicator and the SEL competency generate the assessment and instruction.	Design the assessment based on the objectives. Ask yourself the question, "What can my students do to show me they have met the standard?"
1.5.1 <u>Describe</u> the relationship between healthy behaviors *such as impulse control, self-discipline, and self-motivation* and personal health. (Joint Committee on National Health Education Standards, 2007, p. 24)	1.5.1 Students <u>describe</u> the relationship between healthy behaviors such as *controlling impulses, being self-disciplined and self-motivated and how each affects* personal health.

(continues)

Table 4.6 Lesson Objectives, Assessment, and Instruction *(continued)*

Step 1 – Lesson Objectives	Step 2 – Assessment
7.5.2 <u>Demonstrate</u> a variety of healthy practices and behaviors such as *impulse control, self-discipline, and self-motivation,* to maintain or improve personal health. (Joint Committee on National Health Education Standards, 2007, p. 35)	7.5.2 Students <u>demonstrate</u> healthy practices and behaviors such as *one way to control impulses, be self-disciplined, and be self-motivated* to maintain or improve personal health.
SEL-Self-management: Impulse control, Self-discipline, Self-motivation	Students demonstrate impulse control. Students demonstrate self-discipline. Students demonstrate self-motivation.

Step 3 – Instruction
Design the instruction so that students learn the content, skill, and competency to be successful on the assessment. Ask yourself the question, "What do I need to teach so that the students will be successful when assessed?"

Step 3 – Instruction

1. Define
   a. Identify: To recognize a particular person or an object.
   b. Demonstrate: To show how something is accomplished.
   c. Impulse control: The ability to resist a strong, sudden urge.
   d. Self-discipline: A person's capacity to control his/her behavior.
   e. Self-motivation: The ability to encourage one's self to accomplish a task.
2. 1.5.1 <u>Describe</u> the relationship between healthy behaviors *such as impulse control, self-discipline, and self-motivation* and personal health.
   a. Place students in groups and equip each student with a white board or piece of paper.
   b. Ask the students to think of a time when they were tempted to do something they knew they shouldn't do and write it down. For example, eat a cookie.
   c. Ask, "If you were told not to eat a cookie before supper but you really wanted it ...."
      1) "What would you do?" Would you wait and get permission, or would you take the cookie?
      2) "Would you eat the cookie if you knew you wouldn't get caught?"
      3) "Would you take the cookie if your parents/guardian didn't tell you not to?"
   d. In groups, using the **Worksheet 4.2 Effects of Controlling/Not Controlling Impulses on Personal Health**, ask the students to discuss the relationship between controlling impulses and not controlling impulses and how each affects personal health.

<u>Note</u>: The children may list more short-term effects. **Table 4.7** lists long-term effects.
   e. To reinforce and practice impulse control, Play the Freeze Game.
      <u>Note</u>. Students who are "out" stand around the play areas and move in place/stop to the

Table 4.7 Effects of Controlling/Not Controlling Impulses

Effect of Controlling Impulses	Long-Term Effect of Not Controlling Impulses
In control of behavior	Drop out of school
Feel good about self for resisting the urge to give into the impulse.	Drug abuse
Able to stand in line	Teen pregnancy
Able to wait for their turn	(Randy M. Page., 2015, p. 68)
Able to think before they act	
Have better critical thinking skills	
Able to tolerate frustration	
Contributes to academic success (Very Well Family, 2020)	

Data from Very Well Family. (2020, April). The Importance of Teaching Children Impulse Control. Retrieved from Very Well Family: https://www.verywellfamily.com/the-importance -of-teaching-children-impulse-control-1095019?print; Randy M. Page., T. S. (2015). Promoting Health and Emotional Well-Being in Your Classroom. Burlington, MA: Jones and Bartlett Learning, p. 68.

music until the game is over. This maintains total engagement and more physical activity for all students.

1) When the music is playing, move and dance around the room.

2) When the music stops, freeze in place and do not move until the music resumes.

3) If a student moves before the music begins, they are out.

4) Increase the challenge by offering the students an incentive to move when they are frozen such as, no homework, extra snack, etc.

5) Discuss

    a) How difficult was it to freeze, especially when there was an extra incentive?

    b) What inner strength did you use to stop when the music stopped? (Self-control)

    c) How did you motivate yourself to freeze? (desire to succeed)

    d) How did focusing on freezing helped you demonstrate impulse control and self-control? (Centervention, 2020)

3. 7.5.2 <u>Demonstrate</u> a variety of healthy practices and behaviors such as *impulse control, self-discipline, and self-motivation* to maintain or improve personal health.

    a. Use **Worksheet 4.3 Impulse Control Tools** to identify and demonstrate strategies to control impulses and demonstrate self-discipline and self-motivation.

4. Read the practice prompt. Students will answer the reflection questions and discuss.

Practice Prompt: Aubrey

Aubrey has a problem with controlling her behavior. She is trying to control herself but sometimes she loses it.

The other day, she was very hungry because she got up late and skipped breakfast so she could make the bus. She didn't pack any snacks and was very jittery. She had trouble concentrating on her work and couldn't sit still. She kept looking at the clock, hoping it would hurry to lunch time.

Finally, the class lined up for lunch. She ran to the front of the line, but Aiden was there, and he told her to go back. She said, "No!" and pushed him aside. When she tried to take his place, the other classmates started complaining and told the teacher. Aubrey stomped her feet and yelled at her peers to leave her alone. Aubrey is in big trouble.

Mrs. Tranquil asked the aide to take the children to lunch and asked Aubrey to have lunch with her at the quiet table. Mrs. Tranquil asked Aubrey what happened. Aubrey explained she was very hungry and made a bad choice to push Aiden aside. Everyone is going to be mad at her. She feels sick and wants to go home. Mrs. Tranquil reminded Aubrey that everyone in the class cares about one another and controlling her impulses is very important for learning and keeping friends. She also reminded Aubrey that taking the time to eat breakfast and packing a snack is really important.

Aubrey planned to apologize to Aiden after lunch. Mrs. Tranquil reminded her to motivate herself to take control because that is what is best for her. She also encouraged her to discipline herself to take deep breaths when she gets upset, say positive things to herself, visualize something pleasant, go to the Break Space if she needs to be by herself for a while, and ask for help when she feels that she is losing control.

After lunch, Aubrey felt much better. She was motivated to apologize to Aiden and was grateful that her classmates forgave her.

Tomorrow is another day and Aubrey plans to eat breakfast and bring her coping skills to school!

5. Use the review questions in **Table 4.8** to help the children understand the relationship between impulse control, self-discipline, and self-motivation.

6. End of class review. Ask the students to put away their materials then ask review questions.

    a. How does impulse control affect personal health? (1.5.2)

    b. How does self-discipline affect personal health? (1.5.2)

    c. How does self-motivation affect personal health? (1.5.2)

    d. Demonstrate one healthy impulse-control strategy. (7.5.2)

7. Exit ticket (Self-Management: Impulse control, self-discipline, self-motivation)

Today, I started to.........without thinking but then I did............instead!

Grades 6-8: Self-Management: Impulse Control, Self-Discipline, Self-Motivation

Lesson Overview: Impulse Control and Texting. In this lesson, students learn the importance of being motivated to use self-discipline to control their impulses when texting.

The subcompetencies of impulse control, self-discipline, and self-motivation are combined in

Table 4.8 How Impulse Control Affects the Components of Health and How to Control Impulses

Question	Answer
What happened when Aubrey did not control her impulses? (1.5.2)	Aubrey ran to the front of the line and pushed Aiden away. The classmates yelled at her and told the teacher.
How did that lack of control affect Aubry's personal health?	Aubrey felt very bad because everyone was mad at her. However, the teacher invited Aubrey to lunch, and they discussed what happened and what Aubrey needs to do to be motivated to have the self-discipline to control her impulses.
How is Aubrey going to demonstrate *one way to control impulses, be self-disciplined, and be self-motivated* to maintain or improve personal health? (7.5.2)	Aubrey plans to ■ Apologize to Aiden after lunch. ■ Motivate herself to do what is best for her, control her impulses. ■ Discipline herself to take deep breaths when she gets upset, say positive things to herself, visualize something pleasant, go to the Break Space if she needs to be by herself for a while, and ask for help when she feels that she is losing control.
SEL-Self-management: Impulse control, self-discipline, self-motivation How did Aubrey demonstrate impulse control? How did Aubrey demonstrate self-discipline?	Aubrey demonstrated impulse control when she disciplined herself to take deep breaths when she got upset, said positive things to herself, visualized something pleasant, went to the Break Space to be by herself for a while.
How did Aubrey demonstrate self-motivation?	Aubrey motivated herself to do what is best for her and to control her impulses.

this lesson framework because a student needs to be motivated to exercise self-discipline over his/her impulses.

Resources:

- Consensogram: www.theteachertoolkit.com/index .php/tool/consensogram
- The Blessing and Curses of Impulsiveness: https://www.psychologytoday.com/us/blog /teen-angst/201510/the-blessings-and-curses -impulsiveness

Materials needed:

- **Worksheet 4.4 Impulse Control, Self-Discipline, Self-Motivation Consensogram**

Table 4.9 provides an overview of the lesson objectives, assessment, and instruction for this lesson.

Table 4.9 Lesson Objectives, Assessment, and Instruction

Step 1 – Lesson Objectives	Step 2 – Assessment
The verb of the *infused* performance indicator and the SEL competency generate the assessment and instruction.	Design the assessment based on the objectives. Ask yourself the question, "What can my students do to show me they have met the standard?"
1.8.7 <u>Describe</u> the benefits of and barriers to practicing healthy behaviors *when struggling with impulse control when texting.* (Joint Committee on National Health Education Standards, 2007, p. 25)	1.8.7 Students <u>describe</u> *two* benefits and *two* barriers to practicing healthy behaviors *when struggling with impulse control when texting.*
7.8.2. <u>Demonstrate</u> healthy practices and behaviors that maintain or improve the health of self and others *such as using the THINK process when texting.* (Joint Committee on National Health Education Standards, 2007, p. 35)	7.8.2 Students <u>demonstrate</u> the THINK process when texting.

SEL-Self-management: Impulse control, Self-discipline, Self-motivation	Students demonstrate how to motivate self to be disciplined to control impulses when using social media.

Step 3 – Instruction

Design the instruction so that students learn the content, skill, and competency to be successful on the assessment. Ask yourself the question, "What do I need to teach so that the students will be successful when assessed?"

Step 3 – Instruction

1. Define
   a. Describe: To use words that help others envision the physical attributes of a person, place, or thing.
   b. Demonstrate: To show how something is accomplished.
   c. Impulse control: The ability to resist a strong, sudden urge.
   d. Self-discipline: A person's capacity to control his/her behavior.
   e. Self-motivation: The ability to encourage one's self to accomplish a task.

2. 1.8.7 <u>Describe</u> the benefits of and barriers to practicing healthy behaviors *when struggling with impulse control when texting.*
   a. <u>Note:</u> The consensogram may be implemented in a variety of ways. **Worksheet 4.4 Impulse Control, Self-Discipline, Self-Motivation Consensogram** is used individually or in a group. Another option is to place three columns on the board and after reading the statement, students either individually or as a group consensus, place a mark in one of the columns. Additionally, label three sheets of newsprint (Agree, Not sure, Disagree), read the statements, and students place a circle sticker in the column of their choice. Regardless of the mode, enjoy a discussion about the benefits and barriers to being impulsive.
   b. Using **Worksheet 4.4 Impulse Control, Self-Discipline, Self-Motivation Consensogram**, discuss the benefits and barriers to impulsive behavior.
   c. Answers to the consensogram
      1) True
      2) True
      3) False. Being impulsive is a barrier to practicing healthy behaviors because the person does not consider all the pros and cons of all the options.
      4) True

   5) False. Being impulsive is a benefit because it allows a person to act quickly and go after an opportunity or react to an emergency.
   6) True
   7) False. An impulsive person may experience barriers to practicing healthy behaviors because he/she may be out of control and unstable.
   8) True
   9) False. Exercise helps control impulsivity.
   10) False. Mindfulness does help control impulses.

3. 7.8.2 <u>Demonstrate</u> healthy practices and behaviors that maintain or improve the health of self and others *such as using the THINK process when texting.*
   a. The THINK process (Collaborative for Academic Social Emotional Learning, 2020)
      1) T – Is it true?
      2) H – Is it helpful?
      3) I – Is it inspiring?
      4) N – Is it necessary?
      5) K – Is it kind?
   b. On the board, write, The Negative Results of Impulsive Texting and The Positive Results of Impulsive Texting. Using post-its, students respond and post the note on the board under the appropriate heading. As the notes are posted, group them into similar topics. Review and comment.
   c. In small groups, role play students impulsively texting. Before the student sends the text, a peer asks the THINK questions, the benefits of sending the text, and the possibly harmful effects of sending the text. Continue to role play and brainstorm alternative choices to sending hurtful texts.

4. Read the practice prompt. Students answer the reflection questions, discuss.

Practice Prompt: Maddy

Finally, Maddy's mother and father bought her a phone so she can call if she misses the bus, is staying afterschool, or going to a friend's house. Maddy is very excited because she can finally text and use the apps her friends talk about.

Sometimes, Maddy gets herself in trouble because she acts before she thinks. Knowing this, her parents warned her about using social media, and in particular, texting.

Well, today the coach made the cut for track and field. Maddy made it but Merri did not. Maddy thinks it is because she has put on weight and can't run fast anymore. Maddy was about to text her friends the news when Jerri came by and asked her what she was doing. Maddy told her she was going to tell everyone that Merri didn't make the team because she has put on so much weight.

"What!! Don't send that text, Maddy!!" "Why?" asked Maddy. "Everyone will want to know who made the team." "Right," said Merri, "but how do you think Merri will feel when she reads it?"

Let's THINK it through. "Is what you are saying **t**rue?" asked Jerri. "Is the text **h**elpful to Merri?" "Will it **i**nspire her to try again for the team?" "Is what you want to text, **n**ecessary?" "Are your words **k**ind?"

Maddy didn't think about any of those things. She felt really badly because she was texting just because she was excited that she could use her phone to tell her friends about something that happened. "You are right, Jerri. I am glad you stopped me. I didn't think. The text would be very unkind and hurtful. If I sent it, none of you would ever trust me again."

That was a close call. Maddy is trying hard to control her behavior. She is motivated to improve her relationships with her friends, gain the confidence of her parents, and discipline herself to control those pesky impulses. She is learning to think and pause before she acts. When she is fighting her impulses, she practices deep breathing and tries a few mindfulness activities.

Maddy still struggles but is working hard and disciplining herself not to give in to her impulses.

5. Use the review questions in **Table 4.10** to help the children understand the benefits of and barriers to impulse texting and how to use the THINK method when texting.

6. End of class review. Ask the students to put away their materials then ask review questions.
   a. What are two benefits of controlling impulses? (1.8.7)

Table 4.10 The Benefits of and Barriers to Impulse Texting and How to Use the THINK Method When Texting

Question	Answer
What are *two* benefits and *two* barriers of practicing healthy behaviors to Maddy *when struggling with impulse control when texting.* (1.8.7)	Benefits to practicing healthy behaviors when texting. ■ Maddy will gain the confidence of her parents. ■ Her friends will trust her. Barriers to practicing healthy behaviors when texting. ■ Maddy is impulsive and acts before she thinks. ■ Maddy was excited to text her friends about who made the team but didn't think about what she was saying and the effects it would have on Merri.
How did Maddy <u>demonstrate</u> the THINK process when texting? (7.8.2) T – Is it true? H – Is it helpful? I – Is it inspiring? N – Is it necessary? K – Is it kind?	Maddy's friend, Jerri, went through each of the steps to help Maddy understand that sending the text would be a big mistake. T – Think - "Is what you are saying **t**rue?" asked Jerri. H – Is it helpful? "Is the text **h**elpful to Merri?" I – Is it inspiring" "Will it **i**nspire her to try again for the team?" N – Is it necessary? "Is what you want to text **n**ecessary?" K– Is it kind? "Are your words **k**ind?"

SEL-Self-management: Impulse control, self-discipline, self-motivation	Impulse control
How did Maddy demonstrate how to motivate herself to be disciplined to control impulses when using social media?	■ She is learning to think and pause before she acts. ■ When she is fighting her impulses, she practices deep breathing and tries a few mindfulness activities. Self-Discipline ■ Maddy is trying hard to identify when her impulses are being pesky and to discipline herself to control them. Self-Motivation. Maddy is motivated to ■ Improve her relationships with her friends ■ Gain the confidence of her parents ■ Discipline herself to control those pesky impulses.

    b. What are two barriers to controlling impulses? (1.8.7)

    c. Demonstrate the THINK steps. (7.8.2)

7. Exit ticket (Self-Management: Impulse control, self-discipline, self-motivation)

How can a teen be motivated to discipline themselves to control their impulsive behavior?

Grades 9–12: Self-Management: Impulse Control, Self-Discipline, Self-Motivation

Lesson Overview: Controlling Impulses and Sexual Relationships. In this lesson, students learn the importance of being motivated to use self-discipline to control their sexual impulses.

27.4% of high school teens (28.4% girls; 26.3% boys) are currently sexually active. (Centers for Disease Control and Prevention, 2020)

45.7% of teens (50.4% girls; 40% of boys) did not use a condom during their last sexual intercourse. (Centers for Disease Control and Prevention, 2020)

Impulsive teens make quick decisions without thinking of the consequences. These teens are more prone to early sexual activity and drug dependency. Teens who prefer an immediate smaller reward over a larger but delayed reward (temporal discounting paradigm) are more prone to seek immediate gratification resulting in greater likelihood of engaging in risky behaviors. (Khurana, 2012)

Materials needed:

- **Worksheet 4.5 The Benefits of and Barriers to Practicing a Variety of Healthy Sexual Behaviors**
- **Worksheet 4.6 Analyzing the Role of Individual Responsibility in Enhancing Sexual Health**

Table 4.11 provides an overview of the lesson objectives, assessment, and instruction for this lesson.

Table 4.11 Lesson Objectives, Assessment, and Instruction

Step 1 – Lesson Objectives	Step 2 – Assessment
The verb of the *infused* performance indicator and the SEL competency generate the assessment and instruction.	Design the assessment based on the objectives. Ask yourself the question, "What can my students do to show me they have met the standard?"
1.12.7 <u>Compare</u> and <u>contrast</u> the benefits of and barriers to practicing a variety of healthy behaviors *regarding sexual relationships*. (Joint Committee on National Health Education Standards, 2007, p. 25)	1.12.7 <u>Compare</u> and <u>contrast</u> three benefits of and three barriers to practicing a variety of healthy behaviors *regarding sexual relationships*.
7.12.1 <u>Analyze</u> the role of individual responsibility in *controlling impulses* and enhancing *sexual* health. (Joint Committee on National Health Education Standards, 2007, p. 35)	7.12.1 Students <u>analyze</u> *three ways* of taking individual responsibility *to control impulses* and enhance *sexual* health.

(continues)

Table 4.11 Lesson Objectives, Assessment, and Instruction   *(continued)*

Step 1 – Lesson Objectives	Step 2 – Assessment
SEL-Self-management: Impulse control, self-discipline, self-motivation	Students demonstrate how to motivate self to be disciplined to control impulses when in a sexual relationship.

Step 3 – Instruction
Design the instruction so that students learn the content, skill, and competency to be successful on the assessment. Ask yourself the question, "What do I need to teach so that the students will be successful when assessed?"

Step 3 – Instruction

1. Define
   a. Analyze: To scrutinize something or someone in order to understand how it or they work(s).
   b. Compare/Contrast: Analysis of what is similar and what is different about two situations or two people.
   c. Impulse control: The ability to resist a strong, sudden urge.
   d. Self-discipline: A person's capacity to control his/her behavior.
   e. Self-motivation: The ability to encourage one's self to accomplish a task.
2. 1.12.7 <u>Compare</u> and <u>contrast</u> the benefits of and barriers to practicing a variety of healthy behaviors regarding controlling sexual impulses.
   a. Distribute **Worksheet 4.5 The Benefits of and Barriers to Practicing a Variety of Healthy Sexual Behaviors** (**Figure 4.2**) and provide time for the students to discuss and write down the benefits of and barriers to controlling sexual impulses. Discuss.
3. 7.12.1 <u>Analyze</u> the role of individual responsibility in controlling impulses and enhancing *sexual* health.
   a. Use **Worksheet 4.6 Analyzing the Role of Individual Responsibility in Enhancing Sexual Health** to help students understand the role of the individual to control impulses, demonstrate self-discipline and self-motivation.
   b. <u>Note</u>: When students complete the worksheet, discuss and review the evidence of personal responsibility.
      1) Be informed about male and female sexuality, pregnancy, and sexually transmitted infections.
      2) Set limits on expressing affection. Abstinence and safer sex are options.
      3) Communicate limits with your partner so there is mutual understanding and respect.

   4) Talk with a trusted adult about controlling impulses and being responsible.
   5) Keep dates low pressure by attending parties where adults are present or date in groups.
   6) Date someone who has similar values, commitment to setting limits, prevention of sexually transmitted infections and pregnancy.
   7) Avoid alcohol and drugs. Use makes controlling impulses more difficult and increases involvement in high risk behaviors.

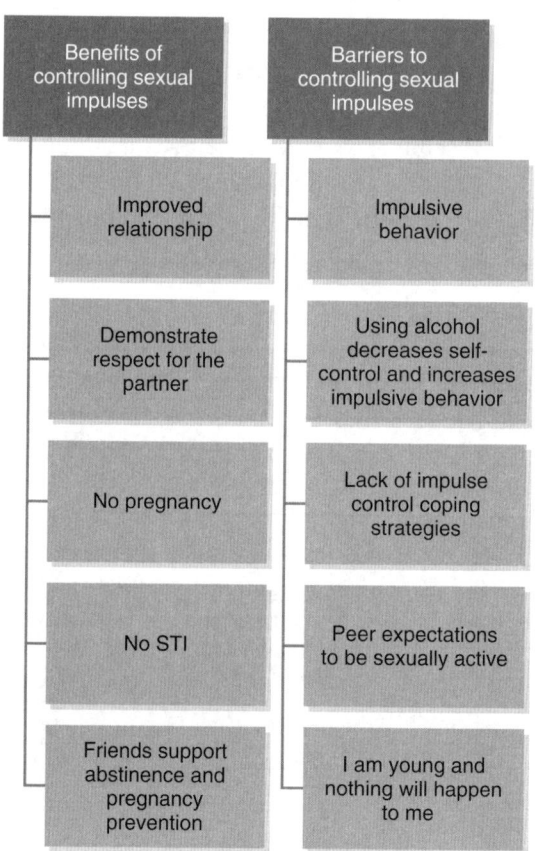

Figure 4.2 Benefits and Barriers to Controlling Sexual Impulses.

8) Avoid being alone at home or in an isolated place with your date. Impulse control is harder to manage in those environments. Adapted from: (Mary H. Bronson, 2009)

c. Strategies to control impulses

1) When you feel an emotional outburst erupting, breathe deeply through the nose and exhale through the mouth.

2) Monitor the impulses by becoming aware of when they occur and when they do not occur. This helps to slow down choices and curb the impulsive behavior.

3) Monitor the impulses of your friends. By identifying impulsive behavior in others, it may be easier to identify and monitor personal impulsive behavior. (Damico, 2020)

4. Read the practice prompt, students answer the reflection questions and discuss.

Practice Prompt: Libby and Larry

Libby and Larry are friends and they are worried about their peers. The high school is diverse in many ways. They see couples of the opposite sex, the same sex, and a variety of other pairs. The students are noted for being independent and "doing their thing" regardless of the consequences. They have also experienced the increase in teen pregnancy and STI infections and want to do something about it.

They approached their health teacher, Mr. Safetti, to talk about impulse control and safer sex. Mr. Safetti challenged the students with the prompt below and several discussion questions to reflect on the benefits of and barriers to controlling sexual impulses and the role of personal sexual responsibility.

A couple at the high school, Alondra and Anton, do not think much about the future. They like to respond to the moment and their feelings. They like being "free spirits" and encourage their friends to behave the same way. As a result, they are not monogamous, thinking this way of living increases their creativity.

Recently, they had a scare. Itching and oozing took them to the teen clinic where they were diagnosed with chlamydia. The doctor gave them a prescription and told them to use a condom every time they were intimate. Suddenly, being a "free spirit" was a problem for them and their partners.

Anton, decided that being impulsive has not worked out for him. He saw what happened to himself and has observed that his "free spirit" friends are putting themselves at risk for all sorts of unhealthy things. He has decided to change his behavior; he broke up with Alondra and is striving to think before he acts. He is trying to be aware of his triggers and when challenged, he pauses and practices his deep breathing. He has also learned that it is easier to discipline himself if he does not hang out with the "spirits."

It was difficult for Anton to change his behavior, but he is motivated to take care of himself. Being impulsive came naturally to him. But after seeing how being impulsive was not good for him, he is disciplining himself and making progress in changing. He has made new friends and has a new partner who is respectful, thoughtful, and fun to be with.

---

5. Use the review questions in **Table 4.12** to help the students understand the benefits of and barriers to practicing healthy sexual behaviors and ways to control sexual impulses.

6. End of class review. Ask the students to put away their materials then ask review questions.

a. What are two benefits of controlling impulses? (1.12.7)

b. What are two barriers to controlling impulses? (1.12.7)

c. What is one way to control impulses and enhance sexual health? (7.12.3)

7. Exit ticket (Self-Management: Impulse control, self-discipline, self-motivation)

a. What is one way a teen can be motivated to discipline themselves to control their impulsive behavior?

Self-Management: Stress Management

"Yoga is a powerful medium for developing the personality of children and making them capable of facing the present-day challenges and problems." (Hagen, 2004)

Yoga improves children's emotional and physical well-being. Teaching yoga in schools helps children develop resilience, and improves mood and self-regulation skills relating to emotions and stress. (Hagen, 2004)

PreK-2

Lesson Overview: Practicing Yoga and Other Strategies to Cope with Stress. In this lesson, children learn healthy ways to cope with stress.

Table 4.12 The Benefits of and Barriers to Practicing Healthy Sexual Behaviors and Ways to Control Sexual Impulses

Question	Answer
What were three benefits of and three barriers to Anton practicing a variety of healthy behaviors regarding sexual relationships? (1.12.7)	Three benefits of Anton practicing healthy behaviors. ■ Disciplined to be more in control of his impulses. ■ Motivated to be healthier and as a result has made new friends. ■ Has a new partner who is respectful, thoughtful, and fun. Three barriers to Anton practicing healthy behaviors. ■ Did not think much about the future. ■ Was a "free spirit." ■ Believed that being a "free spirit" increased his creativity.

How did Anton analyze his individual responsibility to control his impulses and enhance his sexual health? (7.12.3)	■ After being diagnosed with chlamydia, Anton decided that being a "free spirit" was not good for his health.
	■ Anton is striving to
	  • Think before he acts
	  • Take deep breaths to control his impulses
	  • Monitor and track when he is impulsive so he can remove himself from those situations.
	  • Learn from his impulsive friends so he doesn't repeat their mistakes.

SEL-Self-management: Impulse control, self-discipline How did Anton motivate himself to be disciplined to control impulses when in a sexual relationship?	Impulse control/self-discipline ■ Anton has disciplined himself to be more in control of his impulses by deep breathing; monitoring, tracking, and curbing his impulses; and learning the dangers of impulsive behavior from watching his friends.
SEL-Self-management: Self-motivation	Self-motivation. ■ Anton is motivated to be healthier and as a result has made new friends and has a new partner.

Modeling is one of the steps of skill building. To enhance yoga instruction, model the breathing and poses yourself or choose from many excellent videos on the Internet.

Resources:

- Johns Hopkins 15-minute Mindfulness video. The visual includes fish swimming in tropical, warm water. https://www.youtube.com/watch?v=V1-0JJJw_IQ

- Horse Stance: https://svasthaayurveda.com/yoga-pose-of-the-month-horse-stance/
- Yoga poses: https://kidshealth.org/en/kids/yoga-home.html

Materials needed:

- **Worksheet 4.7 How to Decrease Stress**

   Table 4.13 provides an overview of the lesson objectives, assessment, and instruction for this lesson.

Table 4.13 Lesson Objectives, Assessment, and Instruction

Step 1 – Lesson Objectives	Step 2 – Assessment
The verb of the *infused* performance indicator and the SEL competency generate the assessment and instruction.	Design the assessment based on the objectives. Ask yourself the question, "What can my students do to show me they have met the standard?"
1.2.1 Identify that healthy behaviors *such as practicing yoga and other strategies to cope with stress,* affect personal health. (Joint Committee on National Health Education Standards, 2007, p. 24)	1.2.1 Students identify *two* ways healthy behaviors *such as practicing yoga and other strategies to cope with stress* affects personal health.

7.2.1 <u>Demonstrate</u> healthy practices and behaviors, *practicing yoga and other strategies*, to maintain or improve personal health. (Joint Committee on National Health Education Standards, 2007, p. 35)	7.2.1 Students <u>demonstrate</u> healthy practices and behaviors, *such as mindful belly breathing and three yoga poses*, to maintain or improve personal health.
SEL-Self-management: stress management	Students identify and demonstrate *mindful belly breathing and three yoga poses to cope with stress and* maintain or improve personal health.

Step 3 – Instruction

Design the instruction so that students learn the content, skill, and competency to be successful on the assessment. Ask yourself the question, "What do I need to teach so that the students will be successful when assessed?"

Step 3 – Instruction

1. Define
   a. Identify: To recognize a particular person or an object.
   b. Demonstrate: To show how something is accomplished.
2. 1.2.1 <u>Identify</u> that healthy behaviors *such as practicing yoga and other stress reduction strategies* affect personal health.
   a. Ask the students the meaning of stress. What does it feel like? What does it do to your body? Is all stress bad? What can you do to get rid of the stress?
      1) Stress is something that causes your body to have a headache, bellyache, or unable to concentrate. You may have trouble eating, sleeping, and become cranky.
      2) <u>Note</u>: Put a happy face on the board to explain eustress. Good stress (Eustress) helps us get ready for something or accomplish a task such as making a presentation in class or completing a project.
      3) <u>Note</u>: Put a frowny face on the board to explain distress Bad stress occurs when something is bothering you for a long time. For example: Parents arguing or separating, or a family member is sick. (Kidshealth, 2020)
   b. Explain how yoga and other strategies affect personal health.
      1) Yoga calms the body through exercise and breathing.
      2) Talking to a parent, friend, teacher, counselor helps figure out the problem. They may make suggestions to feel better.
      3) Meditation helps calm the body by relaxing the mind. (Kidshealth from Nemours, 2020)

3. 7.2.1 <u>Demonstrate</u> healthy practices and behaviors *such as practicing yoga and other strategies* to maintain or improve personal health.
   a. Model stretching your body while breathing in. Relax the stretch and breathe out. Follow with student practice. Ask how the stretching makes the students feel.
      1) Calmer
      2) More relaxed
   b. Yoga and breathing exercises. Practice each strategy then ask the children how it makes them feel.
      1) Belly (Balloon) Breathing **Figure 4.3**
         a) Sit in a comfortable position with one hand on the belly.
         b) With the mouth closed, and the jaw relaxed, inhale through the nose, allowing your belly to expand. Imagine the lower part of the lung filling up first, then the rest of the lung inflating.

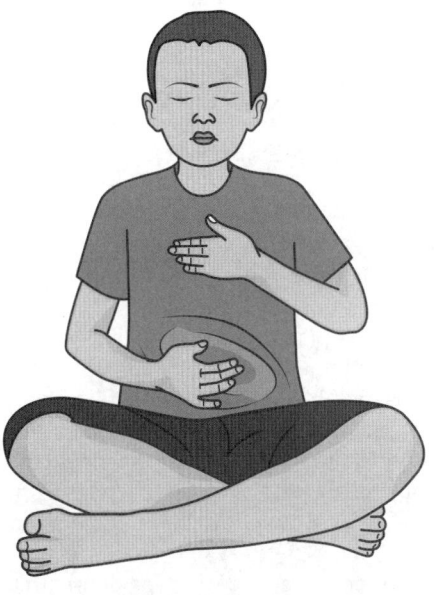

Figure 4.3 Belly (balloon) Breathing.

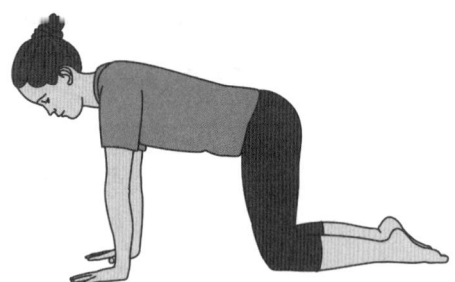

Figure 4.4 Table Pose.

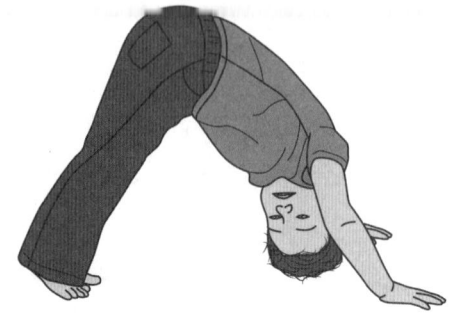

Figure 4.5 Downward-Facing Dog.

c) Slowly exhale imagining the air leaving the lung. Let the belly flatten.
d) Repeat 4–5 times. (Kidshealth from Nemours, April)

2) Table Pose **Figure 4.4**
a) Begin on your hands and knees.
b) Line up your hands under your shoulders and your knees under your hips.
c) Spread your fingers wide apart.
d) Keep your back flat and be careful not to drop your head
e) Hold the pose for a couple of breaths then gently bring yourself to a seated position. (Namaste Kid, 2020)

3) Downward-Facing Dog **Figure 4.5**
a) Begin on hands and knees in Table Pose.
b) Curl your toes under, straighten your knees, and lift your hips.
c) Keep your head between your arms.
d) When you are ready, lower your knees to the mat. (Namaste Kid, 2020)

4) Horse Stance **Figure 4.6**
a) Place arms at the side with the elbows, slightly bent.

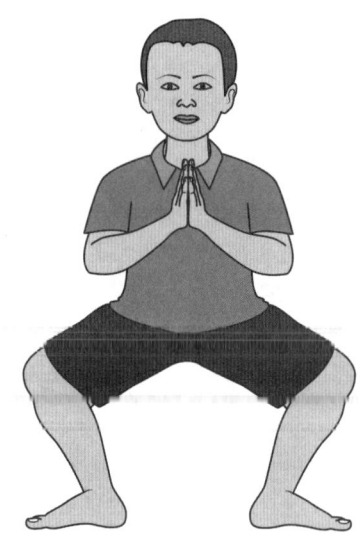

Figure 4.6 Horse Stance.

b) Place feet wide apart as if you were riding a horse.
c) Straighten the back
d) Pretend to sit a little bit.

4. Read the practice prompt, students answer the reflection questions, discuss.

Practice Prompt: Linette

Linette is stressed and she is only in the second grade! School work is hard for her and she doesn't have many friends. Mom and Dad are always fighting so she goes to her Nonnie's house on the weekends. She is having trouble sleeping and her belly hurts. She cries a lot but doesn't know why.

On Saturday, Linette and Nonnie went for a walk by the beach then to the playground. While swinging, Nonnie asked Linette what was on her mind. Linette told her grandmother she was worried her parents were getting a divorce. It was all she could think about.

Nonnie used to be a health teacher so she had an idea. "Let's relax tonight by doing yoga!" Nonnie said. "What is that?" Linette asked. "Well, we stretch our bodies and practice a special type of breathing and I guarantee we will both feel better."

That evening Nonnie and Linette practiced balloon breathing. Nonnie told her that balloon breathing is also Mindfulness activity. Linette practiced other mindfulness activities in health class, so she knew about them. First, Nonnie blew up a balloon to show Linette how the lungs fill with air. She then let the air out of the balloon slowly to show how to exhale. They tried it and pictured themselves walking the beach being very peaceful and happy. They both began to relax.

They watched a video of the Table Pose and Downward Facing Dog and tried each. Then they pretended they were riding a horse and held the pose for a short time. They had such fun and they both felt very refreshed and relaxed.

Linette loves to visit Nonnie. She is great fun and knows all sorts of things to help her be healthy.

Table 4.14 Benefits of Practicing Yoga to Decrease Stress

Question	Answer
What two ways did Linette identify to help her cope with stress? (1.2.1)	■ Balloon breathing (mindfulness) helped her relax. ■ Talking to her grandmother helped Linette figure out what was causing her stress. ■ Doing yoga with her grandmother caused Linette to feel very refreshed and relaxed.
How did belly breathing (mindfulness) improve Linette's personal health? (7.2.1) Which three yoga poses did Linette and her grandmother demonstrate that helped improve her health? (7.2.1)	The belly breathing (mindfulness) helped Linette and her grandmother picture themselves walking the beach and being very peaceful and happy. Yoga poses ■ Table Pose ■ Downward-Facing Dog ■ Horse Pose

SEL-Self-management: Stress management
 	
How did Linette identify and demonstrate *mindful belly breathing and three yoga pose, to cope with stress and* maintain or improve personal health?
	■ Linette practiced Balloon Breathing and that helped her relax.
	■ Linette and her grandmother practiced several yoga poses and they both felt refreshed and relaxed.
	  • Table Pose
	  • Downward-Facing Dog
	  • Horse Pose

5. Use the review questions in **Table 4.14** to help the children understand how yoga and belly breathing affect health and how to practice each to reduce stress.
6. End of class review. Ask the students to put away their materials then ask review questions.
   a. How does yoga and balloon breathing help reduce stress? (1.2.1)
   b. Demonstrate the Table Pose (7.2.1)
   c. Demonstrate the Downward-Facing Dog Pose (7.2.1)
   d. Demonstrate the Horse Pose (7.2.1)
7. Exit ticket (Self-Management: Stress management)

   Worksheet 4.7 How to Decrease Stress

Grades 3–5: Self-Management: Stress Management

Lesson Overview: Using Stress Reduction Strategies to Cope with Stress. In this lesson, students learn stress reduction strategies and how they affect personal health.

About 14% of children (ages 8–12) say they worry a lot or a great deal (American Psychological Association, 2012; Smith, 2020).

Children are exposed to many outward stimuli from the Internet, social media, and various forms communication technology that all compete for attention. In addition, children are pressured to achieve academically.

Including yoga in instruction is a practice that helps students deal with stress and self-regulate. It helps children listen to their bodies, feelings, and ideas. (Hagen, 2004)

Resources:

• Belly Breathing-Inner Explorer: https://www .youtube.com/watch?v=d91xVuDpUUU&feature =youtu.be

Materials needed:

• **Worksheet 4.8 Belly Breathing**

Table 4.15 provides an overview of the lesson objectives, assessment, and instruction for this lesson.

Table 4.15 Lesson Objectives, Assessment, and Instruction

Step 1 – Lesson Objectives	Step 2 – Assessment
The verb of the *infused* performance indicator and the SEL competency generate the assessment and instruction.	Design the assessment based on the objectives. Ask yourself the question, "What can my students do to show me they have met the standard?"

(continues)

Table 4.15 Lesson Objectives, Assessment, and Instruction *(continued)*

Step 1 – Lesson Objectives	Step 2 – Assessment
1.5.1 <u>Describe</u> the relationship between healthy behaviors, *such as using stress-reducing strategies* and personal health. (Joint Committee on National Health Education Standards, 2007, p. 24)	1.5.1 Students <u>describe</u> the relationship between *three stress-reducing strategies* and personal health.
7.5.2 Demonstrate a variety of healthy practices and behaviors, *such as stress reduction strategies*, to maintain or improve personal health. (Joint Committee on National Health Education Standards, 2007, p. 35)	7.5.2 Students <u>demonstrate</u> *how to stretch, how to breathe, three yoga positions, and three relaxation techniques* to maintain or improve personal health.
SEL-Self-management: Stress management	Students <u>describe</u> the relationship between *three stress-reducing strategies* and personal health. Students <u>demonstrate</u> *how to stretch, how to breathe, three yoga positions, and three relaxation techniques* to maintain or improve personal health.

Step 3 – Instruction
Design the instruction so that students learn the content, skill, and competency to be successful on the assessment. Ask yourself the question, "What do I need to teach so that the students will be successful when assessed?"

Step 3 – Instruction

1. Define
   a. Describe: To use words that help others envision the physical attributes of a person, place, or thing.
   b. Demonstrate: To show how something is accomplished.
2. 1.5.1 <u>Describe</u> the relationship between healthy behaviors *such as belly breathing* and personal health. Using **Worksheet 4.8 Belly Breathing**, discuss the benefits of belly breathing.
   a. Demonstrate belly breathing followed by a student practice.
   b. Belly (Balloon) breathing
      1) Lie on a comfortable surface.
      2) Put both hands on the belly. An alternative is to place a toy on the belly so the children can see the up and down movement.
      3) Keep the mouth closed and take a slow breath in through the nose.
      4) Imagine as you breathe in that there is a balloon in your belly and you are trying to fill it up with air.
      5) Encourage the children to keep breathing in until they think the balloon in their belly has enough air inside. Don't encourage the children to breathe in too much as because they may find it hard to stay relaxed.
      6) Children should feel their belly move up.

7) When the children feel the belly balloon is full of air, encourage them to imagine they have let go of the balloon and the air is rushing out.
8) Guide the children to breathe out slowly through their mouth (with pursed lips).
9) They should feel their belly moving down.
10) Repeat 4–5 times. (Children Inspired by Yoga, 2020)
   c. Ask the following questions.
      1) Was belly breathing relaxing? Why is belly breathing a good way to get air into your lungs?
         a) Answer: Belly breathing is relaxing because the deep breaths cause the heart and lungs to slow down. Belly breathing is a very efficient and relaxed way of getting enough air into the lungs.
      2) Does the slow movement of air in and out of the lungs remind you of something you do every day?
         a) Answer: The movement mimics sleep, digesting food, or resting.
      3) If you practiced belly breathing frequently through the day, do you think it gives you more energy?
         a) Answer: The exercise boosts energy level when performed throughout the

day. More oxygen is provided to the muscles.

    4) Why is it important to take the time to stop what you are doing, and belly breathe?

        a) Answer: Belly breathing supports the life skill of being able to relax. (Children Inspired by Yoga, 2020)

3. 7.5.2 Demonstrate a variety of healthy practices and behaviors *such as stress-reduction strategies* to maintain or improve personal health.

  a. <u>Note:</u> There are a variety of strategies below. Select the ones that best meet the needs of your students.

  b. To assess the social-emotional status of your students, ask them to describe how they are feeling using weather analogies. For example: "Today, I feel like a snowstorm. The wind is blowing from all directions and the snow is piling up. I feel cooped up." Explain that today's lesson provides ways to cope when we are stressed. Ask how they can make themselves feel better.

  c. Mindfulness

    1) The Bell Listening activity (helps children connect to the present moment and their perceptions)—Ring a bell and ask the children to listen carefully. Ask them to stay silent and raise their hand when they no longer hear the sound. Ask the children to stay silent and listen to the other sounds around them. Reflect on the activity.

    2) The Art of Touch (helps children isolate their senses and focus on separate, specific experiences.) Give each child an object to touch such as a ball, a feather, a soft toy, a stone, etc. Children close their eyes and describe what it feels like to a partner. Partners swap items and repeat. (Alternative: Children close their eyes first then receive the toy and describe it to their partner. The partner tries to identify the item.) (Mindfulness4U, 2020)

  d. Yoga positions

    1) Cow Pose **Figure 4.7**

        a) Start from all fours in a "tabletop" position. Place the knees under the hips and wrists under the shoulders or slightly forwards of them.

        b) Spread the fingers and press them to the mat.

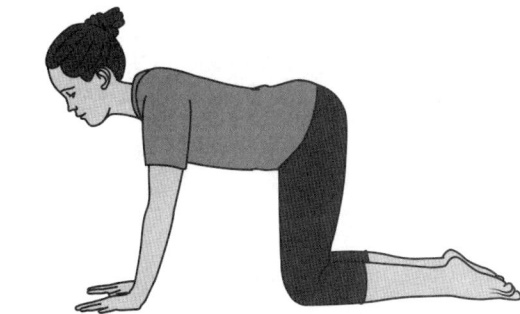

Figure 4.7 Cow Pose.

        c) When inhaling, lower the belly; lift the chest with the tailbone pointing up; and then look up.

        d) Exhale and come back to the neutral "tabletop" position. (Ekhart Yoga, 2020)

    2) Cat Pose **Figure 4.8**

        a) Start from all fours in a "tabletop" position. Place the knees under the hips and wrists under the shoulders or slightly forwards of them.

        b) Spread the fingers and press them to the mat.

        c) During the exhale, pull the belly in, lift the side waists, round the spine, and release the head toward the floor.

        d) Actively press the floor away and feel the stretch in the back of the body.

        e) Inhale and come back to the neutral starting position. (Ekhart Yogo, 2020)

    3) Child's Pose **Figure 4.9**

        a) Sit on the heels, knees spread, and bring the head toward the floor.

        b) Stretch the arms out to the front, by your side, or underneath the forehead.

        c) Breathe.

        d) Stay in the pose from 30 seconds to several minutes.

        e) To exit the pose, exhale and roll up the spine or come back to sitting with a straight spine. (Ekhart Yogo, 2020)

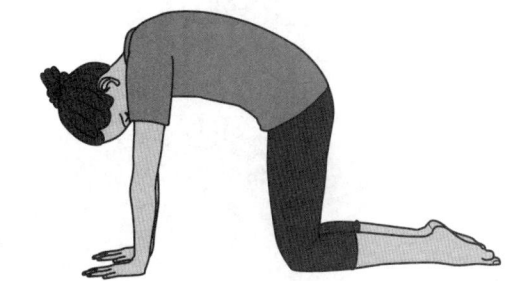

Figure 4.8 Cat Pose.

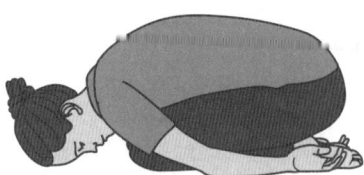

Figure 4.9 Child's Pose.

4) Easy Pose **Figure 4.10**
a) Sit on the mat with the sitting bones on the front edge of a firm cushion or folded blanket.
b) Cross the shins parallel to the mat, bringing each foot more or less beneath the opposite knee.
c) Press the sitting bones down to find length in the spine. Firm the shoulder blades in.
d) Place the hands on the lap or knees with palms up (more open) or down (calming).
e) Try to switch the cross of the legs each time you come into the pose. (Ekhart Yoga, 2020)

5) Hero Pose **Figure 4.11**
a) From all fours, bring the knees closer together and separate the feet slightly wider than hip distance apart.
b) Press the top of the feet down and slowly lower the hips back until eventually sitting on the mat between the heels.
c) Draw the navel in and up, ground through the sitting bones and extend through the crown of the head.
d) Stay for 5–10 breaths
e) Come out of the pose by placing the hands in front and lifting the hips back up to all fours.

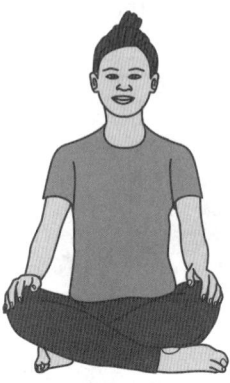

Figure 4.10 Easy Pose.

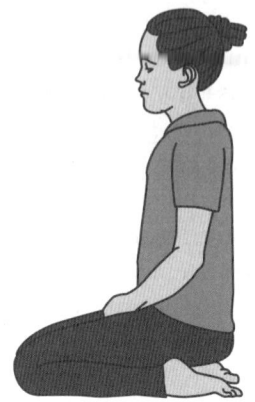

Figure 4.11 Hero Pose.

e. Relaxation techniques
1) The Squish and Relax Activity (Progressive relaxation exercise): Children lie on the floor with their eyes closed. Squish the muscles for a few seconds then release. Start with the toes and feet, then the leg muscles, stomach, hands, shoulders, and head. Reflect on the activity. (Mindfulness4U, 2020)
4. Read the practice prompt, students answer the reflection questions, and discuss.

Practice Prompt: Josie

Josie is new to this country. His parents brought him here from his native country because it was no longer safe to live there. Josie only knows how to speak in his native language and is finding school impossible. In his home country, he loved science and did very well in school. Here, every day is stressful. He just wants to stay home with his grandmother and tend the backyard garden.

The ESL teacher encourages him to be patient and has reminded him of the progress he has made since September. He knows she is right, but every day is a difficult day.

In his health class, the teacher demonstrated different ways to stretch, a special way to breathe, and three yoga poses: The Easy Pose, Child Pose, and the Hero Pose. He was able to do the poses by watching the teacher and his classmates. The stretches felt really good and the deep breathing started to relax him. He liked the exercise where he tightened then relaxed his muscles from his toes to his head. At least in this class, he could do what everyone else was doing and that made him feel good.

Josie plans to teach these exercises to his family tonight because they are also very stressed.

Table 4.16 Using a Variety of Stress-reducing Strategies and Their Effect on Personal Health

Question	Answer
How did Josie describe the relationship between *three stress-reducing strategies and his* personal health? (1.5.1)	The stretching, deep breathing, and yoga poses helped Josie feel relaxed and good about himself because, although he doesn't understand English very well, he was able to do all the exercises by watching his teacher and his classmates.
Which three stress reduction strategies did Josie demonstrate in class that helped improve his personal health? (7.5.2)	<ul><li>Belly Breathing</li><li>The Squish and Relax Strategy</li><li>The Easy Pose</li><li>The Child Pose</li><li>Hero Pose</li></ul>
SEL-Self-management: Stress management How did Josie describe the relationship between *three stress-reducing strategies and his* personal health?	The stretching, deep breathing, and yoga poses helped Josie feel relaxed and good about himself because, although he doesn't understand English very well, he was able to do all the exercises by watching his teacher and his classmates.
Which three stress-reduction strategies did Josie demonstrate in class that helped improve his personal health?	<ul><li>Belly Breathing</li><li>The Squish and Relax Strategy</li><li>The Easy Pose</li><li>The Child Pose</li><li>Hero Pose</li></ul>

5. Use the review questions in **Table 4.16** to help the children understand how stress-reduction strategies affect personal health.
6. End of class review. Ask the students to put away their materials then ask review questions.
   a. How do stress reduction strategies affect personal health? (1.5.1)
   b. Demonstrate belly breathing (7.5.2)
   c. Demonstrate the Squish and Relax Strategy (7.5.2)
   d. Demonstrate the Easy Pose (7.5.2)
   e. Demonstrate Child's Pose (7.5.2)
   f. Demonstrate the Hero Pose (7.5.2)
7. Exit ticket (Self-Management: Stress management)
   Worksheet 4.9 How Am I Feeling Now?

Grades 6–8: Self-Management: Stress Management

Lesson Overview: Effect of Anxiety and Anxiety-reducing Strategies. In this lesson, students learn the effects of anxiety on the components of wellness and strategies to overcome anxiety.

Anxiety is a normal reaction to stress. However, when anxiety becomes overwhelming, it interferes with well-being.

About 14% of children (ages 8–12) say they worry a lot or a great deal (American Psychological Association, 2012) and 31.9% have symptoms of anxiety disorders. (Merikangas et al., 2010). Systematic, effective, and efficient interventions for managing stress and reducing anxiety could have major benefits for school children, their families, and school staff. (Smith, 2020)

Resources:

- Teenshealth by Nemours: https://kidshealth.org/en/teens/anxiety-tips.html

Materials needed:

- **Worksheet 4.10 Effects of Anxiety on the Components of Wellness**
- **Worksheet 4.11 How Practicing Anxiety-Reducing Strategies Promotes Wellness**
- **Worksheet 4.12 How Practicing Anxiety-Reducing Strategies Enhances the Components of Wellness**

Table 4.17 provides an overview of the lesson objectives, assessment, and instruction for this lesson.

Table 4.17 Lesson Objectives, Assessment, and Instruction

Step 1 – Lesson Objectives	Step 2 – Assessment
The verb of the *infused* performance indicator and the SEL competency generate the assessment and instruction.	Design the assessment based on the objectives. Ask yourself the question, "What can my students do to show me they have met the standard?"
1.8.2. <u>Describe</u> the interrelationships *of anxiety* to emotional, intellectual, physical, and social health in adolescence. (Joint Committee on National Health Education Standards, 2007, p. 25)	1.8.2 <u>Describe</u> *two* interrelationships *of anxiety* to emotional, intellectual, physical, and social health in adolescence.
7.8.2 <u>Demonstrate</u> a variety of healthy practices and behaviors *such as anxiety-reduction strategies* to maintain or improve the health of self and others. (Joint Committee on National Health Education Standards, 2007, p. 35)	7.8.2 Students <u>demonstrate</u> *three anxiety-reducing strategies* to maintain or improve the health of self and others.
SEL-Self-management: Stress management	<u>Describe</u> *two* interrelationships *of anxiety* to emotional, intellectual, physical, and social health in adolescence. Students <u>demonstrate</u> *three anxiety-reducing strategies* to maintain or improve the health of self and others.

Step 3 – Instruction

Design the instruction so that students learn the content, skill, and competency to be successful on the assessment. Ask yourself the question, "What do I need to teach so that the students will be successful when assessed?"

Step 3 – Instruction

1. Define
   a. Describe: To use words that help others envision the physical attributes of a person, place, or thing.
   b. Demonstrate: To show how something is accomplished.
   c. Stress: An emotional, intellectual, social, or physical tension a person experiences.
   d. Eustress: Stress that results in positive effects on the person's health, feelings, and ability to complete tasks.
   e. Distress: State of mind in which the person feels anxious, nervous, and upset.
   f. Anxiety: An apprehensive feeling about what is happening or what may happen.
2. 1.8.1 Describe the interrelationships *of anxiety* to emotional, intellectual, physical, and social health in adolescence. Use **Worksheet 4.10 Effects of Anxiety on the Components of Wellness**
   a. Directions
      1) Place the graphic organizer and the cut-up signs of teen anxiety in a baggie.
      2) Provide time for the students to align the signs of anxiety to the components of wellness. Discuss.
   b. Signs of teen anxiety **Table 4.18**

3. 7.8.2 <u>Demonstrate</u> a variety of healthy practices and behaviors *such as anxiety-reduction strategies* that maintain or improve the health of self and others.
   a. Use **Worksheet 4.11 How Practicing Anxiety-Reducing Strategies Promotes Wellness** as an alternative
   b. <u>Note</u>: Set up five stations around the classroom. On each station, provide information about dealing with anxiety. Students move from one station to another reading the information and adding their thoughts about coping strategies that work for them. Mats may enhance the participation in the deep breathing and yoga station. Discuss.

      This engaging activity is also a good introduction into an advocacy project where students take each of the strategies, make a public service announcement or video, and post or broadcast to the student population. The information could also be used for a teacher or parent education program, led by students.
   c. Activity stations
      1) **Station 1: Learn and practice how to relax.** Daily practice of relaxation strategies effects the brain and are helpful in reducing anxiety. Try these easy strategies and add other strategies that work for you.

Table 4.18 Signs of Teen Anxiety

Increased heart rate	Increased breathing	Avoiding friends	Problems with family
Less involvement in extracurricular activities	Unable to concentrate on schoolwork	Spending more time alone	Frequent headaches
Stomach aches	Excessive fatigue	Changes in eating habits	Not feeling well but no signs of sickness
Trouble falling asleep	Trouble staying asleep	Not feeling refreshed after sleeping	Absenteeism
Decrease in grades	Feeling overwhelmed with schoolwork load	Procrastination	Not completing school assignments

Data from Katie Hurley, L. (2018, September 26). 6 Hidden Signs of Teen Anxiety. Retrieved from PSYCOM: https://www.psycom.net/hidden-signs-teen-anxiety/

Easy Yoga Pose (see Figure 4.10):
a) Sit on the mat with the sitting bones on the front edge of a firm cushion or folded blanket.
b) Cross your shins parallel to the mat, bringing each foot more or less beneath the opposite knee.
c) Press your sitting bones down to find length in the spine. Firm your shoulder blades in.
d) Place your hands on your lap or knees with palms up (more open) or down (calming).
e) Try to switch the cross of your legs each time you come into the pose. (Ekhart Yogo, 2020)
Maintain the Easy Yoga pose and try the Four Square Breathing strategy.

Four square breathing: 1: Inhale for four seconds; 2: Hold the breath for four seconds; Exhale slowly for four seconds; Hold the position for four seconds (**Figure 4.12**).

Reflection: Your strategy.
2) **Station 2: Sleep, Diet, and Exercise** (**Table 4.19**)
3) **Station 3: Connection suggestions.** Spending time with people we feel close to contributes to a sense of security and support. Having fun and sharing experiences and ideas contributes to happiness and helps us to be less upset about other things. It is helpful to talk to someone who cares and will listen when you are worried or nervous about something. When someone listens, it helps us feel understood and helps us cope in a healthy way.

a) Who is a member of your connection net?
b) What fun things do you do when feeling anxious or stressed?
c) Reflection:
4) **Station 4: Connection with nature.** Taking a walk by the beach, in the woods, or at a park; bike riding, snow shoeing; skiing; surfing; or wherever and however you enjoy nature is a great way to relax. Enjoying nature with a trusted friend, family member, or trusted adult also helps us connect with others.
a) How do you connect with nature?
b) How does being with nature affect your anxiety or stress?
c) Reflection:
5) **Station 5: Concentrate on the positive.** When negative or anxiety-provoking thoughts are in your head, acknowledge them then make a choice to get rid of them and think positive. Focus on what

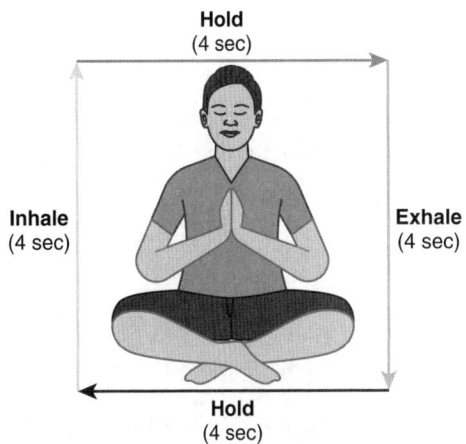

Figure 4.12 Four Square Breathing.

Table 4.19 Station 2: Sleep, Diet, and Exercise Recommendations

Recommended Sleep	Recommended Diet		Recommended Exercise
8–10 hours of sleep (Teens Health from Nemours, 2020)	Eat nutritious foods ■ 2,800 calories for boys ■ 2,200 calories for girls Appropriate portions from the five food groups (vegetables, fruits, grains, protein, dairy)		60 minutes each day (Connolly, 2018, p. 421)
Your sleep:	Your diet:		Your exercise

Reflection:

is good, beautiful, and positive. Acknowledge the small things in life that you enjoy. Dream, wish, and imagine good things that can happen. (Teenshealth by Nemours, 2020)

   a) What is one way you can concentrate on the positive?

   b) Reflection:

4. Read the practice prompt. students answer the reflection questions and discuss.

Practice Prompt: Ceiri

"7th grade is really hard!" said Ceiri. It is not the schoolwork that is hard but all the social stuff that happens. If she participates in class, as she likes to do, some peers call her a nerd. If she is quiet, she becomes frustrated because she likes to participate. She has a few friends but not one close, best friend.

Sometimes, she deliberatly stays in the bathroom in the morning so she misses the bus and her mom has to drive her. Not taking the bus relieves a lot of anxiety because she doesn't have to cope with the other peers.

Riding the bus home is another story. She usually sits alone and by the time she gets home, she has a headache and is very grumpy. She tries to do her homework right away but can't because she is so aggrevated. She checks social media to see if anyone is talking about her then after supper, she starts her homework. By then, she is tired and doesn't always finish the assignments. Her grades are beginning to slip.

Lunchtime is difficult because she is not sure where she will sit each day. Sometimes, her regular table is full and she just walks around looking for an empty seat. It seems like everyone is looking at her. Lately, she eats in the nurse's office. The nurse understands Ceiri's anxieties and tries to help her.

One day, Mrs. Cucino, the health teacher, came into the nurse's office during lunch and saw Ceiri

there. She asked, "How come you are here and not in the lunch room?" Ceiri explained and the nurse added that there are many other students who have similar anxieties.

Mrs. Cucino sat down with Ceiri and showed her some simple exercises to help relieve anxiety. They sat in the Easy Yoga Pose and practiced the four square breathing technique. It felt weird at first but then she enjoyed it. The nurse even joined in and they all had a good laugh when they were done.

They had a nice conversation about eating healthy and getting enough sleep to help control the anxiety. They recommended getting out and going for a walk either with friends or family. Ceiri's neighbor goes to her school. She doesn't know her very well but she is nice. Maybe she will ask the neighbor to go for a walk around the neighborhood.

Ceiri agreed that she could try letting negative thoughts go and concentrate on the positive. Mrs. Cucino and the nurse recommended thinking about things that she enjoys and focus on them rather than negative things.

They also told her there are many other students in school that have the same problem and that both Mrs. Cucino and the nurse have made the same suggestions to them. Ceiri asked that maybe they could meet and have lunch in the office.

Ceiri understands herself better now. She doesn't want the axiety to affect her anymore and plans to take steps to cope. She knows it won't be easy but she is willing to try. She knows she has Mrs. Cucino and the nurse to go to if she needs help.

5. Use the review questions in **Table 4.20** to help the children understand how anxiety reduction strategies affect personal health.

6. End of class review. Ask the students to put away their materials then ask review questions.

   a. What are two ways anxiety affects personal health? (1.8.2)

Table 4.20 Effects of Anxiety on the Components of Wellness and Anxiety Reduction Strategies

Question	Answer
How did Ceiri's anxiety affect her emotional, intellectual, physical, and social health? (1.8.2)	Ceiri's Emotional health ■ Suffered because she felt she could not be herself. Ceiri's Intellectual health ■ Her grades were slipping and she did not complete homework. Ceiri's Physical health ■ Ceiri experienced headaches and stomach aches at the end of the day after riding home on the bus. Ceiri's Social health ■ Ceiri's social health suffered at lunch when she had nowhere to sit and on the bus when she chose to sit alone.
Which *three anxiety-reducing strategies* did *Ceiri use* to maintain her health? (7.8.2)	■ Four square breathing ■ Easy yoga pose ■ Planning to eat healthy and get enough sleep ■ Planning to reach out to a neighbor to go for a walk ■ Concentrating on positive thoughts
SEL-Self-management: Stress management How did Ceiri's anxiety affect her emotional, intellectual, physical, and social health?	Ceiri's emotional health ■ Suffered because she felt she could not be herself. Ceiri's intellectual health ■ Her grades were slipping, and she did not complete homework. Ceiri's physical health ■ Ceiri experienced headaches and stomach aches at the end of the day after riding home on the bus. Ceiri's social health ■ Ceiri's social health suffered at lunch when she had nowhere to sit and on the bus when she chose to sit alone.

b. How much sleep should a teen your age be getting? (7.8.2)

c. Give an example of a balanced diet. (7.8.2)

d. How much exercise should a teen your age be getting? (7.8.2)

e. Why is it important to have connections with friends and family? (7.8.2)

f. Why is it important to connect with nature? (7.8.2)

g. Why is it important to think positive? (7.8.2)

h. Demonstrate Four Square Breathing (7.8.2)

i. Demonstrate the Easy Pose (7.8.2)

7. Exit ticket (Self-Management: Stress management)

Worksheet 4.12 How Practicing Anxiety-Reducing Strategies Enhances the Components of Wellness.

For each component of wellness, write down one way anxiety-reducing strategies help us be healthier.

Grades 9–12: Self-Management: Stress Management

Lesson Overview: Using Mindfulness to Cope with Stress and Anxiety. In this lesson, students propose ways to reduce health problems related to stress and anxiety and learn to practice mindfulness.

Seven in 10 teens, from across gender, racial, and socio-economic lines; and demographic groups; see anxiety and depression as a problem.

Sixty-one percent of teens say they feel a lot of academic pressure; 29% feel a pressure to look good; 28% feel pressure to fit in socially; 21% feel pressured to be involved in extracurricular activities and be good at sports; 50% feel that drugs and alcohol are a problem among their peers; only 4% feel pressure to use drugs; and 6% feel pressured to use alcohol. (Pew Research Center, 2019, p. 2)

Anxiety is a reaction to stress and as skills based health educators, we provide the content, skill, and SEL competency to help students cope with anxiety and stress in a healthful way

Resources:

• Mindful eating exercise with a raisin: https://mynutritionclinic.com.au/wp-content/uploads/2016/12/Mindful-eating-with-a-raisin.pdf

Materials needed:

• **Worksheet 4.13 On a Roll Activity**
• **Worksheet 4.14 Mindfulness Practice**

Table 4.21 provides an overview of the lesson objectives, assessment, and instruction for this lesson.

Step 3 – Instruction

1. Define
    a. Propose: To present a new idea for serious consideration and discussion by other people.
    b. Demonstrate: To show how something is accomplished.
    c. Anxiety: An apprehensive feeling about what is happening or what may happen.
    d. Mindfulness: The conscious ability of a person to concentrate on their feelings, ideas, and experiences at all times.

2. 1.12.5 Propose ways to reduce or prevent injuries and health problems *related to stress and anxiety*.

Worksheet 4.13 On a Roll Activity

a. The questions below relate to stress and anxiety and how to reduce them. Students work in pairs or groups. The sets are expandable to six. One student rolls the die and answers a question from that numbered pile. If the response is incorrect, another player in the group takes the question, explains the correct answer, and puts it in a pile to be asked again during the next round. The rounds continue until all questions are answered correctly. With more than two students, take turns answering the questions.

Note: Use your imagination to creatively ask the questions. An electronic alternative to review content is to use Kahoot or Quizlet. They are electronic formatives that students enjoy using when reviewing or previewing health content.

b. If the student rolls a #1 or #4, ask the following questions about teen stress and anxiety. (Pew Research Center, 2019)
    1) Sixty-one percent of teens aged 14–17 say their Number 1 source of stress is …. (pressure to get good grades)
    2) Twenty-eight percent of teens feel a lot of _____ pressure to fit in. (social)

Table 4.21 Lesson Objectives, Assessment, and Instruction

Step 1 – Lesson Objectives	Step 2 – Assessment
The verb of the *infused* performance indicator and the SEL competency generate the assessment and instruction.	Design the assessment based on the objectives. Ask yourself the question, "What can my students do to show me they have met the standard?"
1.12.5 Propose ways to reduce or prevent injuries and health problems *related to stress and anxiety*. (Joint Committee on National Health Education Standards, 2007, p. 25)	1.12.5 Propose three ways to reduce or prevent injuries and health problems *related to stress and anxiety*.
7.12.2 Demonstrate a variety of healthy practices and behaviors *such as mindfulness* that maintain or improve the health of self and others. (Joint Committee on National Health Education Standards, 2007, p. 35)	7.12.2 Students demonstrate *three mindfulness strategies* to maintain or improve the health of self and others.
SEL-Self-management: Stress management	Propose three ways to reduce or prevent injuries and health problems *related to stress and anxiety*. Students demonstrate *three mindfulness strategies* to maintain or improve the health of self and others.

Step 3 – Instruction
Design the instruction so that students learn the content, skill, and competency to be successful on the assessment. Ask yourself the question, "What do I need to teach so that the students will be successful when assessed?"

3) Fifty percent of teens believe that _____ and _____ use are major problems with people in their age group. (drugs, alcohol)

4) What is your major source of stress and anxiety? (answers will vary)

c. If the student rolls a #2 or a #5, ask the following questions about how to reduce anxiety and stress resulting from using social media? (Heitler, 2020)

1) Why does social media lead to high levels of anxiety? (on average, teens spend 4 hours a day on social media. Constant social comparisons contribute to worry and anxiety about not being good enough.)

2) How does social media decrease socialization? (Instead of spending time with friends in person, which builds social connections and in turn builds self-confidence, the electronic device replaces the socialization.)

3) Do electronic devices lead to compulsive behavior? (Compulsive behavior: Actions that a person takes repeatedly although the results are generally negative. Some teens constantly/compulsively check their device frequently through the day.)

4) What is one way to reduce anxiety resulting from the use of social media? (answers will vary)

d. If the student rolls a #3, ask the true/false questions about stress. (American Psychological Association, 2019)

1) T F Signs of stress and anxiety include being grumpy, short-tempered, and argumentative. (True)

2) T F Being stressed or anxious does not affect sleep. (False. Teens may complain of being tired all the time, sleep more than usual, or have trouble falling asleep)

3) T F Teens who are stressed or anxious tend to eat too much or too little. (True)

4) T F Stressed and anxious teens only show psychological symptoms, not physical symptoms. (False. Stress often has physical symptoms such as headaches, stomachaches, and frequent trips to the nurse.)

e. If the student rolls a #6, ask the questions about Proposals to reduce stress/anxiety.

1) A teen should have _____ hours of sleep each night.
a) 8, b) 10, c) 12, d) 5   (10 hours)

2) A teen should have _____ minutes of exercise each day.
a) 30, b) 25, c) 60, d) 80   (60 minutes)

3) Talking with a _____ helps put stress and anxiety into perspective.
a) trusted adult, b) family member, c) guidance counselor, d) all
(Trusted adult)

4) Taking time to have _____ is an important way to reduce stress and anxiety. Maybe it is a movie, a game, being with friends, biking, etc.   (Fun)

5) Getting out into _____ is a great way to relieve stress and anxiety and improve overall well-being. It may be a park, a beach, the woods, etc.   (Nature)

6) _____ about your experiences by journaling is a great way to get the feelings out, relieve stress and anxiety and improve well-being. (Writing)

3. 7.12.2 Demonstrate a variety of healthy practices and behaviors, *such as mindfulness*, that maintain or improve the health of self and others.

a. Note: In this portion of the lesson, brainstorm practices and behaviors that help manage stress and anxiety. Then proceed to the skill of practicing mindfulness.

b. Benefits of mindfulness: Teens who practice mindfulness experience less stress than those who do not practice this stress/anxiety reducing strategy. (American Psychological Association, 2019)

c. Mindfulness strategies.

1) Note: Explain that mindfulness is a skill and needs to be practiced. Mindfulness helps train our attention and helps us to pay attention to what we are doing. Consequently, it helps to manage stress and anxiety. When we concentrate hard on something, we are practicing mindfulness. (playing music, dancing, participating in physical activity, cooking, playing a strategic game, etc.)

2) Note: Model the mindful breathing and eating strategy then provide time for the students to practice the other exercises using **Worksheet 4.14 Mindfulness Practice.** (KidsHealth from Nemours, 2020)

3) Mindful breathing: Model the strategy and then provide time for the students to practice.
   a) Sit in a relaxed, comfortable position. Close your eyes and think of something to focus on such as an object or a word.
   b) Pay attention to each breath that you inhale and exhale. Pay attention to the rise and fall of your belly as you breathe.
   c) Spend a few minutes just paying attention to your breath going in and out of your body.
   d) When your mind wanders. It is OK. Just guide your attention back to your breathing. (Nemours. Children's Health System, 2020)
   e) **Alternate mindful breathing: Four square breathing:** 1: Inhale for four seconds; 2: Hold the breath for four seconds; Exhale slowly for four seconds; Hold the position for four seconds.

4) Mindful eating. Use the five senses to demonstrate how to eat mindfully. Follow with student practice. Note: Students bring a snack that is safe for them, being "mindful" of food allergies.
   a) Sense of touch: Hold the food in your hands and notice how it feels.
   b) Sense of smell: Place the food near the nose and smell it. Is there a smell to the food?
   c) Sense of sight: Look at the food. What does it look like? Is it smooth? (Apple) What is the shape? (round, square, oval, etc.)
   d) Sense of taste: Taste the food. Take the time to notice how it feels in the mouth, on the tongue, and against the teeth. Take the time to enjoy the flavor and texture of the food. (TeensHealth from Nemours, 2020)
   e) Sense of hearing: Does the food make any noise when eating it? (crunch, etc.)
   f) How does mindful eating enhance personal health?

5) Mindful walking. Mindful walking focuses on the experience of walking and being aware of the body and surroundings.
   a) Walk at a natural pace. With each step, pay attention to the lifting and falling of the foot, movement in your legs, and shifting of body weight from side to side.
   b) Sense of sound. Notice the sounds in the environment. Rather than labeling the sounds, just acknowledge them.
   c) Sense of smell. Pay attention to smells you encounter.
   d) Sense of sight. Observe the different colors, objects, people, animals, or anything else that attracts your attention.
   e) Maintain a sense of awareness of your surroundings as you walk, acknowledging that there is nothing to do other than walk and be aware.
   f) As the walk is nearing completion, pay attention to the movement of your body. (feet, legs, arms, etc.)
   g) At the end of the walk, reflect on the difference between mindful walking and walking without the awareness of the body and surroundings. (Bertin, 2017)

6) Mindful driving. Mindful driving helps the driver remain focused rather than distracted.
   a) Before starting the car, pay attention to how your body feels in the driver's seat. Is the seat comfortable? Are you comfortable?
   b) Take in a slow breath and settle into the seat. Make adjustments to the seat to be comfortable and to the mirrors so you can see clearly.
   c) Fasten your seat belt. Using positive self-talk, remind yourself to pay attention while driving and plan to drive safely.
   d) Take a slow breath and start the car. Be mindful of the surroundings. Are there people nearby? Do you see other cars?
   e) As you drive, be mindful of situations that require you to speed up, slow down, or stop.
   f) If you become distracted, remind yourself that you are driving and refocus your attention to the road. (TeensHealth from Nemours, 2020)

4. Read the practice prompt. Students answer the reflection questions and discuss.

Practice Prompt: Marcus

"Well, I have lost my driving privilege again!" Marcus texted to his friend, Piero. "What did you do now, Marcus?" asked Piero. Marcus explained that he was late for work at the pizza restaurant. He was tired and grumpy because he didn't get enough sleep. He jumped in the car, put on his seat belt, turned on the radio, and quickly moved into traffic. His mother used the car in the morning and adjusted the mirrors so she could see but Marcus didn't take the time to change them. He moved into the right lane because he didn't see anyone there and "Boom!" he hit the car next to him.

Piero tried to help his friend feel better by talking with him. Piero also lost his driving privileges because he was in an accident. He and Marcus are similar because they both are very busy with school, sports, and working. They often complain of being tired and not having any time to themselves.

In health class, Mrs. Vega started a new self-management unit and began with stress management. Her first lesson was on reducing stress and anxiety by using mindfulness. The boys were very surprised to learn how many teens suffer from stress and anxiety. It was good to learn that they are not alone.

Mrs. Vega proposed several ways to reduce stress including getting enough sleep, eating healthy, enjoying nature, being physically active, and writing down the personal reaction to stress. The boys had to keep a log of trying to comply with each of the ways to reduce stress. They found that getting enough sleep, eating healthy, and being physically active worked for them.

When the boys heard part of the unit was mindful driving, they were interested. They learned that mindfulness is just being aware of what they are doing, just like the concentration they have when playing their sports.

Marcus asked his mom if they could take a ride together. He showed her how to be a mindful driver starting with getting into the driver's seat, taking a deep breath, putting on the seatbelt, fixing the mirrors, being aware of how he is feeling, other drivers, and the driving conditions. His mother was impressed and agreed to let him use the car again but only if he practices mindful driving and gets enough sleep.

What a difference mindfulness has made on the boys. They are calmer and find it much easier to concentrate on schoolwork and whatever it is they are doing at the moment. They know know that being distracted happens but they know to redirect their thoughts to the activity at hand.

Neither Marcus nor Piero have been in any accidents lately. Life is good!

5. Use the review questions in **Table 4.22** to help the children understand how stress-reduction strategies affect personal health.
6. End of class review. Ask the students to put away their materials then ask review questions.
   a. What are three ways to reduce or prevent injuries and health problems related to stress and anxiety? (1.12.5)
   b. Demonstrate four square breathing. (7.12.2)
   c. Demonstrate how to mindfully eat. (7.12.2)
   d. Demonstrate how to mindfully walk. (7.12.2)
7. Exit ticket (Self-Management: Stress management)

   Worksheet 4.15 A Personal Plan to Cope with Stress and Anxiety

Section 2. Setting and Achieving Personal and Educational Goals/ Organizational Skills

(Collaborative for Academic Social Emotional Learning, 2020)

Goal setting is an important life skill. The National Health Education Standards guide goal setting skill development PreK–12. Achieving a realistic goal enhances emotional well-being. Young children learn to set goals such as tying their shoes to putting

Table 4.22 Proposal of Ways to Reduce Injuries Related to Stress and Anxiety and the Use of Mindfulness

Question	Answer
How can *Marcus* reduce or prevent injuries and health problems *related to stress and anxiety?* (1.12.5)	<ul><li>Get 10 hours of sleep each night.</li><li>Get 60 minutes of physical activity each day.</li><li>Talk to a trusted adult when stressed/anxious.</li><li>Connect with nature.</li><li>Get outside.</li><li>Take time to have fun.</li><li>Write down thoughts when stressed or anxious.</li></ul>

(continues)

Table 4.22 Proposal of Ways to Reduce Injuries Related to Stress and Anxiety and the Use of Mindfulness
(continued)

Question	Answer
Which *three mindfulness strategies* did Marcus demonstrate to maintain or improve the health of self and others? (7.12.2)	<ul><li>Mindful driving</li><li>Getting enough sleep</li><li>Eating healthy</li><li>Being physically active</li></ul>
SEL-Self-management: Stress management How can *Marcus* reduce or prevent injuries and health problems *related to stress and anxiety?* (1.12.5)	<ul><li>Get 10 hours of sleep each night.</li><li>Get 60 minutes of physical activity each day.</li><li>Talk to a trusted adult when stressed/anxious</li><li>Connect with nature</li><li>Get outside</li><li>Take time to have fun</li><li>Write down thoughts when stressed or anxious.</li></ul>
Which *three mindfulness strategies* did Marcus demonstrate to maintain or improve the health of self and others? (7.12.2)	<ul><li>Mindful driving</li><li>Getting enough sleep</li><li>Eating healthy</li><li>Being physically active</li></ul>

away their belongings. As students mature, more guidance is needed how to set short- and long-term goals. (Randy M. Page , 2015, p. 65) In the classroom, involve the students in setting goals and provide guidance, support, and recognition for when the goals are reached.

In the lessons below, SMART Goals have been modified to a SMARTHR goal model by adding the elements of H: Who can help and R: Reflection.

PreK–2 Self-Management: Goal Setting

Lesson Overview: Goal Setting to Eat Healthy and Increase Physical Activity

In this lesson, students learn how physical activity affects their health, how to set a short term goal to eat healthy and become more physically active, and who can help them set a goal.

Young children have the ability to set and achieve goals with support and guidance. Teaching goal setting also teaches accountability and perseverance. (Alyssa, 2020) Achieving goals helps children increase their self-esteem and self-confidence as they identify, adopt, and maintain healthy behaviors.

In addition to subcompetency of goal setting, this section also includes organizational skills because students plan and track progress to reaching a goal.

Resources:

- RMC: PreK–2 Goal Setting: https://www.rmc.org /what-we-do/training-expertise-to-create-healthy -schools/health-education/goal-setting/

Materials needed:

- **Worksheet 4.16 Benefits of Physical Activity on Physical Health**
- **Worksheet 4.17 Goal Setting**

Table 4.23 provides an overview of the lesson objectives, assessment, and instruction for this lesson.

Table 4.23 Lesson Objectives, Assessment, and Instruction

Step 1 – Lesson Objectives	Step 2 – Assessment
The verb of the *infused* performance indicator and the SEL competency generate the assessment and instruction.	Design the assessment based on the objectives. Ask yourself the question, "What can my students do to show me they have met the standard?"
1.2.1 <u>Identify</u> that healthy *physical activity* behaviors *affect* personal health. (Joint Committee on National Health Education Standards, 2007, p. 24)	1.2.1 <u>Identify</u> *five* healthy *physical activity* behaviors *and how they affect* personal health.

6.2.1 <u>Identify</u> a short-term personal health goal and take action toward achieving the goal. (Joint Committee on National Health Education Standards, 2007, p. 34).	6.2.1 <u>Identify</u> *one* short-term health goal for *healthy eating and getting adequate exercise* and take action to achieve the goal.
6.2.2 <u>Identify</u> who can help when assistance is needed to achieve a personal health goal. (Joint Committee on National Health Education Standards, 2007, p. 34)	6.2.2 <u>Identify</u> *one person* who can help when assistance is needed to achieve the personal health goal *of eating healthy and getting adequate exercise.*
SEL-Self-management: Goal setting; organizational skills	<u>Identify</u> *five* healthy *physical activity* behaviors *and how they affect* personal health. <u>Identify</u> *one* short-term health goal for *healthy eating and getting adequate exercise* and take action to achieving the goal. <u>Identify</u> *one person* who can help when assistance is needed to achieve the personal health goal *of eating healthy and getting adequate exercise.*

Step 3 – Instruction

Design the instruction so that students learn the content, skill, and competency to be successful on the assessment. Ask yourself the question, "What do I need to teach so that the students will be successful when assessed?"

Step 3 – Instruction

1. Define
   a. Identify: To recognize a particular person or an object.
   b. Goal: An achievement that is reached following the completion of established criteria.
   c. Short-term goal: A step taken to achieve a goal.
2. 1.2.1 Identify that healthy behaviors *such as healthy eating and exercise* affect personal health.
   a. Ask the following questions to determine the amount of student physical activity. Use a white board, smile/frown faces, sticky notes, Kahoot, or any form of formative tools.
   b. Positive responses indicate physical activity.
   c. Questions
      1) Do you play outside several times a day or inside where you are free to move?
      2) Do you spend less than two hours a day in front of a screen? (not counting schoolwork)
      3) Do you move for at least 60 minutes each day?
      4) When actively playing, do you sweat and breathe quickly?

d. Use **Worksheet 4.16 Benefits of Physical Activity on Physical Health** to identify how physical activity affects personal health.
3. 6.2.1 Identify a short-term personal health goal and take action toward achieving the goal.
   a. Show the children a picture of a symbol of a goal, such as a soccer goal.
   b. Ask the children to identify the symbol and explain what happens when a ball goes into the net. (goal); Ask, "How do athletes score a goal?" (work as a team, *take turns kicking the ball* (short term goal))
   c. Ask, "Who can identify an example of a personal health goal?"
   d. Ask, "What are some small steps that will help you reach your goal?" (short-term goals)
4. 6.2.2 Identify who can help when assistance is needed to achieve a personal health goal.
   a. Ask, "Who can help you reach your goal?" (trusted adult, friend, teacher, neighbor, etc.)
   b. Model the goal-setting steps (**Figure 4.13**).
   c. Use **Worksheet 4.17 Goal Setting** to help the children set a personal health goal.
5. Read the practice prompt. Students answer the reflection questions and discuss.

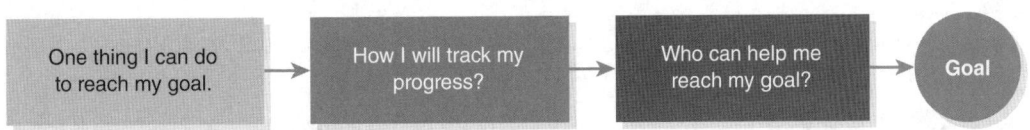

Figure 4.13 Steps of Goal Setting.

Practice Prompt: Amanda

Amanda is so bored! The pandemic has kept her out of school, away from her friends, and stuck in the house!

She misses her classmates, lunch time, recess, her teacher, and learning in the classroom.

She logs into the school website and her mother or father helps her complete her lessons. She is sitting a long time and misses going out to play. She gets squirmy and has trouble sitting still in front of the computer. She is doing all her work but feels like she needs to move.

Her health teacher, Mr. Allen, decided that it was time for a goal-setting unit on finding ways to be active for 60 minutes each day while being inside. He first showed slides of children riding bicycles, dancing, walking, practicing soccer or basketball, and other activities. He identified how being physically active helps children maintain healthy weight, get sick less, have stronger bones and muscles, develop their brains, be more creative, and feel good about themselves.

For her physical activity assessment, Amanda decided to exercise to her Wii video. Other students chose PBS or YouTube videos. Mr. Allen approved the ideas and gave each student the Goal-Setting worksheet.

Amanda put 60 minutes of activity at the top of the steps. On the first step, she said she is using Wii to exercise at different times each day for a total of 60 minutes. On the second step, she is keeping track of her progress by putting red (she didn't exercise), yellow (she exercised but not for 60 minutes), and green (she completed 60 minutes of exercise that day) stickers next to the day and drawing what she did or didn't do to reach her goal. On the third step, she drew a picture of her mom exercising with her. It really helped Amanda meet her goal by having someone exercising with her.

She was so pleased at the end of the week. She reached her goal! By exercising each day, she found that she was able to sit longer and complete her school work and she felt much better! She drew a picture of herself and her mom dancing to reflect on how pleased she was with her self.

6. Use the review questions in **Table 4.24** to help the children understand how stress-reduction strategies affect personal health.
7. End of class review. Ask the students to put away their materials then ask review questions.
   a. What are three ways physical activity affects personal health? (1.2.1)
   b. Give an example of a personal health goal and how to keep track of progress. (6.2.1)
   c. Who can help a child reach their goal? (6.2.2)
8. Exit ticket (Self-Management: Goal setting, organizational skills)

Before transitioning to new content, tell the students they are going to walk laps around

Table 4.24 Effects of Physical Activity on Personal Health and Setting a Goal to Eat Healthy and Get Adequate Exercise

Question	Answer
What were the four healthy *physical activity* behaviors *Mr. Allen showed the class? Explain how they affect* personal health. (1.2.1)	Physical activities ▪ Riding bicycles ▪ Dancing ▪ Playing basketball ▪ Walking ▪ Practicing soccer Physical activity helps children ▪ Maintain a healthy weight ▪ Get sick less often ▪ Have stronger bones and muscles ▪ Develop their brains and be more creative ▪ Feel good about themselves
What was one short-term health goal that Amanda set for *getting adequate exercise?* (6.2.1)	Amanda used Wii to exercise at different times each day for a total of 60 minutes.
Who helped Amanda reach her goal? (6.2.2)	Amanda's mom exercised with her. Having company while exercising helped Amanda to meet her goal.

SEL-Self-management: Goal setting	Amanda used Wii to exercise at different times each day for a total of 60 minutes
<u>Identify</u> one short-term health goal for *healthy eating and getting adequate exercise* and take action to achieving the goal. (6.2.1)	
<u>Identify</u> one person who can help when assistance is needed to achieve the personal health goal *of eating healthy and getting adequate exercise.* (6.2.2)	Amanda's mom exercised with her. Having company while exercising helped Amanda meet her goal.
SEL-Self-management: Organizational skills	Organizational skills were assessed during 6.2.1 when Amanda placed red, yellow, or green circles next to the days she exercised. This tracking helped Amanda organize and acknowledge progress in reaching her goal of 60 minutes of exercise each day.

the room and practice goal setting. During the first lap, the children state one personal goal. The second lap, they identify how they plan to reach the goal. On the third lap, the children explain how they are going to keep track of their progress. On the fourth lap, the children will think of someone who can help them reach their goal.

Grades 3–5: Self-Management: Goal Setting

Lesson Overview: Goal Setting to Use MyPlate to Eat Healthy

In this lesson, students learn the relationship between using MyPlate to eat healthy and personal health and how to set a SMARTHR goal to eat healthy.

This lesson introduces nutrients, the benefits of eating foods from the five food groups, and how to set a goal to use MyPlate to plan meals.

Organizational skills are embedded in SMARTHR goal setting. Students must design a plan to meet the goal and keep track of progress.

Resources:

- MyPlate videos: https://www.choosemyplate.gov/resources/videos
- <u>MyPlate games:</u> https://www.choosemyplate.gov/browse-by-audience/view-all-audiences/children/kids/games
- Dairy Council of California-MyPlate 5 Food Group, video: https://youtu.be/7GGUeqS3_7c

Materials needed:

- **Worksheet 4.18 Sorting Food Groups, Nutrients, and Effect on the Body**
- **Worksheet 4.19 Grades 3–5 SMARTHR Goal Setting**

Table 4.25 provides an overview of the lesson objectives, assessment, and instruction for this lesson.

Table 4.25 Lesson Objectives, Assessment, and Instruction

Step 1 – Lesson Objectives	Step 2 – Assessment
The verb of the *infused* performance indicator and the SEL competency generate the assessment and instruction.	Design the assessment based on the objectives. Ask yourself the question, "What can my students do to show me they have met the standard?"
1.5.1 <u>Describe</u> the relationship between healthy behaviors *such as using MyPlate to eat healthy* and personal health. (Joint Committee on National Health Education Standards, 2007, p. 24)	Students <u>describe</u> *three* relationships between healthy behaviors *such as using MyPlate to eat healthy* and personal health.
6.5.1 Set a personal health goal *to use MyPlate to eat healthy* and track progress toward its achievement. (Joint Committee on National Health Education Standards, 2007, p. 34).	Students use the SMARTHR goal-setting model to set a personal health goal *about using MyPlate to plan to eat healthy* and track progress toward its achievement.
6.5.2 Identify resources to assist in achieving the personal health goal *of using MyPlate to eat healthy.* (Joint Committee on National Health Education Standards, 2007, p. 34)	Students identify a resource to assist in achieving the personal health goal *of using MyPlate to eat healthy.*

(continues)

Table 4.25 Lesson Objectives, Assessment, and Instruction *(continued)*

Step 1 – Lesson Objectives	Step 2 – Assessment
SEL-Self-management: Goal setting, organizational skills	The goal is to use MyPlate to eat healthy for one week. The organizational skill is using the SMARTHR goal worksheet to plan and track progress toward the goal.

Step 3 – Instruction
Design the instruction so that students learn the content, skills, and competency to be successful on the assessment. Ask yourself the question, "What do I need to teach so that the students will be successful when assessed?"

Step 3 – Instruction

1. Define
   a. Describe: To use words that help others envision the physical attributes of a person, place, or thing.
   b. Identify: To recognize a particular person or an object.
   c. Goal: An achievement that is reached following the completion of established criteria.
   d. Short-term goal: A step taken to achieve a goal.
   e. Nutrients: What we get from food to help our bodies grow strong and stay healthy.
2. 1.5.1 Describe the relationship between healthy behaviors *such as using MyPlate to eat healthy* and personal health.
   a. Show the MyPlate poster of the types of foods found in each food group (**Figure 4.14**): https://in02200641.schoolwires.net/cms /lib/IN02200641/Centricity/Domain/541 /eatsmartposter.pdf#:~:text=Eat%20Smart %20To%20Play%20Hard%20Use%20 MyPlate%20to,for%20foods%20with%20 added%20sugars%20or%20solid%20fats.
   b. Show the video Dairy Council of California: MyPlate 5 Food Group, video: https://youtu .be/7GGUeqS3_7c
   c. Use **Worksheet 4.18 Sorting Food Groups, Nutrients, and Effect on the Body** (**Table 4.26**)
3. Set a SMARTHR goal to eat healthy
   a. 6.5.1 Set a personal health goal *to use MyPlate to eat healthy* and track progress toward its achievement.
   b. 6.5.2 Identify resources to assist in achieving the personal health goal *of using MyPlate to eat healthy*.

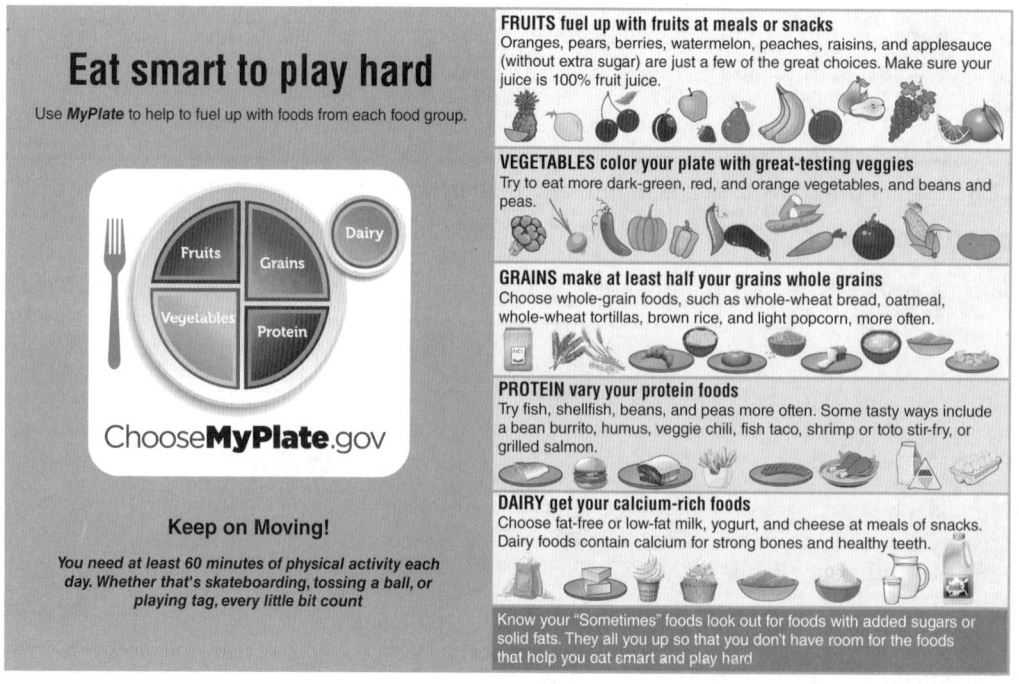

Figure 4.14 Eat Smart to Play Hard.

Data from: U.S. Department of Agriculture. Eat Smart to Play Hard poster. https://fns-prod.azureedge.net/sites/default/files/resource-files/eatsmartposter.pdf. Accessed April 12, 2021. http://teamnutrition.usda.gov

Table 4.26 Food Groups, Nutrients, and Effect on the Body

MyPlate Food Groups	Serving Size	Nutrients	Effect on Personal Health
Fruits	1.5 cups	Vitamin C Potassium	Vitamin C helps the body and skin heal Potassium helps keep the heart healthy and muscles heal faster.
Vegetables	2 cups	Vitamin A, Fiber	Vitamin A builds healthy eyes and skin. Fiber makes us feel full
Meat	5 ounces	Protein Iron	Builds strong muscles Iron carries oxygen to cells in the body
Grains	5 ounces (half/ whole grain)	Vitamin B Fiber	Vitamin B gives us energy Fiber makes us feel full
Dairy	3 cups	Vitamin A, Protein	Builds strong bones, muscles, and teeth

Data from Dairy Council of California. (2020, May 5). My Plate 5 Food Group video. Retrieved from YouTube: https://www.youtube.com/watch?v=7GGUeqS3_7c&feature=youtu.be

c. Model how to set a SMARTHR goal.
  1) Use **Worksheet 4.19 Grades 3–5 SMARTHR Goal Setting** to help the students plan to eat foods from the five food groups each day for one week.
4. Read the practice prompt. Students answer the reflection questions and discuss.

Practice Prompt: Joel

Joel is learning to set goals about nutrition in health class. He saw a video about the colorful MyPlate and the five food groups. He has heard about goal setting but didn't think it was something a child does.

Joel's classroom teacher, Mrs. Cohn, always tries to collaborate with Mr. Pateneau to keep instruction consistent across disciplines. She reminds the class that, in science, they also set classroom goals when they plan steps to meet the goal of finishing their science project.

During the next health class, Mr. Pateneau told the students they were going to learn about the value of eating foods from the five food groups and how to set a personal goal to plan meals using MyPlate.

The class watched a colorful and musical video about the five food groups and how they keep the body healthy. Mr. Pateneau told the children to write down the vegetables they like to eat as they watched the video. He hung up large sticky notes around the room. Each had a different food group listed at the top. At the end of the video, the children went to the sticky note and wrote down the foods they eat from each of the groups on the sticky notes.

Mr. Pateneau reviewed the results then explained how each group keeps the body healthy. Joel was glad to learn that milk builds strong bones and muscles because he loves milk! Joel doesn't like vegetables very much so he knows he has to eat more because he wants keep his eyes and skin healthy. Joel's mom makes spaghetti and meatballs often so he knows he gets enough grains for energy and protein to build and strong muscles. His family doesn't buy much fresh fruit because it is very expensive but he thinks he gets enough vitamin C to help his body and skin heal if he gets injured and enough of the mineral, potassium, to keep his heart healthy.

Then things got challenging. Mr. Pateneau demonstrated how to set a SMARTHR goal then challenged each of the students to set their own goal of using MyPlate to plan healthy, balanced meals for one week.

Joel asked his mom and dad to help because he is not the one who buys groceries so, together, they figured out the foods they needed for one week to plan healthy meals. Joel's mom loved the assignment because it reminded her about the nutrients in different foods and how they keep the body healthy.

Each day, Joel checked off his calendar and put either a smiley, uncertain face, or frowny face, depending on if he met his goal for that day.

Mr. Pateneau liked the work his students completed and rewarded them with another video about nutrition that had a story, fun characters, delicious-looking food, and great music!

Mr. Pateneau rocks!

Table 4.27 Using MyPlate to Set a SMARTHR Goal to Eat Healthy

Question	Answer
What *three* relationships did *Joel discover* between healthy behaviors *such as using MyPlate to eat healthy* and personal health? (1.5.1)	■ Joel was glad to learn that milk builds strong bones and muscles because he loves milk! ■ Joel's mom makes spaghetti and meatballs often so he knows he gets enough grains for energy and protein to build and strong muscles. ■ Joel knows he has to eat more vegetables because he wants keep his eyes and skin healthy. ■ Joel thinks he gets enough vitamin C to help his body and skin heal if he gets injured and enough of the mineral, potassium, to keep his heart healthy.
Students use the SMARTHR goal-setting model to set a personal health goal *about using MyPlate to plan to eat healthy* and track progress toward its achievement. (6.5.1) *Who did Joel identify* to help when assistance is needed to achieve the personal health goal *of using MyPlate to plan to eat healthy?* (6.5.2)	**S** – Joel set a SMARTHR goal by using MyPlate to plan healthy, balanced meals for one week. **M** – Joel believes the goal is attainable, with help from his parents. **A** – Joel wants to reach his goal in one week. **R** – The goal is relevant because Joel wants to keep his body healthy by eating foods from the five food groups. **T** – Joel wants to reach his goal in one week. **H** – Joel asked his mom and dad to help because they buy the groceries. **R** – Joel reached his goal with Mr. Paterneau's guidance and his parent's support.
SEL-Self-management: Goal setting skills Students set a SMARTHR goal to use MyPlate to eat healthy for one week. SEL-Self-management: Organizational skills The organizational skill is using the SMARTHR goal worksheet to plan and track progress toward the goal.	Joel set a SMARTHR goal to use MyPlate to plan healthy meals for one week. He checked off his calendar each day and put either a smiley, uncertain face, or frowny face depending on if he met his goal for that day. (6.5.1) He asked his mom and dad for help because they bought the groceries. (6.5.2) Organizational skills were assessed during 6.5.1 when Joel placed red, yellow, or green circles in the calendar next to the days he reached his goal. This tracking helped Joel organize and acknowledge progress in reaching his SMARTHR goal using MyPlate to plan to eat healthy.

5. Use the review questions in **Table 4.27** to help the children understand the relationship between eating healthy and personal health and how to set personal health goals.
6. End of class review. Ask the students to put away their materials then ask review questions.
   a. What are *three* relationships between *using MyPlate to eat healthy* and personal health? (1.5.1)
   b. What is an example of a personal health goal? What is a good strategy to keep track of progress? (6.5.1)
   c. Who can help you to achieve a personal health goal *of using MyPlate to plan to eat healthy?* (6.5.2)
7. Exit ticket (Self-Management: Goal setting, organizational skills)

What are the steps of setting a SMARTHR goal? How does using SMARTHR help with organizational skills?

Grades 6–8: Self-Management: Goal Setting

Lesson Overview: Goal Setting to Eat Breakfast

In this lesson, students learn the benefits of and barriers to eating breakfast. They use the SMARTHR goal setting to set a goal to eat breakfast for one week.

Fifty-three to 59.2% of middle school students did not each breakfast on all seven days prior to the survey. (Centers for Disease Control and Prevention, 2020)

The percentage range of middle school students who did not eat breakfast during the seven days prior to the survey was 8.7% to 15.5%. (Centers for Disease Control and Prevention, 2020)

Organizational skills are embedded in the SMARTHR goal setting model. Students design a plan to meet the goal and use the template to keep track of progress.

Resources:

- Make Small Changes: https://www.choosemyplate.gov/node/5760

Materials needed:

- **Worksheet 4.20 Benefits of and Barriers to Eating Breakfast and Overcoming Barriers**
- **Worksheet 4.21 Grades 6–8 SMARTHR Goal Setting**

Table 4.28 provides an overview of the lesson objectives, assessment, and instruction for this lesson.

Step 3 – Instruction

1. Define
   a. Describe: To use words that help others envision the physical attributes of a person, place, or thing.
   b. Assess: To evaluate for significance, meaning, or quality.
   c. Goal: An achievement that is reached following the completion of established criteria.
2. 1.8.7 Describe the benefits of and barriers to practicing healthy behaviors, *such as eating breakfast.*
   a. <u>Note</u>: Place large sticky notes on the wall. Label them: Benefits of Eating Breakfast,

Table 4.28 Lesson Objectives, Assessment, and Instruction

Step 1 – Lesson Objectives	Step 2 – Assessment
The verb of the *infused* performance indicator and the SEL competency generate the assessment and instruction.	Design the assessment based on the objectives. Ask yourself the question, "What can my students do to show me they have met the standard?"
1.8.7 <u>Describe</u> the benefits of and barriers to practicing healthy behaviors, *such as eating breakfast*. (Joint Committee on National Health Education Standards, 2007, p. 25)	1.8.7 Students <u>describe</u> *three* benefits of and *three* barriers to eating breakfast.
6.8.1 Assess personal health practices *regarding eating breakfast.* (Joint Committee on National Health Education Standards, 2007, p. 34).	6.8.1 Students assess *how often they eat breakfast for one week and the effect of not eating on their health* then use the SMARTHR goal setting worksheet to record the assessment.
6.8.2 Develop a goal to adopt, maintain, or improve a personal health practice *such as eating breakfast each day.* (Joint Committee on National Health Education Standards, 2007, p. 34)	6.8.2 Use the SMARTHR goal-setting worksheet to set a goal to eat breakfast each day.
6.8.3 Apply strategies and skills needed to attain a personal health goal. (Joint Committee on National Health Education Standards, 2007, p. 34)	6.8.3 Use the SMARTHR goal setting worksheet to apply strategies and skills needed to attain the goal of eating breakfast each day.
6.8.4 Describe how personal health goals vary with changing abilities, priorities, and responsibilities. (Joint Committee on National Health Education Standards, 2007, p. 34)	6.8.4 Use the SMARTHR goal-setting worksheet to reflect on why/why not the goal was reached.
SEL-Self-management: Goal setting SEL-Self-management: Organizational skills	The goal is to set a SMARTHR goal to eat breakfast for one week. Organizational skills are enhanced by using the SMARTHR goal worksheet to plan and track progress toward the goal of eating breakfast each day.
Step 3 – Instruction	
Design the instruction so that students learn the content, skill, and competency to be successful on the assessment. Ask yourself the question, "What do I need to teach so that the students will be successful when assessed?"	

Barriers to Eating Breakfast, Strategies to Overcome the Obstacles.

b. In groups, using **Worksheet 4.20 Benefits of and Barriers to Eating Breakfast and Overcoming Barriers**, students brainstorm a response to each of the categories, summarize then record the responses on the sticky note.

c. Discuss each of the summaries.
  1) Benefits of eating breakfast
    a) Teens who eat breakfast have a lower body mass index than teens who never eat breakfast or only ate breakfast on occasion.
    b) Teens who eat breakfast have better concentration and more energy.
    c) Cereals and whole wheat breads contain fiber, which helps with weight control and is linked to lower cholesterol levels.
    d) Breakfast foods may be high in calcium (milk, yogurt), which helps build strong bones and teeth.
    e) Breakfast foods may be high in vitamin D (eggs, milk, yogurt), which is very good for boosting immunity.
  2) Barriers to eating breakfast
    a) Teens go to bed late. In the morning, they do not take the time to eat.
    b) Teens may feel too tired or nauseous to eat.
    c) Teens think skipping breakfast will help them lose weight.

  3) Strategies to overcome the barriers
    a) Go to bed earlier and get up earlier.
    b) Set up quick and easy breakfast items the night before such as yogurt, breakfast/granola bars, fresh fruit, dried fruit.
    (Healthy Children Magazine, 2020)
    c) Prepare breakfast the night before and heat it up in the morning. (waffles, pancakes, hard boiled eggs, etc.)
    d) Buy prepackaged, nutritious, balanced, breakfast foods that just need a quick warm up.

3. The National Health Education goal-setting performance indicators are below. They are included on the SMARTHR model.
4. (6.8.1-6.8.4) **Worksheet 4.21 Grades 6–8 SMARTHR Goal Setting**
  a. Discuss why it is important to be able to set goals.
  b. Model how to set a personal goal using the SMARTHR goal-setting template.
5. Using **Worksheet 4.21 Grades 6–8 SMARTHR Goal Setting**, individually or in groups, set a SMARTHER goal to eat breakfast every day for one week.
  a. Formatively assess student work and provide effective feedback.
  b. Students share how they plan to reach their goals.
6. Read the practice prompt. Students answer the reflection questions and discuss.

Practice Prompt: Jannie

Jannie is hungry and it is just first period! Jannie babysits her neighbor's Kindergarten child after school until the mom gets home, around 7:00 PM. When Jannie gets home, she eats whatever the family had for dinner but probably eats too much because she is so hungry.

After supper, she checks her social media then starts her homework. Sometimes, she doesn't turn out the lights until 11:00 PM. Her alarm is set for 6:00 AM but she hits the snooze alarm a few times before she gets out of bed. She takes a quick shower and gets dressed.

She is hungry but doesn't have time to eat. She runs to the bus stop, hoping she will not miss the bus. Once at school, she is tired, grumpy, and cannot concentrate. She knows something isn't right but she doesn't know what.

In health class, Mrs. Monroe is teaching a goal-setting lesson about eating breakfast. She began by asking students if they ate breakfast in the last three days. Jannie only ate breakfast one time. Sixty percent of the students did not eat breakfast at all. Jannie was shocked. There are a lot of hungry students in the school!

Mrs. Monroe explained the many benefits of eating breakfast (lower body mass index than teens who never eat breakfast; better concentration and more energy; cereals and whole wheat breads contain fiber, which helps with weight control and linked to lower cholesterol levels; breakfast foods may be high in calcium (milk, yogurt), which helps build strong bones and teeth; breakfast foods may be high in vitamin D (eggs, milk, yogurt), which is very good for boosting immunity. Jannie's mouth was watering just thinking about eating breakfast.

Jannie and her friends gave lots of reasons why they do not eat breakfast such as getting up too late, no time to make breakfast, and eating in the morning makes some teens sick. Mrs. Monroe wrote down all of the reasons. As a group, they came up with ways to overcome each one.

Mrs. Monroe then challenged the class to set a goal to eat breakfast every day. First, she modeled how to set a SMARTHR goal, then gave the students time to work on a goal of their own. Jannie enjoyed working on the goal because the worksheet was very organized and help her stay organized while she was

planning. She particularly enjoyed having to think through the steps to meet her goal. The smaller steps made it easier than just trying to tackle one big goal.

Jannie did it! With her mom's help, she prepared food the night before and warmed it up in the morning. It was very quick and she feels so much better!

Now, a big challenge....How shall she reward herself?

7. Use the review questions in **Table 4.29** to help the students to understand the benefits of and barriers to eating breakfast and using the steps of SMARTHR goal setting to eat breakfast every day.

8. End of class review. Ask the students to put away their materials and then ask review questions.
   a. What are *three* benefits of and *three* barriers to eating breakfast that Jannie experienced. (1.8.7)

Table 4.29 Benefits of and Barriers to Eating Breakfast and Using SMARTHR Goal to Eat Breakfast

Question	Answer
What were *three* benefits of and *three* barriers to eating breakfast that Jannie experienced? (1.8.7)	Benefits of eating breakfast ■ Lower body mass index ■ Better concentration and more energy ■ Cereals and whole wheat breads contain fiber, which help with weight control and linked to lower cholesterol levels ■ Breakfast foods may be high in calcium (milk, yogurt), which helps build strong bones and teeth ■ Breakfast foods may be high in vitamin D (eggs, milk, yogurt), which is very good for boosting immunity. Barriers to eating breakfast ■ Getting up too late ■ No time to make breakfast ■ Eating in the morning makes some teens sick
How often did the students in Jannie's class eat breakfast in the past three days? What was the effect of not eating on their health? (6.8.1)	Jannie ate breakfast only one time. Sixty percent of the students did not eat breakfast at all. When Jannie did eat breakfast, she was tired, grumpy, and couldn't concentrate.
How did Jannie use the SMARTHR goal-setting worksheet to set a goal to eat breakfast each day? (6.8.2–6.8.4)	**S** – Jannie's goal was to eat breakfast every day for one week. (6.8.2) **M** – Jannie measured her success by keeping track of the number of times she ate breakfast. **A** – Jannie believes the goal is attainable as long as she has help from her mom and goes to bed earlier and gets up earlier. **R** – The goal is relevant because when she does not eat breakfast, she is grumpy and cannot concentrate. (6.8.3) **T** – Jannie knows she has to try for one week to meet her goal. **H** – Her mom helped her prepare food the night before. **R** – Jannie feels good she achieved her goal. (6.8.4)
SEL-Self-management: Goal setting SEL-Self-management: Organizational skills	Jannie set a SMARTHR goal to eat breakfast every day for one week. Jannie enjoyed working on the goal because the worksheet was very organized and helped her stay organized while she was planning. She particularly enjoyed having to think through the steps to meet her goal. The smaller steps made it easier than just trying to tackle one big goal.

b. How do you use the SMARTHR template to set a personal goal of healthy snacking? (6.8.1–6.8.4)

9. Exit ticket (Self-Management: Goal setting, organizational skills)

How does making SMARTHR help develop organizational skills?

Grades 9–12: Self-Management: Goal Setting

Lesson Overview: Goal Setting to Be with Friends and Not Drink

This lesson explores the dangers of drinking alcohol, particularly binge drinking, and setting a SMARTHR goal to be with friends but not drink.

29.2% of high school students drank alcohol at least one day during the 30 days prior to the survey. (Centers for Disease Control and Prevention, 2020)

13.7% of high school students report current binge drinking (4+ drinks in a row for girls; 5+ drinks in a row for boys.) (Centers for Disease Control and Prevention, 2020)

Organizational skills are embedded in SMARTHR goal setting. Students must design a plan to meet the goal and keep track of progress.

Resources:

- How does alcohol affect the teenage brain? https://www.alcohol.org/teens/binge-drinking-facts/

Materials needed:

- **Worksheet 4.22 Analyze Susceptibility to Injury, Illness, or Death if Drinking Alcohol and Binge Drinking.**

Table 4.30 provides an overview of the lesson objectives, assessment, and instruction for this lesson.

Step 3 – Instruction

1. Define
   a. Analyze: To scrutinize something or someone in order to understand how it or they work(s).
   b. Goal: An achievement that is reached following the completion of established criteria.

Table 4.30 Lesson Objectives, Assessment, and Instruction

Step 1 – Lesson Objectives	Step 2 – Assessment
The verb of the *infused* performance indicator and the SEL competency generate the assessment and instruction.	Design the assessment based on the objectives. Ask yourself the question, "What can my students do to show me they have met the standard?"
1.12.8 <u>Analyze</u> the personal susceptibility to injury, illness, or death if engaging in unhealthy behaviors *such as drinking alcohol and binge drinking.* (Joint Committee on National Health Education Standards, 2007, p. 25)	1.12.8 Students <u>analyze</u> their susceptibility to injury, illness, or death if engaging in unhealthy behaviors *such as drinking alcohol and binge drinking.*
6.12.1 Assess personal health practices and overall health status *regarding alcohol use and binge drinking.* (Joint Committee on National Health Education Standards, 2007, p. 34).	6.12.1 Students assess their use of alcohol and participating in binge drinking.
Use the SMARTHR goal-setting worksheet to set a goal to be with friends but not drink alcohol. (6.12.2–6.12.4)	(6.12.2–6.12.4) Students use the SMARTHR goal setting model to set a goal to be with friends but not drink alcohol.
SEL-Self-management: Goal setting	Students set a goal using the SMARTHR Goal-Setting model.
SEL-Self-management: Organizational skills	Organizational skills are enhanced by using the SMARTHR goal worksheet to plan and track progress toward the goal of eating breakfast each day.

Step 3 – Instruction
Design the instruction so that students learn the content, skill, and competency to be successful on the assessment. Ask yourself the question, "What do I need to teach so that the students will be successful when assessed?"

2. 1.12.8 Analyze the personal susceptibility to injury, illness, or death if engaging in unhealthy behaviors *such as drinking alcohol and binge drinking*

   a. <u>Note</u>: **Use Worksheet 4.22 Analyze Susceptibility to Injury, Illness, or Death if Drinking Alcohol and Binge Drinking** for the analysis. The puzzle does not take long to complete. Once complete, discuss (either in small share groups or as one large group) and summarize the four major topics: binge drinking data, consequences of underage drinking, teens who drink are more likely to experience…, and risks of binge drinking.

   b. Binge drinking for girls is defined as four drinks in a row and for boys, five drinks in a row.

   c. Consequences of underage binge drinking
      1) School problems such as higher absences and poor or failing grades.
      2) Physical problems such as hangover or illnesses.
      3) Legal problems such as arrest for driving or physically hurting someone while drunk.
      4) Social problems such as fighting and not participating in youth activities.
      5) Binge drinking may result in unintended pregnancy, sexually transmitted infections, car crashes, falls, burns, and alcohol poisoning.
      6) Teens who drink are more likely to experience higher risk of suicide and homicide, misuse of other drugs, change in brain development, and death from alcohol poisoning.

3. 6.12.1-6.12.4 Model how to set a personal goal using the SMARTHR goal setting model.

4. Use **Worksheet 4.23 Grades 9–12 SMARTHR Goal Setting** to help the students set a goal to be with friends but not drink alcohol or binge drink.

5. Read the practice prompt. Students answer the reflection questions and discuss.

Practice Prompt: Dimetri

School is closed because of the pandemic. Dimetri completes his remote assignments in the morning and has most of the afternoon to himself. His parents are working from home and there is little privacy.

After the new year until the middle of March, Dimetri and his friends had parties every weekend. They are a close group and enjoy spending time together. Often, the parents were out for the evening or the weekend and they had the house to themselves. There was a lot of drinking and weed smoking. Dimetri started drinking this year and he noticed he was drinking more and more. One time, they were playing a drinking game. He kept losing and had to drink five shots in a row. Dimetri didn't remember much after that except he got in a fight with Derek because he was flirting with Derek's girlfriend. Dimetri's girlfriend, Elsa, dumped him and he went into the bathroom and threw up. It was gross.

The same night, a few of his friends all piled into one car and took off. Not long after, the driver crashed into another car. No one was injured but he won't be driving again for a long time.

Lately, he is thinking a lot about his drinking. He doesn't like how he feels when he is drinking and he realizes there are a lot of negative consequences. He likes school and enjoys sports and doesn't want to jeapordize either. He only drinks when he is with his friends and he wonders if he can hang out with them without drinking.

In health class, Mrs. Walker taught a goal-setting unit. He challenged the students to set a personal health goal. Dimetri's goal is to party with his friends without drinking.

He assessed how frequently he drank and decided it was too much and too dangerous. He wanted to be able to party but not drink. He used the SMARTHR goal-setting model to see if he could come up with a goal that would work for him.

He knows what his goal is "He wants to be able to party but not drink." It is easy to measure because either he drinks or he doesn't! He believes the goal is attainable if he puts his mind to it. He might socialize with smaller groups that don't drink to make it easier rather than attend larger parties. Also, his girlfriend forgave him and said she would help him if he was tempted to drink. The goal is realistic because he has a plan. He is trying not to drink for three weekends so keeping track will be easy.

At the end of three weeks, Dimetri did pretty well. He did have one beer but his girlfriend reminded him of his goal and he put it down. He is grateful she is helping him. His long-term plan is to party with friends who do not drink.

Dimetri and Elsa are celebrating by going to the movies by themselves. A real date!

Table 4.31 Analyzing Susceptibility to Injury When Drinking Alcohol and Setting a SMARTHR Goal Not to Drink with Friends

Question	Answer
What was Dimetri's assessment of his drinking behavior? (1.12.8)	He didn't like how he felt when he was drinking and he realized there were a lot of negative consequences. He likes school and enjoys sports and doesan't want to jeapordize either. ■ Drank alcohol on the weekend. ■ Lost at a drinking game and drank five drinks in a row. ■ Fought with his friend. ■ His girlfriend broke up with him. ■ He threw up from drinking.
How did Dimetri set a SMARTHR goal to not drink for three weeks?	Dimetri assessed that he was drinking too much and too often. (6.12.1) **S** – Dimetri set a goal to be able to party with his friends but not drink. (6.12.3) **M** – Dimetri will easily measure the goal each time he parties and does/does not drink. **A** – Dimetri believes the goal is attainable if he puts his mind to it. **R** – The goal is realistic and relevant because he could party with a smaller group who do not drink; his girlfriend forgave him and told him she would help; his plan will help him achieve the goal. (6.12.3) **T** – Dimetri wants to party and not drink for three weekends to see if he can do it. **H** – Dimetri's girlfriend is going to help him if he gets tempted to drink. **R** – At the end of three weekends, he started to drink a beer but his girlfriend reminded him that he set a goal not to drink and he put the beer down. His long-term plan is to party with friends who do not drink. (6.12.4)
SEL-Self-management: Goal setting	Dimetri used the SMARTHR model to set a goal to party with friends without drinking.
SEL-Self-management: Organizational skills	Organizational skills are enhanced by using the SMARTHR goal worksheet to plan and track progress toward the goal of partying with friends and not drinking.

6. Use the review questions in **Table 4.31** to help the students to analyze susceptibility to illness or injury when drinking alcohol and binge drinking and setting a goal to not drink when with friends.
7. End of class review. Ask the students to put away their materials and then ask review questions.
   a. How did Dimetri analyze his susceptibility to illness or injury because of his drinking? (1.12.8)

   b. How would a teen use the SMARTHR goal model to set a personal health goal of not vaping? (6.12.1–6.12.4)
8. Exit ticket (Self-Management: Goal setting, organizational skills)

   How does using the SMARTHR Goal-Setting Model help improve organizational skills?

Sample Lesson Plan for Self-Management: Using Yoga and Belly Breathing to Reduce Stress

Note: To maintain the time frame of the lesson, maintain the functional health information about stress (Standard 1 and Self-management: stress management) and the belly breathing exercise (Standard 7 and Self-Management: Stress Management). As time permits, select one or two other Yoga poses.

Unit: *State the unit of the lesson.*	Practicing Healthy Behaviors
Topic: *State the topic of the lesson.*	Practicing Yoga and other Strategies to Cope with Stress
Grade level: *State the grade level of the lesson.*	PreK–2

Time allotment: *State the time allotted for the lesson.*	40 minutes
Lesson summary: *Provide a summary of the lesson.*	In this lesson, children learn healthy ways to cope with stress.
Risk behavior data: *Provide time rationale for this lesson by accessing the risk behavior that the lesson reduces.*	None available
Standards and SEL Competency to reduce the risk factor(s): *List the standard 1 and skills standards and the SEL competency/sub-competency.*	1.2.1 <u>Identify</u> that healthy behaviors affect personal health. 7.2.1 <u>Demonstrate</u> healthy practices and behaviors to maintain or improve personal health. SEL – Self-Management: Stress Management
Objectives: *The objectives are the infused performance indicators and SEL competency.*	1.2.1 <u>Identify</u> that healthy behaviors, *such as practicing yoga and other strategies to cope with stress,* affect personal health. 7.2.1 <u>Demonstrate</u> healthy practices and behaviors, *such as mindful belly breathing and three yoga poses,* to maintain or improve personal health. SEL – Self-Management: Stress Management
Lesson assessment: *Design an assessment for each infused performance indicator and SEL competency.*	1.2.1 Students <u>identify</u> two ways healthy behaviors *such as practicing yoga and other strategies to cope with stress* affects personal health. 7.2.1 Students <u>demonstrate</u> healthy practices and behaviors, *such as mindful belly breathing and three yoga poses,* to maintain or improve personal health. SEL – Self-Management: Stress Management ■ Students identify and demonstrate *mindful belly breathing and three yoga poses, to cope with stress and* maintain or improve personal health.
Lesson instruction: *Provide a detailed description of how content, skill, and SEL competency are taught, "bell to bell."*	Review/Preview 　Ask students if they know what Yoga is. 　Ask students if they have ever tried Yoga. 　Explain that Yoga is a good way to help their bodies relax. Lesson Objectives 　Explain the infused performance indicators, including the meaning of the verbs, and SEL competency/subcompetency and how the students will demonstrate proficiency. 　For example: We are going to learn about stress and ways to move our bodies to help ourselves relax when we feel tense.
	Lesson 1.　1.2.1 <u>Identify</u> that healthy behaviors, *such as practicing yoga and other stress-reduction strategies,* affect personal health. 　　a.　Ask the students the meaning of stress. What does it feel like? What does it do to your body? When is stress bad for your body? When is stress good for your body? What can you do to get rid of the bad stress? 　　　1)　Stress is something that causes your body to have a headache, bellyache, or unable to concentrate. You may have trouble eating, sleeping, and become cranky. 　　　2)　<u>Note</u>: Put a happy face on the board to explain eustress (good stress). Eustress helps us to get ready for something or accomplish a task such as making a presentation in class or completing a project. 　　　3)　<u>Note</u>: Put a frowny face on the board to explain distress (bad stress). Distress occurs when something is bothering you for a long time. For example: parents arguing or separating or a sick family member. (Kidshealth, 2020)

    h Explain how Yoga and other strategies affect personal health
       1) Yoga calms the body through exercise and breathing.
       2) Talking to a parent, friend, teacher, or counselor helps figure out the problem. They may make suggestions to feel better.
       3) Meditation helps calm the body by relaxing the mind. (Kidshealth from Nemours, 2020)

2. 7.2.1 Demonstrate healthy practices and behaviors, such as practicing Yoga and other strategies, to maintain or improve personal health.
    a. Practice stretching your body while breathing in. Relax the stretch and breathe out. Follow with student practice. Ask how the stretching makes the students feel.
       1) Calmer
       2) More relaxed
    b. Yoga and breathing exercises. Practice each strategy then ask the children how it makes them feel.
       1) Belly (Balloon) Breathing
          a) Sit in a comfortable position with one hand on the belly.
          b) With the mouth closed and the jaw relaxed, inhale through the nose, allowing your belly to expand. Imagine the lower part of the lungs filling up first, then the rest of the lung inflating.
          c) Slowly exhale, imagining the air leaving the lung. Let the belly flatten.
          d) Repeat 4–5 times. (Kidshealth from Nemours, April)
       2) Table Pose
          a) Begin on your hands and knees.
          b) Line up your hands under your shoulders and your knees under your hips.
          c) Spread your fingers wide apart.
          d) Keep your back flat and be careful not to drop your head.
          e) Hold the pose for a couple of breaths then gently bring yourself to a seated position. (Namaste Kid, 2020)
       3) Downward-Facing Dog
          a) Begin on hands and knees in Table Pose.
          b) Curl your toes under, straighten your knees, and lift your hips.
          c) Keep your head between your arms.
          d) When you are ready, lower your knees to the mat. (Namaste Kid, 2020)
       4) Horse Stance:
          a) Place arms at the side with the elbows slightly bent.
          b) Place feet wide apart as if you were riding a horse.
          c) Straighten the back.
          d) Pretend to sit a little bit.

3. 7.5.2 Demonstrate a variety of healthy practices and behaviors such as *impulse control, self-discipline, and self-motivation* to maintain or improve personal health.
    a. Use **Worksheet 4.3 Impulse Control Tools** to identify and demonstrate strategies to control impulses demonstrate self-discipline and self-motivation.

4. Read the practice prompt then ask the students the re-enforcement questions.

> ## Practice Prompt: Linette
>
> Linette is stressed and she is only in the second grade! School work is hard for her and she doesn't have many friends. Mom and dad are always fighting so she goes to her Nonnie's house on the weekend. She is having trouble sleeping and her belly hurts. She cries a lot but doesn't know why.

On Saturday, Linette and Nonnie went for a walk by the beach then to the playground. While swinging, Nonnie asked Linette what was on her mind. Linette told her grandmother she was worried her parents were getting a divorce. It was all she could think about.

Nonnie used to be a health teacher so she had an idea. "Let's relax tonight by doing yoga!" Nonnie said. "What is that?" Linette asked. "Well, we stretch our bodies and practice a special type of breathing and I guarantee we will both feel better."

That evening, Nonnie and Linette practiced balloon breathing. Nonnie told her that balloon breathing is also a mindfulness activity. Linette practiced other mindfulness activities in health class, so she knew about them. First, Nonnie blew up a balloon to show Linette how the lungs fill with air. She then let the air out of the balloon slowly to show how to exhale. They tried it and pictured themselves walking on the beach, being very peaceful and happy. They both began to relax.

They watched a video of the Table Pose and Downward-Facing Dog and tried each. Then they pretended they were riding a horse and held the pose for a short time. They had such fun and they both felt very refreshed and relaxed.

Linette loves to visit Nonnie. She is great fun and knows all sorts of things to help her be healthy.

5. Use the following review questions to help the children review healthy ways to cope with stress.

Question	Answer
What two ways did Linette identify to help her cope with stress? (1.2.1)	<ul><li>Balloon breathing (mindfulness) helped her to relax.</li><li>Talking to her grandmother helped Linette figure out what was causing her stress.</li><li>Doing yoga with her grandmother caused Linette to feel very refreshed and relaxed.</li></ul>
How did belly breathing (mindfulness) improve Linette's personal health? (7.2.1)	The belly breathing (mindfulness) helped Linette and her grandmother picture themselves walking on the beach and being very peaceful and happy.
Which three yoga poses did Linette and her grandmother demonstrate that helped improve her health? (7.2.1)	Yoga poses<ul><li>Table Pose</li><li>Downward-Facing Dog</li><li>Horse Pose</li></ul>
SEL-Self-management: Stress management How did Linette identify and demonstrate *mindful belly breathing and three yoga poses, to cope with stress and* maintain or improve personal health?	<ul><li>Linette practiced Balloon Breathing and that helped her relax.</li><li>Linette and her grandmother practiced several yoga poses and they both felt refreshed and relaxed.<ul><li>Table Pose</li><li>Downward-Facing Dog</li><li>Horse Pose</li></ul></li></ul>

	6. End of class review. Ask the students to put away their materials and then ask review questions. a. How does Yoga and balloon breathing help reduce stress? (1.2.1) b. Demonstrate the Table Pose (7.2.1) c. Demonstrate the Downward-Facing Dog Pose (7.2.1) d. Demonstrate the Horse Pose (7.2.1) 7. Exit ticket (Self-Management: Stress management) **Worksheet 4.7 How to Decrease Stress**
Materials: *List the materials used to plan and implement the lesson, including formative assessments.*	**Worksheet 4.7 How to Decrease Stress**
Resources: *What resources were used to plan and implement the lesson?*	Emotion Regulation Activity: Calm Down tools: https://media.centervention.com/pdf/GRIN-Smart-Not-Smart-Calm-Down-Strategies.pdf
Differentiated instruction: *Which modifications are being made for students with disabilities and English learners?*	Students work in groups, specifically designed to support students with disabilities or English learners.
Sample student products: *Provide exemplars of how other students successfully complete this assignment.*	Show previously completed worksheets.
Collaboration: *Are the students completing the activity individually, in pairs, in groups, etc.?*	Students work in groups of four to pair up or work as a group.
Teacher reflection: *What can I do to improve this lesson next time it is taught?*	It will vary.

References

ACT for Youth. (2020). *Self-management*. Retrieved from ACT Youth: http://actforyouth.net/youth_development/professionals/sel/self-management.cfm

Alyssa. (2020). *Goal setting for elementary students*. Retrieved from Alyssa Teaches: https://alyssateaches.com/goal-setting-for-elementary-students/

American Psychological Association. (2019). *How to help children and teens manage their stress*. Retrieved from American Psychological Association https://www.apa.org/topics/children-teens-stress

Armstrong, T. (2019). *Mindfulness in the classroom: Strategies for promoting concentration, compassion, and calm*. Alexandria: ASCD.

Bertin, M. (2017). *A daily mindful walking practice*. Retrieved from Mindful: Healthy Mind, Healthy Life https://www.mindful.org/daily-mindful-walking-practice/

Bronson, M. H. (2009). *Glencoe Health*. Woodland Hills, CA: McGraw Hill.

CASEL. (2019). *What is SEL?* Retrieved from CASEL https://casel.org/what-is-sel/

Centers for Disease Control and Prevention. (2020). *2019 Middle School YRBS-Middle School Students—Did not eat breakfast on all 7 days prior to the survey*. Retrieved from Center for Disease Control and Prevention https://nccd.cdc.gov/youthonline/App/Results.aspx?TT=B&OUT=0&SID=MS&QID=QNBK7DAY&LID=LL&YID=RY&LID2=&YID2=&COL=&ROW1=&ROW2=&HT=&LCT=&FS=&FR=&FG=&FA=&FI=&FP=&FSL=&FRL=&FGL=&FAL=&FIL=&FPL=&PV=&TST=&C1=&C2=&QP=&DP=&VA=CI&CS=Y&SYID=&EYID=&SC=&SO=

Centers for Disease Control and Prevention. (2020). *High School YRBS, 2019 Results, Did not wear a condom*. Retrieved from Centers for Disease Control and Prevention https://nccd.cdc.gov/youthonline/App/Results.aspx?TT=B&OUT=0&SID=HS&QID=H63&LID=LL&YID=RY&LID2=&YID2=&COL=&ROW1=&ROW2=&HT=&LCT=&FS=&FR=&FG=&FA=&FI=&FP=&FSL=&FRL=&FGL=&FAL=&FIL=&FPL=&PV=&TST=&C1=&C2=&QP=&DP=&VA=CI&CS=Y&SYID=&EYID=&SC=&SO=

Centers for Disease Control and Prevention. (2020). *High School YRBS, Sexual behaviors*. Retrieved from Centers for Disease Control and Prevention https://nccd.cdc.gov/youthonline/App/QuestionsOrLocations.aspx?CategoryId=C04

Centers for Disease Control and Prevention. (2020). *High School YRBS 2019 Results, Sexually active*. Retrieved from Centers for Disease Control and Prevention https://nccd.cdc.gov/youthonline/App/Results.aspx?TT=B&OUT

=0&SID=HS&QID=H61&LID=LL&YID=RY&LID2=&YID2
=&COL-&ROW1=&ROW2=&HT=&LCT=&FS=&FR
=&FG=&FA=&FI=&FP=&FSL=&FRL=&FGL=&FAL=&FIL
=&FPL=&PV=&TST=&C1=&C2=&QP=&DP=&VA
=CI&CS=Y&SYID=&EYID=&SC=&SO=

Centervention. (2017). *Impulse control intro lesson: Freeze game*. Retrieved from Centervention https://media.centervention .com/pdf/1000-Impulse-Control-Intro-Lesson-Freeze-Game .pdf

Children Inspired by Yoga. (2020). *Belly Breathing*. Retrieved from Children Inspired by Yoga https://childreninspiredbyyoga .com/blog/2018/03/belly-breathing-anxiety/

Collaborative for Academic and Social Emotional Learning. (2020). *CASEL Competencies*. Retrieved from CASEL https://casel.org/wp-content/uploads/2019/12/CASEL -Competencies.pdf

Collaborative for Academic Social Emotional Learning. (2020). *www.casel.org/.../08/Sample-Teaching-Activities-to-Support -Core-Competencies-8-20-17.pdf*. Retrieved from CASEL.org www.casel.org/.../08/Sample-Teaching-Activities-to-Support -Core-Competencies-8-20-17.pdf

Connell, G. (2016). *Setting (almost) SMART goals with my students*. Retrieved from Scholastic.com https://www.scholastic.com /teachers/blog-posts/genia-connell/setting-almost-smart-goals -my-students/

Connolly, M. (2018). *Skills-based health education*, (2nd ed.). Burlington: Jones and Bartlett.

Courtney Ward. (2020). *Lesson plans*. Retrieved from https:// learningwardinstruction.wordpress.com/character-ed/self -control-bubbles/

Dairy Council of California. (2017). *My Plate 5 Food Group video*. Retrieved from YouTube https://www.youtube.com /watch?v=7GGUeqS3_7c&feature=youtube

Damico, P. (2020). *Strategies to Curb Teen Impulsivity*. Retrieved from Paradigm Malibu https://paradigmtreatment.com/strategies -to-curb-teen-impulsivity/

Ekhart Yogo. (n.d.). *Cat Pose*. Retrieved from Ekhartyoga https:// www.ekhartyoga.com/resources/yoga-poses/cat-pose

Ekhart Yogo. (n.d.). *Child's Pose*. Retrieved from Ekhartyoga https:// www.ekhartyoga.com/resources/yoga-poses/childs-pose

Ekhart Yoga. (n.d.). *Cow Pose*. Retrieved from Ekhart Yoga: https:// www.ekhartyoga.com/resources/yoga-poses/cow-pose

Ekhart Yogo. (n.d.). *Easy Pose*. Retrieved from Ekhartyoga https:// www.ekhartyoga.com/resources/yoga-poses/easy-pose

Frey, N., Fisher, D., & Smith, D. (2019). *All learning is social and emotional: Helping students develop essential skills for the classroom and beyond*. Alexandria: ASCD.

Hagen, I., & Nayar, U. S. (2004). Yoga for children and young people's mental health and well-being: Research review and reflections on the mental health potentials of Yoga. *Frontiers in Psychiatry, 5*(35), 1–6.

Healthy Children Magazine. (2012). *The case for eating breakfast*. Retrieved from Healthy Children.org healthychildren.org /English/healthy-living/nutrition/Pages/The-Case-for-Eating -Breakfast.aspx

Heitler, S. (2020). *High schools and college student anxiety: Why the epidemic?* Retrieved from Psychology Today https://www.psychologytoday.com/us/blog/resolution-not -conflict/201806/high-school-and-college-student-anxiety -why-the-epidemic

Hurley, K. (2018). *6 Hidden signs of teen anxiety*. Retrieved from PSYCOM https://www.psycom.net/hidden-signs-teen -anxiety/

Joint Committee on National Health Education Standards. (2007). *National Health Education Standards*, (2nd ed.). American Cancer Society.

Khurana, A., Romer, D., Betancourt, L. M., Brodsky, N. L., Giannetta, J. M., & Hallam, H. (2012). Early adolescent sexual debut: The mediating role of working memory ability, sensation seeking, and impulsivity. *Developmental Psychology, 48*(5), 1416–1428.

KidsHealth from Nemours. (2015). *Stress*. Retrieved from Kidshealth from Nemours https://kidshealth.org/en/kids/stress .html

KidsHealth from Nemours. (2017). *Mindfulness*. Retrieved from KidsHealth from Nemours https://teenshealth.org/en/kids /mindfulness.html

KidsHealth from Nemours. (2018). *Yoga for lowering stress*. Retrieved from https://kidshealth.org/en/kids/yoga-stress.html: https://kidshealth.org/en/kids/yoga-stress.html

KidsHealth from Nemours. (n.d.). *Yoga: Meditation and Breathing*. Retrieved from Kidshealth from Nemours https://kidshealth .org/en/teens/meditation.html?WT.ac=ctg

Mindfulness4U. (2020). *10 Mindfulness activities for kids*. Retrieved from Mindfulness4U: https://mindfulness4u.org /mindfulness-activities-children/

Morin, A. (2020). *The importance of teaching children impulse control*. Retrieved from Very Well Family https://www .verywellfamily.com/the-importance-of-teaching-children -impulse-control-1095019?print

My Learning Tools. (2020). *Self managment*. Retrieved from My Learning Tools https://mylearningtools.org/self-management/

Namaste Kid. (2020). *Downward Facing Dog*. Retrieved from Namaste Kid https://www.namastekid.com/teaching-tools /downward-facing-dog/

Namaste Kid. (2020). *Table Pose*. Retrieved from Namaste Kid https://www.namastekid.com/teaching-tools/table-pose/

Nemours. Children's Health System. (2017). *Teens. Mindful Exercises*. Retrieved from Nemours. Children's Health System https://kidshealth.org/Nemours/en/teens/mindful-exercises .html

Page, R. M., Page, T. S. (2014). *Promoting health and emotional well-being in your classroom*. Burlington, MA: Jones and Bartlett.

Pew Research Center. (2019). *Most US Teens See Anxiety and Depression as a Major Problem Among Their Peers*. Pew Research Center.

PIco, I. (2019). *The Wheel of Emotions, by Robert Plutchick*. Retrieved from PsicoPico https://psicopico.com/en/la-rueda -las-emociones-robert-plutchik/

RMC Health. (2020). *Goal Setting*. Retrieved from RMC Health https://www.rmc.org/what-we-do/training-expertise-to-create -healthy-schools/health-education/goal-setting/

School Social Work Association of America. (2020). *10 Session Impulse Control Workshop*. Retrieved from School Social Work Association of http://sswaaorganization.org/userfiles /file/2011-Conference-Handouts/G49-WK.pdf

Smith, B. H. (2020). Promoting mind–body health in schools: Interventions for mental health professionals; school-based yoga for managing stress and anxiety. *American Psychological Association*, 201–216.

Teenshealth by Nemours. (2016). *5 Ways to deal with anxiety*. Retrieved from TeensHealth by Nemours https://kidshealth .org/en/teens/anxiety-tips.html

TeensHealth from Nemours. (2017). *Mindfulness exercises*. Retrieved from TeensHealth https://teenshealth.org/en/kids /mindful-exercises.html

Teens Health from Nemours, (2019). *How much sleep do I need?* Retrieved from TeensHealth from Nemours https://kidshealth .org/en/teens/how-much-sleep.html

Transforming Education. (2014). *Introduction to self-managment.* Retrieved from Transforming Education https://www .transformingeducation.org/wp-content/uploads/2019 /04/Introduction_to_Self-Management_Handout_Final_CC .pdf

Transforming Education. (2020). *Self-management: Sample strategies.* Retrieved from Transforming Education https://www .transformingeducation.org/wp-content/uploads/2018 /07/2018_Self-Management-Strategies_website.pdf

Understood. (2020). *The 3 types of self-control.* Retrieved from Understood https://www.understood.org/en/friends-feelings /common-challenges/self-control/the-3-types-of-self-control ?_ul=1*q4cwmp*domain_userid*YW1wLUdnNFdocGNScm 9xUmlvQ1dXNmVRRVE

Your Dictionary. (2020). *Goal Setting.* Retrieved from Your Dictionary https://www.yourdictionary.com/goal-setting

YTS Your Therapy Source. (2017). *Self regulation: 10 FUN self control games to practice self regulation skills (no equipment needed).* Retrieved from YTS Your Therapy Source: https:// www.yourtherapysource.com/blog1/2017/05/16/games -practice-self-regulation-skills/

Chapter 4—Appendix A

Self-Management: Scope, Sequence, Content, SEL–Competency/Subcompetencies

<u>Note:</u> This page is organized by grade span, Standard 1, skill standards, the HECAT content areas, and SEL– Competency/Subcompetencies.

The HECAT content areas include: AOD – Alcohol and Other Drugs; HE – Healthy Eating; MEH – Mental/ Emotional Health; PHW – Personal Health and Wellness; PA – Physical Activity; S – Safety; SH – Sexual Health; T – Tobacco; V – Violence Prevention

Impulse Control, Self-Discipline, Self-Motivation

Grade Span	Standard 1	Skill	HECAT Content Areas and Specific Content	SEL Competency and Subcompetencies
PreK–2	1.2.2 <u>Recognize</u> that *impulse control* affects multiple components of health.	7.2.1 <u>Demonstrate</u> healthy practices and behaviors, *such as impulse control*, to maintain or improve personal health.	Mental/Emotional Health: Impulse control, self-discipline, self-motivation	SEL–Self-management: Impulse control, self-discipline, self-motivation
3–5	1.5.2 Identify examples of *how* emotional, intellectual, physical, and social health *are affected by impulse control, self-discipline, and self-motivation.*	7.5.2 Demonstrate a variety of healthy practices and behaviors such as *impulse control, self-discipline, and self-motivation,* to maintain or improve personal health.	Mental/Emotional Health: Impulse control, self-discipline, self-motivation	SEL–Self-management: Impulse control, self-discipline, self-motivation
6–8	1.8.7 <u>Describe</u> the benefits of and barriers to practicing healthy behaviors *when struggling with impulse control when texting.*	7.8.2. <u>Demonstrate</u> healthy practices and behaviors that maintain or improve the health of self and others *such as using the THINK process when texting.*	Mental/Emotional Health: Impulse control, self-discipline, self-motivation; social media	SEL–Self-management: Impulse control, self-discipline, self-motivation
9–12	1.12.7 <u>Compare</u> and <u>contrast</u> the benefits of and barriers to practicing a variety of healthy behaviors regarding *sexual relationships.*	7.12.1 <u>Analyze</u> the role of individual responsibility in *controlling impulses* and enhancing *sexual* health.	Mental/Emotional Health: Impulse control, self-discipline, self-motivation; sexuality	SEL–Self-management: Impulse control, self-discipline, self-motivation

Stress Management				
PreK–2	1.2.1 <u>Identify</u> that healthy behaviors, *such as practicing Yoga to cope with stress*, affect personal health	7.2.1 <u>Demonstrate</u> healthy practices and behaviors, *such as practicing Yoga*, to maintain or improve personal health.	Personal Health and Wellness: Stress management; Yoga	SEL–Self-management: Stress management
3–5	1.5.1 <u>Describe</u> the relationship between healthy behaviors, *such as using stress reducing strategies*, and personal health.	7.5.2 Demonstrate a variety of healthy practices and behaviors, *such as stress reduction strategies*, to maintain or improve personal health.	Personal Health and Wellness: Stress management-Stress reduction strategies	SEL–Self-management: Stress management
6–8	1.8.2 Describe the interrelationships *of anxiety* to emotional, intellectual, physical, and social health in adolescence.	7.8.2 Demonstrate a variety of healthy practices and behaviors, *such as anxiety reduction strategies*, to maintain or improve the health of self and others.	Personal Health and Wellness: Stress management; anxiety	SEL–Self-management: Stress management
9–12	1.12.5 Propose ways to reduce or prevent injuries and health problems *related to stress and anxiety*.	7.12.2 Demonstrate a variety of healthy practices and behaviors, *such as mindfulness*, that maintain or improve the health of self and others.	Personal Health and Wellness: Stress management; mindfulness	SEL–Self-management: Stress management
Setting and Achieving Personal and Educational Goals/Organization Skills				
PreK–2	1.2.1 Identify that healthy *physical activity* behaviors *affect* personal health.	6.2.1 Identify a short-term personal health goal and take action toward achieving the goal. 6.2.2 Identify who can help when assistance is needed to achieve a personal health goal.	Physical Activity: -Goal setting to increase physical activity and enhance organizational skills.	SEL–Self-management: Goal setting, organizational skills
3–5	1.5.1 Describe the relationship between healthy behaviors *such as using MyPlate to eat healthy* and personal health.	**S – Specific**: 6.5.1 Set a personal health goal *to use MyPlate to eat healthy* and track progress toward its achievement. **M- Measurable** **A – Attainable** **R – Realistic and Relevant** (6.5.1 Set a personal health goal *to use MyPlate to eat healthy* and track progress toward its achievement.) **T – Time bound** **Help – Resources needed** (6.5.2 Identify resources to assist in achieving the personal health goal *of using MyPlate to eat healthy*.) **R - Reflection**	Healthy Eating: Using MyPlate to set goals for healthy eating.	SEL–Self-management: Goal setting, organizational skills

(continues)

Impulse Control, Self-Discipline, Self-Motivation *(continued)*

Grade Span	Standard 1	Skill	HECAT Content Areas and Specific Content	SEL Competency and Subcompetencies
Setting and Achieving Personal and Educational Goals/Organization Skills				
6–8	1.8.7 <u>Describe</u> the benefits of and barriers to practicing healthy behaviors, *such as eating breakfast*.	**S – Specific** (6.8.1 Assess personal health practices) 6.8.2 Develop a goal to adopt, maintain, or improve a personal health practice. **M – Measurable** **A – Attainable** **R – Realistic** (6.8.4 Describe how personal health goals vary with changing abilities, priorities, and responsibilities.) **T – Time Phased** **H – Help Needed** (6.8.3 Apply strategies and monitor progress in achieving a personal health goal.) **R – Reflection**	Healthy Eating: Use SMARTHR goals to set a goal to eat breakfast every day.	SEL–Self-management: Goal setting, organizational skills
9–12	1.12.8 <u>Analyze</u> the personal susceptibility to injury, illness, or death if engaging in unhealthy behaviors *such as drinking alcohol and binge drinking*.	**S – Specific** (6.12.1 Assess personal health practices and overall health status *regarding alcohol use and binge drinking*.) 6.12.2 Develop a plan to attain a personal health goal that addresses strengths, needs, and risks *relating to drinking alcohol and binge drinking*. **M – Measurable** (6.12.3 Implement strategies and monitor progress in achieving a personal health goal *relating to drinking alcohol and binge drinking*) **A – Attainable** (6.12.3 Implement strategies and monitor progress in achieving a personal health goal *relating to drinking alcohol and binge drinking*) **R – Realistic** (6.12.4 Formulate an effective long-term personal health plan *relating to drinking alcohol and binge drinking*.) **T – Time Phased** **H – Help Needed** **R – Reflection**	Alcohol, Tobacco, and Other Drugs: Use SMARTHR goal to be able to go to a party and not drink.	SEL–Self-management: Goal setting, organizational skills

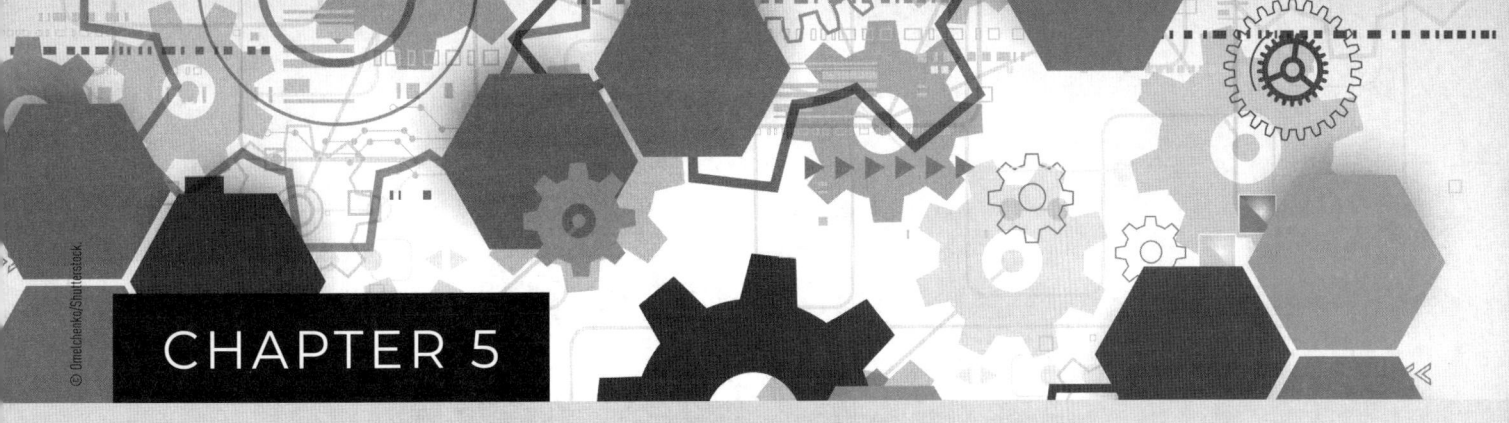

CHAPTER 5

Teaching Social Awareness

LEARNING OBJECTIVES

Upon finishing this course, students will be able to:

- Plan skills-based health (SBH)/SEL lessons using backwards design and practice prompts.
- Incorporate the subcompetencies of social awareness into assessment and instruction.

KEY TERMS

Appreciating diversity
Empathy

Perspective taking
Respect for others

Social awareness

Social and Emotional Learning (SEL) Competencies*

- **Social Awareness Figure 5.1**
  - *The ability to take the perspective of and empathize with others, including those from diverse backgrounds and cultures. The ability to understand social and ethical norms for behavior and to recognize family, school, and community resources and supports.* (CASEL, 2019)

Introduction

The CASEL competencies of **social awareness** and relationship skills are linked because they prepare youth to develop positive social skills. Social awareness challenges the student to examine personal social attitudes, norms, and family and community resources. Relationship skills challenge the student to use those skills to establish and maintain healthy relationships with others.

Social awareness and relationship skills are also considered an important factor in the workforce. A Partnership for 21st Century Skills survey of a variety of employers found that four of the five most important skills for high school students to acquire as they enter the work force are associated with social awareness and relationship skills: professionalism, collaboration, communication, and social responsibility. (Transforming Education, 2020)

Being socially aware is important for the functioning of a safe, engaging classroom. When the teacher and the students demonstrate positive, empathetic, respectful behavior, and understand

*A scope and sequence document is included as an appendix at the end of this chapter.

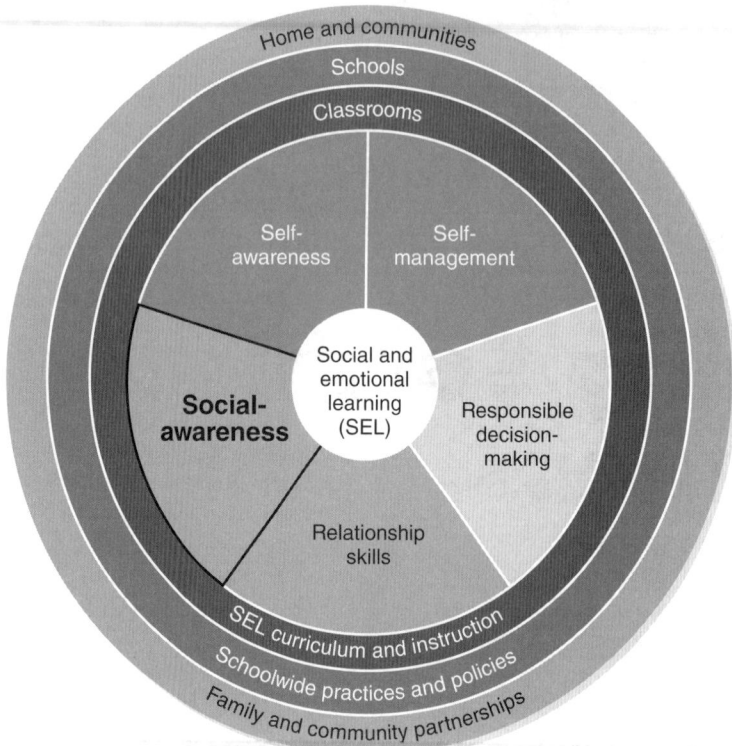

Figure 5.1 The CASEL Framework – Competency on Social Awareness.

that each may differ in perspective or come from a different family culture, they are modeling social awareness.

Students who are socially aware:

- Contribute to a positive classroom environment because they adapt more easily to their environment, empathize with the different perspectives of others, and participate in fewer disruptive behaviors.
- Have better relationships with peers because they have good communication skills and resolve differences as they arise rather than waiting until a conflict erupts.
- Participate in fewer risky behaviors because they have the skill to adapt to new environments, understand the needs and perspectives of their peers, and know where to access family, school, and community resources and support, when needed. (Transforming Education, 2020)

Teachers help students become socially aware through a variety of resources, assessments, and reflections. Challenging, creative, and culturally sensitive activities help the student examine and clarify personal values and attitudes toward others.

When planning lessons, teachers use practice prompts as the daily vehicle to demonstrate and reinforce content, skill, and SEL competencies. The practice prompt includes situations where the student identifies and examines perspective taking, **empathy**, diversity, and respect and learns the content and skills to reinforce the importance of each.

Providing effective feedback to students as they practice helps guide and direct the student to proficiency of the performance indicator and SEL competency. Successful completion of a skill practice gives the student the self-confidence to learn other skills and ultimately develop a growth mindset. (Frey, Fisher, & Smith, 2019, p. 29)

When progressing through each chapter, it becomes evident that the skills and competencies from previous chapters are interwoven in the subsequent chapters. The richness of skills-based health/SEL is a result of a multi-faceted, engaging, age-appropriate, and experiential assessment and instruction that students use to improve relationships and personal health not only in the school setting but in the work place.

Table 5.1 describes the alignment of social awareness to Standard 3 of the National Health Education Standards: Students demonstrate the ability to access valid information and products and services to enhance health. (Joint Committee on National Health Education Standards, 2007, p. 28)

Table 5.1 Alignment of Social Awareness to Standard 2 of the NHES

Competency	Description	Subcompetencies
Social-Awareness	The ability to take the perspective of and empathize with others, including those from diverse backgrounds and cultures. The ability to understand social and ethical norms for behavior and to recognize family, school, and community resources and supports. (Collaborative for Academic and Social Emotional Learning, 2020)	■ Perspective taking ■ Empathy ■ Appreciating diversity ■ **Respect for others**

When a person is socially aware, he examines his relationship with others and reflects on his ability to think beyond himself. He learns to empathize and be respectful of others regardless of perspectives and differences. Socially aware youth also know how to access family, school, and community resources to enhance their health.

Skills-based health/SEL educators use prompts, based on infused performance indicators, to help students become socially aware and demonstrate proficiency in content, skill, and SEL competency.

For example:

Infused performance indicators:

- 1.12.1 Predict how healthy behaviors *such as buying a toy for a child* affects health status. (Joint Committee on National Health Education Standards, 2007, p. 24)
- 3.12.3 Determine the accessibility of *age-appropriate* products and services that enhance *social-emotional* health. (Joint Committee on National Health Education Standards, 2007, p. 26)
- SEL: Social-awareness: Empathy

Daniel lives in a diverse socio-economic community. As the holidays approached, he learned that some children do not receive presents. He always received plenty of toys and clothes as a child and feels badly that some children do not. Daniel remembers the high school toy drive from last year and how good everyone felt when they donated new toys to the children in their community. He wants to participate this year and feel good about helping by buying a toy and donating it to the holiday charity.

The Intergalactic Star series toys are popular this season, but Daniel wants to make sure his selection is safe of a four-year-old boy. In health class, the teacher told him the Consumer Product Safety Commission is an excellent source of information about toy safety. After researching, he learned the toy is safe! He checked the websites of local stores and found one that sells it.

Daniel feels good about himself that he will make a four year old very happy (and safe) this holiday season. (Connolly, 2020, p. 228)

In this example, the lesson taught to the Grade 10 students was based on empathy, included predicting behaviors, and determining the accessibility of an age-appropriate toy to enhance the social-emotional health of a child and the teen who donated a toy.

Preview

Unit Plan

In a skills-based/SEL unit, the planner accesses and analyzes data and selects a Standard 1 and skills performance indicator to reduce the risk factor and infuses them with content. The SEL competency and subcompetency are aligned with the infused performance indicators. Once established, the instructor plans the assessment and instruction. As the content, skill, and competency are taught, the teacher distributes the performance task, which consists of the unit prompt(s), the scoring rubric, back-up materials needed such as supplemental content, self-checks, and any other information the students need to show proficiency in the performance indicators and SEL competency. Students organize and practice for a few days and present their work to the class. This summative assessment is scored with an analytical rubric.

Skills-Based Lesson Plan

The skills-based/SEL lesson plan contains an agenda, the lesson objectives (infused Standard 1 performance indicator and skills indicator, and the SEL competency/subcompetency), a review/preview, the Standard 1 content, the skill, competency, a student-engaging practice prompt, clarifying questions relating to the prompt and learning objectives, a lesson review, and an exit ticket.

Skills-Based Lesson Infrastructure

The sections that follow present <u>infrastructure</u> for a <u>lesson</u>, not a unit. The infrastructure provides the teacher with guidance without interfering with individual creativity. Each begins with an overview, data (when available), and a list of resources. Following the overview, a table initiates backwards design and consists of the infused performance indicators and SEL competencies as the lesson objectives.

Assessments are designed for each of the performance indicators and SEL competency. The prompt and the review questions engage the learner and help the teacher determine if the students met the lesson objectives. An exit question concludes the lesson infrastructure and provides an opportunity for students to reflect on how to use what was taught.

When reading, let your imagination guide your planning. You may need more or fewer lessons to teach the material. You may like an idea and modify it to meet the needs of your students. You may find the worksheets valuable or may prefer to edit them.

When modifying, maintain the integrity of the backwards design. Teach content, skill, and SEL each day. If the lesson infrastructure contains too much material, plan an additional day(s) but maintain the integrity of aligning SEL and teaching content through the infused performance indicators. Refer to the sample lessons at the end of each chapter to understand how to align SEL and teach content through the skill.

Organization

The learning activities for the core competency of social awareness are divided into two sections:

- Taking the perspective of and empathizing with others, respecting others, and recognizing community resources
- **Appreciating diversity**, respecting others, continuing to address challenges, and recognizing community resources. (Collaborative for Academic Social Emotional Learning, 2020)

Each section below contains background information about the subcompetency followed by lesson suggestions and resources.

The NHES is grouped according to the grade spans PreK–2, Grades 3–5, Grades 6–8, and Grades 9–12. The examples follow that structure.

Table 5.2 Social-Awareness by Subcompetencies

Perspective-taking	Empathy
Appreciating diversity	Respect for others

The classroom examples may require the teacher to be creative and adjust instruction to accommodate the age and abilities of the students.

The headings of each section represent a social awareness subcompetency (**Table 5.2**). The practice prompt is aligned with the competency and the infused performance indicators of the National Health Education Standards.

Section 1. Taking the Perspective of and Empathizing with Others, Respecting Others and, Recognizing Community Resources

(Collaborative for Academic Social Emotional Learning, 2020)

Empathy is an important social skill. To be able to recognize the emotions someone else is experiencing and understand how those emotions makes that person feel is the foundation of this section (Randy M. Page., 2015, p. 61) because if a person is empathetic, they are more aware of another person's perspective, they appreciate the differences in others, and are respectful of both.

There are specific classroom strategies that help students develop empathy:

- Design practice prompts that help students identify emotions in others.
- Set time aside to talk about personal emotions and the emotions of others including peers, teachers, and family.
- Acknowledge when students demonstrate empathy.
- Teach how to notice and identify nonverbal cues that show the emotional status of others.
- Control angry reactions and instead, use "I" messages to communicate dissatisfaction.
- Provide classroom tasks that require empathy such as watering plants, taking care of classroom pets, distributing and collecting materials. Being

H Halt! Stop what you are doing and pay attention to the speaker.

E Engage the speaker by focusing on him/her.

A Anticipate. Look forward to what the speaker has to say. You may learn something new.

R Replay. Analyze and restate what is being said to better understand.

Figure 5.2 The HEAR Method of Effective Listening.

Data from Wilson, D. C. (2017, January 4). 4 Proven Strategies for Teaching Empathy. Retrieved from George Lucas Educational Foundation, Edutopia: https://www.edutopia.org/article/4-proven-strategies-teaching-empathy-donna-wilson-marcus-conyers.

responsible helps children think of the needs of others rather than their own. (Frey, Fisher, & Smith, 2019, pp. 109-111)

Taking Perspective of and Empathizing with Others, Respecting Others, and Recognizing Community Resources

As skills-based health/SEL educators, teaching empathy occurs synchronously and seamlessly through instruction.

Affective empathy occurs when one person shares the emotions of another person. For example, smiling when another person smiles or joining in on the physical response of another when he/she jumps up and down and clapping when experiencing a joyful moment. **Perspective taking**, or cognitive empathy, occurs when we imagine ourselves in the situation of another.

There are four specific classroom strategies that facilitate the teaching of affective and cognitive empathy.

1. Model how to be empathetic.
2. Teach how to cope with rather than arguing over different points of view.
3. Use stories (literature) to teach different perspectives.
4. Model active listening using the HEAR method (Wilson, 2017) **(Figure 5.2)**

PreK–2: Social-Awareness: Perspective Taking, Empathy, and Community Resources

Lesson Overview: Empathy for a Friend and Accessing Community Resources

In this lesson, students learn how being able to take perspective, be empathetic and respectful affects the components of health.

Resources:

- Centervention activity: What Makes Me Happy Today? https://www.centervention.com/lesson-about-gratitude-and-happiness/
- Centervention: Empathy Lesson: Identifying Feelings. https://www.centervention.com/charades-kids-feelings-empathy/
- KidsHealth in the Classroom: Empathy. https://classroom.kidshealth.org/prekto2/personal/growing/empathy.pdf
- The Inclusion Lab. https://blog.brookespublishing.com/5-activities-for-building-empathy-in-your-students/

Materials needed:

- **Worksheet 5.1 What Makes Me Happy?**
- **Worksheet 5.2 Dimensions of Health**

Table 5.3 provides an overview of the lesson objectives, assessment, and instruction for this lesson.

Table 5.3 Lesson Objectives, Assessment, and Instruction

Step 1 – Lesson Objectives	Step 2 – Assessment
The verb of the *infused* performance indicator and the SEL competency generate the assessment and instruction.	Design the assessment based on the objectives. Ask yourself the question, "What can my students do to show me they have met the standard?"

(continues)

Table 5.3 Lesson Objectives, Assessment, and Instruction   *(continued)*

Step 1 – Lesson Objectives	Step 2 – Assessment
1.2.2. <u>Recognize</u> *empathy for a friend in each of the* multiple dimensions of health. (Joint Committee on National Health Education Standards, 2007, p. 24)	1.2.2 Students <u>recognize</u> *one* example of empathy for a friend in each of the components of wellness.
3.2.1 <u>Identify</u> trusted adults and professionals *in the school who* help promote health. (Joint Committee on National Health Education Standards, 2007, p. 26)	3.2.1 Students <u>identify</u> a school adult who can help a friend in need.
SEL-Social-awareness: Perspective taking, Empathy, Community resources.	Students recognize empathy in the dimensions of health and identify a school adult who can help a friend in need.

Step 3 – Instruction
Design the instruction so that students learn the content, skill, and competency to be successful on the assessment. Ask yourself the question, "What do I need to teach so that the students will be successful when assessed?"

Step 3 – Instruction

1. Define
   a. Recognize: To identify a person or thing because there is a history of having seen or interacted with that person or thing in the past.
   b. Identify: To recognize a particular person or an object.
   c. Empathy: Imagining the feelings experienced by another even when not personally experienced.
   d. Perspective taking: A person's capability of seeing a situation from several different points of view.
   e. Body language: The nonverbal physical gestures that a person makes to express emotion, whether consciously or subconsciously.
2. 1.2.2. Recognize *empathy in each of the* multiple dimensions of health.
   a. <u>Note</u>: Explain empathy. Demonstrate expressions of emotions and challenge the students to identify the feeling. Identifying the feelings experienced by another helps children develop empathy.
   b. Use **Worksheet 5.1 What Makes Me Happy?** to start the lesson on empathy and dimensions of wellness. The children draw what makes them happy and the emotion they felt when the event happened. Encourage them to include body language as part of the drawing. To demonstrate empathy, the children switch papers with a peer and try to identify the happy event, the emotion expressed, and how they would feel if it were them in the picture.

   c. <u>Note</u>: Explain the three dimensions of health. **Use Worksheet 5.2 Dimensions of Health** to review a variety of examples. Students raise the appropriate triangle to match the example (**Figure 5.3**).
      1) Physical health: Health of your body. Eating healthy meals and getting 60 minutes of physical activity each day promotes physical health.
      2) Mental/emotional health: Health of the mind and expressing feelings in a positive way.
      3) Social Health: Relationships with family and friends. (Meeks, 2020)
   d. Use **Worksheet 5.2 Dimensions of Health** to help the children recognize the components of health. Model the behaviors, including appropriate body language, or provide examples (children having fun together, children stressed, a physically healthy child performing an activity) of behaviors and ask the children to raise the triangle that represents that dimension of health. Once the children recognize the differences between the dimensions, ask them to look at the picture they

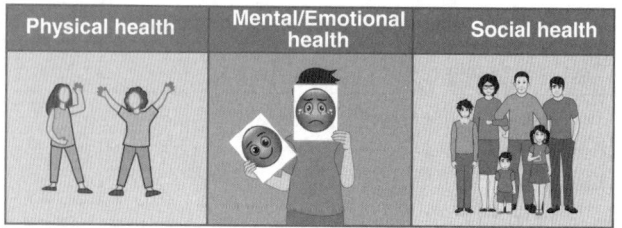

Figure 5.3 Dimensions of Health.

drew of what makes them happy and place the appropriate triangle next to it. Discuss.
3. 3.2.1 <u>Identify</u> trusted adults and professionals *in the school who* help promote health.
   a. Ask the children to identify trusted adults in the school they could go to if they had a problem or wanted to help a friend with one.
   b. Examples: teacher, nurse, guidance counselor, assistant principal, principal, lunch workers, custodians. etc.
4. Read the practice prompt. Students answer the reflection questions and discuss.

Practice Prompt: Daveed

Daveed is Darren's friend. It was almost snack time and Darren was looking forward to sitting with Daveed to talk about the latest video game they are playing. Daveed's head was down on his desk, and he looked sad. Darren asked, "Daveed, Are you OK?" Daveed shook his head. "What is wrong?" Daveed explained his father got very sick last night and his mom took him to the hospital. His mom came home but his dad did not. He is very afraid and worried. Daveed's family is very close and Darren understands why Daveed is so upset. He wants to help and he knows Daveed would do the same for him.

Darren asked if he could tell their teacher, Mrs. Fixall, because she would know what to do. Daveed said, "OK." Mrs. Fixall listened to Darren, called the nurse, and sent the boys to her office. The nurse noticed that Daveed looked pale and upset. She called Daveed's mom and was told that Daveed's dad did go to the hospital last night but is feeling much better and should be home by this evening.

When the nurse shared the news with the boys, they both looked better immediately. Daveed's eyes started to sparkle again, and he was able to smile and say, "Thank you."

5. Use the review questions in **Table 5.4** to help the children understand how to recognize empathy in each of the dimensions of wellness.
6. End of class review. Ask the students to put away their materials then ask review questions.
   a. How would you empathize with someone who is physically upset? (1.2.2)
   b. How would you empathize with someone who is socially upset? (1.2.2)
   c. How would you empathize with someone who is mentally/emotionally upset? (1.2.2)
   d. Who is one person at school that children can go to if they have a problem? (3.2.1)
7. Exit ticket (Social-Awareness: empathy)
   Today, I knew _____ was upset because I saw_____, (empathy) so I told _____. (trusted adult)

Grades 3–5: Social-Awareness: Perspective-Taking, Empathy, and Community Resources

Lesson Overview: Coping with Bullying by Taking Perspective, Being Empathetic, and Accessing Community Resources

In this lesson, students intervene in bullying after taking perspective of the situation, being empathetic toward the victim, and accessing community resources.

31.9% (Female-37.1%; Males-26.8%) to 47.6% (Females-53.3%; Males 41.9%) of middle school students report ever being bullied on school property.

Note: A sample lesson plan for this grade span is found at the end of the chapter.

Resources:

- Arthur: So funny I forgot to laugh (empathy): https://pbskids.org/arthur/friends/so-funny

Table 5.4 Empathy, Perspective Taking, and Recognizing Community Resources

Question	Answer
How did Darren recognize empathy for his friend in each of the components of wellness? (1.2.2)	Physical Health ■ Darren recognized that Daveed's head was down and he looked sad. Darren felt bad and wanted to help his friend. He knew Daveed would do the same for him. Social Health ■ Darren and Daveed are friends. Darren recognized that something was wrong with Daveed and as a good friend, he wanted to help. He asked Daveed for permission to ask the teacher for help.

(continues)

Table 5.4 Empathy, Perspective Taking, and Recognizing Community Resources   *(continued)*

Question	Answer
	Mental/Emotional Health
	■ Darren recognized that Daveed was very upset because his dad was in the hospital and wanted to help him some way.
	■ Darren recognized that Daveed felt much better when he learned his dad was coming home. Seeing Daveed feel better make him feel better.
Who was identified as a trusted school adult who could help Darren and Daveed? (3.2.1)	Darren told Mrs. Fixall that Daveed was upset and she sent the boys to the nurse.
SEL-Social Awareness: Perspective-taking, empathy, recognizing community resources.	
SEL-Social Awareness: Perspective-taking	■ Darren saw that his friend was upset because his head was down, and he looked sad. He knew he had to do something to help. (Perspective taking).
SEL-Social Awareness: Empathy	■ Darren felt bad seeing his friend so upset. (empathy)
SEL-Social Awareness: Recognizing community resources	■ Darren asked permission to go to their teacher to get help (recognizing community resources). Mrs. Fixall sent the boys to the nurse.

- Understood.org. How to show empathy to your students with compassionate curiosity. https://www.understood.org/en/school-learning/for-educators/empathy/using-compassionate-curiosity-to-drive-empathy?_ul=1*8pjd5t*domain_userid*YW1wLUdnNFdocGNScm9xUmlvQ1dXNmVRRVE.
- Understood.org. Teacher to teacher: Use a daily warm-up to build empathy. https://www.understood.org/en/school-learning/for-educators/empathy/teacher-to-teacher-use-a-daily-warm-up-to-build-empathy?_ul=1*1ro98sf*domain_userid*YW1wLUdnNFdocGNScm9xUmlvQ1dXNmVRRVE.
- Mojo-Empathy for students. Episode 1. https://www.bing.com/videos/search?q=children+and+empathy&&view=detail&mid=34D87D42D48D6BF71B7034D87D42D48D6BF71B70&&FORM=VDRVRV
- Mojo: Empathy for students. Episode 2. https://www.bing.com/videos/search?q=children +and+empathy&&view=detail&mid=6810B7CA73335C8733BB6810B7CA73335C8733BB&&FORM=VDRVRV
- Mojo: Empathy for students. Episode 3. https://www.bing.com/videos/search?q=children+and+empathy&&view=detail&mid=8913DE09DAC0B8FE69E28913DE09DAC0B8FE69E2&&FORM=VDRVRV
- Pacer Center's Kids Against Bullying. What is Bullying, The Basics: https://www.pacerkidsagainstbullying.org/what-is-bullying/what-is-bullying-videos/

Materials needed:

- **Worksheet 5.3 Demonstrating How to Be Empathetic toward a Bullying Victim and the Effect it Has on Personal Health.**

Table 5.5 provides an overview of the lesson objectives, assessment, and instruction for this lesson.

Table 5.5 Lesson Objectives, Assessment, and Instruction

Step 1 – Lesson Objectives	Step 2 – Assessment
The verb of the *infused* performance indicator and the SEL competency generate the assessment and instruction.	Design the assessment based on the objectives. Ask yourself the question, "What can my students do to show me they have met the standard?"
1.5.2. <u>Describe</u> the relationship between healthy behaviors, *such as being empathetic toward a bullying victim*, and personal health. (Joint Committee on National Health Education Standards, 2007, p. 24)	1.5.2 Students <u>describe</u> *three* effects on personal health of being empathetic to a bullying victim.

3.5.2 <u>Locate</u> resources from home, school, and community that provide valid health information *about bullying.* (Joint Committee on National Health Education Standards, 2007, p. 28)	3.5.2 Students <u>locate</u> school resources about bullying.
SEL-Social-awareness: Perspective-taking, empathy, and community resources.	Students take perspective of a child being bullied, show empathy, and recognize school resources.

Step 3 – Instruction
Design the instruction so that students learn the content, skill, and competency to be successful on the assessment. Ask yourself the question, "What do I need to teach so that the students will be successful when assessed?"

Step 3 – Instruction

1. Define
   a. Identify: To recognize a particular person or an object.
   b. Empathy: Imagining the feelings experienced by another even when not personally experienced.
   c. Perspective-taking: A person's capability of seeing a situation from several different points of view.
   d. Bullying: The act of intimidating, harassing, manipulating, and/or hurting a vulnerable person.
   e. Locate: To determine exactly where someone or something can be found.
2. 1.5.1 <u>Describe</u> the relationship between healthy behaviors *such as being empathetic* and personal health
   a. Benefits of being empathetic
      1) Improves relationships
      2) Promotes understanding of self
      3) Helps to take perspective of the situations others experience
   b. Model how to show empathy. Example: Set up a role play with a student. Approach the student and say,

   > "Melanie, it is OK. I understand that you are upset because you left your school work at home. You are a responsible student and care about your work. (Empathy) Sometimes I forget things at home, and I know how upsetting it can be." (Perspective taking) Show me your work tomorrow and I'll grade you then. "Thank you," Melanie said with a smile on her face.

   c. Reflect
      1) Ask the children to explain what they observed.
      2) Explain that when we understand the feelings of another and try to help, we are showing empathy.
      3) Explain that when we put ourselves in another person's situation to understand better what is going on, that is taking perspective.
      4) How did the teacher show empathy to Melanie?
      5) How did the teacher take perspective of the situation?
      6) How did the student feel when the teacher told her she could pass in her work tomorrow?
   d. Use **Worksheet 5.3 Demonstrating How to Be Empathetic toward a Bullying Victim and the Effect it Has on Personal Health** to help students learn to be empathetic.
3. 3.5.2 Locate resources from home, school, and community that provide valid health information *about bullying*
   a. Ask the children where they can find information about bullying at school.
      1) Teacher
      2) Classroom/gymnasium
      3) Hallways
      4) Nurse's office
      5) Lunchroom
      6) Offices of the principal/assistant principle.
   b. Ask the children who are the trusted adults in the school they can go to if they are bullied or know someone who is bullied.
4. Read the practice prompt. Students answer the reflection questions and discuss.

Practice Prompt: Eloise

Eloise thought she had friends but all that has changed. The other day, the teacher was leading the class to the gymnasium when three girls behind her started making fun of her clothes. Eloise likes to dress a little differently, preferring colorful dresses to pants. Mrs. Dresser didn't hear the girls, but they were taunting her saying she looked like a cartoon character. They said, "Wait until we are in the gym, that dress won't be so colorful anymore!" They pointed at her and laughed. Eloise thought, "They didn't like what I was wearing last week either!" Eloise is upset but doesn't know what to do to make them stop.

Her line partner, Antoinette, heard the girls and looked back at them and told them to stop. In the gym, Antoinette told Eloise she heard the girls and didn't like what was happening. Eloise was relieved. She told Eloise that she would stay close by in case the girls started taunting her again.

Eloise and Antoinette felt empowered when they made a plan to tell the girls to stop and told them they were going to tell their teachers if they didn't. Once they reminded the girls that Mrs. Dresser taught their class about bullying, told the children that the school policy says bullying is not acceptable, and that bullies would be held accountable for their behavior, the bullying stopped.

Eloise and Antoinette became friends and have a lot of fun together. They sit together on the bus, are partners when they go to their specialist classes (health, PE, music, etc.), eat lunch together, and invite each other to their homes. Together, they proudly told Eloise's parents about the bullying and how they got it to stop.

Eloise feels great that someone understood what she was going through and was willing to help her. Antoinette also feels great because she helped a peer and gained a friend!

(Stop Bullying, 2020)

5. Use the review questions in **Table 5.6** to help the children understand how to recognize empathy in each of the dimensions of wellness.
6. End of class review. Ask the students to put away their materials then ask review questions.
   a. Give an example of how to show empathy toward a bullying victim. (1.5.1)
   b. Who is a resource in the school who can help a bullying victim? (3.5.2)
   c. What document supports children who are victims of bullying in school? (3.5.2)
7. Exit ticket (Social-Awareness: Perspective-taking, empathy, and recognizing school)
   Worksheet 5.4 Empathy Checklist

Table 5.6 How to Take Perspective, Demonstrate Empathy, and Recognize Community Resources

Question	Answer
What were three effects on Eloise's and Antoinette's personal health when Antoinette demonstrated empathy? (1.5.1)	Improved relationships ■ Eloise felt great because she gained a friend. ■ Antoinette felt great because she helped a peer and gained a friend. ■ Antoinette told the bullies to stop and if they didn't, she would tell the teacher. The bullies stopped. Promoted understanding of self ■ Eloise was relieved that Antoinette understood the situation and was willing to help her. ■ Eloise and Antoinette were proud to tell Eloise's parents about how they stopped the bullying. ■ Eloise and Antoinette felt empowered when they make a plan to tell their teacher if the bullying didn't stop. Helped to take perspective of the situations others experience ■ Antoinette told Eloise she heard the girls bullying her and didn't like it. Eloise was relieved. Antoinette told Eloise that she would stay close by in case the girls started taunting her again.
How did Eloise and Antoinette locate school resources about bullying? (3.5.2)	The girls knew Mrs. Dresser already taught their class about bullying, explained that the school policy says bullying is not acceptable, and that bullies would be held accountable for their behavior.

SEL-Social-awareness: Perspective taking, empathy, community resources.	
SEL-Social-awareness: Perspective taking	Antoinette knew that the words from the other peers couldn't make Eloise feel very good. (perspective taking)
SEL-Social-awareness: Empathy	Antoinette realized that Eloise was upset because the girls behind her were (empathy) taunting her.
SEL-Social-awareness: Community resources.	Antoinette and Eloise developed a plan to tell the bullies to stop and if they didn't, Eloise and Antoinette would tell their teacher. (recognizing school resources)

Grades 6–8: Social-Awareness: Perspective-Taking, Empathy, and Community Resources

Lesson Overview: Taking Perspective, Empathizing with, and Recognizing Community Resources for LGBTQ (Lesbian, Gay, Bisexual, Transsexual, and Queer/Questioning) Middle School Students

In this lesson, students describe that being empathetic to LGBTQ students reduces health problems and also learn to use the SPAT technique to check the validity of a website.

Family Acceptance Project research project reported that children were attracted to another person of the same gender at about age 10.

Some students knew they were gay by age 7 or 9.

Students identified as lesbian, gay, or bisexual by about age 13.4. (Ryan, 2009)

Students in a school that provided a Gay/Straight Alliance (GSA) heard anti-LGBTQ remarks less often and had more positive attitudes toward LGBTQ people than students in schools without a GSA. (Greytak, 2016)

GSAs in the middle school benefits school climate and social-emotional health of all students. (Wolpert-Gawrom, 2018)

Resources:

- As an alternative perspective-taking activity, view Susan Boyle: I Dreamed a Dream—Les Misérables. Official Britain's Got Talent 2009 on YouTube. Show the beginning of the video but stop before she sings. Discuss student perspective of Ms. Boyle's talent and ability to perform. Continue viewing the video and discuss whether perspective changed when she finished singing.

Materials needed:

- **Worksheet 5.5 Empathy Self-Test**
- **Worksheet 5.6 Using SPAT to Evaluate a Website**
- **Worksheet 5.7 Sexual Attraction and Orientation Sort**
- **Worksheet 5.8 How to Show Empathy toward Others**

Table 5.7 provides an overview of the lesson objectives, assessment, and instruction for this lesson.

Table 5.7 Lesson Objectives, Assessment, and Instruction

Step 1 – Lesson Objectives	Step 2 – Assessment
The verb of the *infused* performance indicator and the SEL competency generate the assessment and instruction.	Design the assessment based on the objectives. Ask yourself the question, "What can my students do to show me they have met the standard?"
1.8.5. <u>Describe</u> ways to reduce or prevent injuries and other adolescent health behaviors *by being empathetic toward LGBTQ.* (Joint Committee on National Health Education Standards, 2007, p. 24)	1.8.5 Students <u>describe</u> three ways *being empathetic* helps reduce injuries and other adolescent health behaviors *of middle school LGBTQ students.* Include information from the TeensHealth article, Sexual Attraction and Orientation.
3.8.1. <u>Analyze</u> the validity of health information, products, and services *about sexual orientation.* (Joint Committee on National Health Education Standards, 2007, p. 28)	3.8.1 Students <u>analyze</u>, using the SPAT technique, the validity of TeensHealth website information *about sexual orientation.*

(continues)

Table 5.7 Lesson Objectives, Assessment, and Instruction *(continued)*

Step 1 – Lesson Objectives	Step 2 – Assessment
SEL–Social-awareness: Perspective-taking, empathy, and community resources.	Students demonstrate taking perspective of and being empathetic to middle school LBGTQ students, and accessing resources to help LGBTQ students.

Step 3 – Instruction
Design the instruction so that students learn the content, skill, and competency to be successful on the assessment. Ask yourself the question, "What do I need to teach so that the students will be successful when assessed?"

Step 3 – Instruction

1. Define
   a. Describe: To use words that help others envision the physical attributes of a person, place, or thing.
   b. Analyze: To scrutinize something or someone in order to understand how it or they work(s).
   c. Empathy: Imagining the feelings experienced by another even when not personally experienced.
   d. Perspective-taking: A person's capability of seeing a situation from several different points of view.
   e. Sexual orientation: A person's emotional connection and attraction to another person. (Ryan, 2009)
   f. Nonbinary: A person who does not identify as either male or female. (Kenny, LGBTQ youth share their stories, offer advice to adults to end bullying, 2018)
2. 1.8.5. Describe ways to reduce or prevent injuries and other adolescent health problems *by being empathetic toward LGBTQ*.
   a. To determine personal levels of empathy, students complete **Worksheet 5.5 Empathy Self-Test**. "Yes" responses indicate the student shows empathy. "No" responses indicate areas where the students may try to improve.
   b. Steps of showing empathy. After students complete the self-test, divide the class into groups and assign one empathy step to each group. Provide time for the students to discuss how to use the steps to respond to another peer who presents themselves as different. Discuss.
      1) Imagine what it feels like to be in someone else's shoes! Ask yourself, "How would I feel in this situation?" How else can you understand how someone else feels? *This imagining is an example of perspective-taking. Sharing another person's feelings is showing empathy.*
      2) Check on your communication skills. When listening, make eye contact, do not interrupt the speaker, and ask follow-up questions to show the speaker you were trying to understand what the person is experiencing. What other behaviors might show that you are an empathetic listener?
      3) Additional communication skills. To be more attuned to the feelings of another, think about how many times you ask "you" questions instead of making "I" statements. (Teaching Tolerance, 2020) Practice your "I" statements.
3. 3.8.1. Analyze the validity of health information, products, and services *about sexual orientation*.
   a. Copy **Worksheet 5.6 Using SPAT to Evaluate the TeensHealth Website (Table 5.8)**, the TeensHealth article, *Sexual Attraction and Orientation*, and **Worksheet 5.7 Sexual Attraction and Orientation Sort**.
   b. Use **Worksheet 5.6 Using SPAT to Evaluate a TeensHealth website about Sexual Attraction and Orientation** and discuss.
   c. Use **Worksheet 5.7 Sexual Attraction and Orientation Sort** to sort the facts from the TeensHealth article and reinforce the information.
   d. **Use Worksheet 5.8 How to Show Empathy toward Others** to practice empathy skills.
4. Read the practice prompt. Students answer the reflection questions and discuss.

Table 5.8 The SPAT Method of Evaluating Websites

SPAT	Why is it important?
S - Site	
What is the address of the site? What is the content provider type? (.com, .org, .edu, .gov, other)	Provides insight into the motivation and purpose of the website. A .com may have biased information because it is trying to sell a product or service.
P - Publisher	
Look for the contact information for the publisher.	When there is a publisher, you know who is accountable for the content. If there is no publisher, do not trust the content.
A - Audience	
Who is the audience? Do you understand all the words? Are there colors and graphics directed to a particular age group or gender?	Knowing the target audience for the website helps you determine if the website is appropriate.
T - Timeliness	
Look for a publication date, last updated date, or a date created. The date is at the beginning, or at the end, or within the article. (Dr. Elizabeth M. LaRue Ph.D, 2013)	If you are citing statistics, you want to use only current or a range of current dates in order to accurately defend your writing. When writing, use current information or your writing will be inaccurate. Without a date, you do not know when it was written.

Data from Dr. Elizabeth M. LaRue Ph.D, M. (2013, January 10). Website Evaluation Tool. Retrieved from SPAT: http://www.spat.pitt.edu/research.php.

Practice Prompt: Ebon

Ebon is in 7th grade, a good student, and an athlete. He is popular with his male and female friends.

Lately, he is confused because he finds himself dreaming and thinking about boys, not girls. He is hoping these feelings will go away and that they are just part of growing up. Many of his friends talk about sex a lot so he is not the only one who seems preoccupied.

He has observed several of the gay students tormented by others. He felt bad and imagined how difficult it must be to be "out" and bullied. He has also seen "straight" kids bullied because they look "gay." Ebon wanted to say something to his teacher but didn't want anyone to think he was gay.

Sully, a track teammate, is a good friend. He had the feeling something was on Ebon's mind and asked him, "Hey, what is going on? You seem very distracted lately." At first, Ebon told Sully that nothing was wrong but one day while they were waiting for practice to begin, Ebon told Sully he was worried he might be "gay."

Sully laughed until he realized Ebon was serious. He apologized then realized that it took a lot of courage for Ebon to confide in him. If the situation was reversed, he would want Ebon to take him seriously and listen to him so that is what he did.

Sully asked a few questions. "Why do you think you might be "gay?" While Ebon was talking, Sully kept eye contact with him. He didn't interrupt even though he had a million questions. When Ebon finished explaining, Sully asked a few questions just to clarify.

Sully told Ebon, "I've not ever been in this situation before so I am not sure of what to say except you are my friend and it doesn't matter to me if you are gay." Sully told Ebon about the Gay Straight Alliance (GSA) and reminded him that the coach wanted all the team members to do community service and to use the school clubs to meet the requirements.

The boys wanted to know more about GSA before going to a meeting, so they went online to look up the organization. They found it! The gsanetwork.org had all the SPAT elements of a good website they learned about in health class. The address was a .org, the publishing information was at the very bottom of the site and included an address and phone number; the language on the site was clearly for teens; and the publication information was at the very bottom

(continues)

Practice Prompt: Ebon *(continued)*

and included the address, email, telephone number, and copyright date. They now knew a GSA was a real organization they could trust.

Ebon is still reluctant because he doesn't want anyone to think he is "gay." Sully told him that many of their peers belong because they want the school to be more tolerant and that they would fit in just fine.

"You mean, you would come with me?" Ebon asked. Of course, bro. You are my friend. When you are feeling bad, I am feeling bad."

The boys spoke to the GSA advisor and she welcomed them to the club. They are working on an advocacy project, "Athletes for Tolerance," and she thinks they will make an excellent contribution to the group.

---

5. Use the review questions in **Table 5.9** to help the children understand how to recognize empathy in each of the dimensions of wellness.

6. End of class review. Ask the students to put away their materials then ask review questions.

   a. What are three steps for showing empathy toward others? (1.8.5)

   b. How would you analyze a website using the SPAT method? (3.8.1)

7. Exit ticket (Social-Awareness: Perspective taking, empathy, and recognizing school resources)
   Using a sticky note, explain one way to show empathy toward another student.

Grades 9–12: Social-Awareness: Perspective Taking, Empathy, and Community Resources

Lesson Overview: Physical Activity

In this lesson, students take perspective, empathize with, and recognize community resources for students who do not participate in 60 minutes of physical activity each day.

76.8 % (84.6% girls and 69.1% boys) were not physically active at least 60 minutes on all seven days prior to the survey. (Centers for Disease Control and Prevention, 2020)

Table 5.9 How to Take Perspective, Demonstrate Empathy, and Recognize Community Resources

Question	Answer
What are three ways *being empathetic* helps reduce injuries and other adolescent health behaviors *of middle school LGBTQ students?* Include information from the TeensHealth article, *Sexual Attraction and Orientation.* (1.8.5)	■ Ebon described that he felt bad others were being tormented and imagined how difficult it must be to be "out" and be bullied. ■ Sully first laughed when Ebon told him he was worried that he might be "gay" but then realized that it took a lot of courage for Ebon to talk to him and if the situation was reversed, he would want Ebon to take him seriously and listen to him. ■ Sully used good communication skills when Ebon was talking to him. He kept eye contact, didn't interrupt him, and asked follow-up questions. He used "I" statements instead of saying, you....
How did the boys <u>analyze</u>, using the SPAT technique, the validity of TeensHealth website information *about sexual orientation?* (3.8.1)	■ The gsanetwork.org had all the SPAT elements of a good website they learned about in health class. ■ S - The address was a .org. ■ P - the publishing information was at the very bottom of the site and included an address phone number ■ A - the language on the site was clearly for teens ■ T – The timeliness of the website was at the very bottom and included the address, email, telephone number, and copyright date.
SEL–Social-Awareness: Perspective-taking, empathy, and community resources. SEL–Social-Awareness: Perspective-taking SEL–Social-Awareness: Empathy SEL–Social-Awareness: Community resources	 ■ Both Ebon and Sully put themselves in the shoes of others and thereby demonstrated taking perspective. ■ The boys demonstrated empathy, or the sharing of feelings when they realized how hard it must be to "come out." ■ To access resources, Ebon and Sully checked out the GSA organization by going online and using the SPAT method to check its validity.

Resources:

- Brain Bites: The F.I.TT Principle. https://www.youtube.com/watch?v=yAFb0vxopmc&feature=youtu.be
- Open Phys Ed. https://openphysed.org
- Overcoming Barriers to Physical Activity. https://www.cdc.gov/physicalactivity/basics/adding-pa/barriers.html

Materials needed:

- **Sticky notes**
- **Worksheet 5.9 Benefits of and Barriers to Exercising for 60 Minutes each Day**
- **Worksheet 5.10 Using SPAT to Evaluate a Website**
- **Worksheet 5.11 Making a Plan to Become Physically Active**

Table 5.10 provides an overview of the lesson objectives, assessment, and instruction for this lesson.

Step 3 – Instruction

1. Define
   a. Evaluate: To judge a person or thing after methodically examining the situation.
   b. Demonstrate: To show how something is accomplished.
   c. Empathy: Imagining the feelings experienced by another even when not personally experienced.
   d. Perspective taking: A person's capability of seeing a situation from several different points of view.
2. 1.12.7 Compare and contrast the benefits of and barriers to practicing a variety of healthy behaviors *such as being active for 60 minutes each day.*
   a. Divide students into groups of three. Provide six sticky notes to each group. Each person writes down one benefit of exercising for 60 minutes on a sticky note and

Table 5.10 Lesson Objectives, Assessment, and Instruction

Step 1 – Lesson Objectives	Step 2 – Assessment
The verb of the *infused* performance indicator and the SEL competency generate the assessment and instruction.	Design the assessment based on the objectives. Ask yourself the question, "What can my students do to show me they have met the standard?"
1.12.7 Compare and contrast the benefits of and barriers to practicing a variety of healthy behaviors *such as being active for 60 minutes each day.* (Joint Committee on National Health Education Standards, 2007, p. 25)	1.12.7 Students compare and contrast *three* benefits of and *three* barriers to being active for 60 minutes each day.
3.12.1 Evaluate the validity of health information, products, and services *about physical activity.* (Joint Committee on National Health Education Standards, 2007, p. 29)	3.12.1 Students evaluate, using the SPAT technique, the validity of Openpe.org website information *about physical activity.*
7.12.2 Demonstrate a variety of healthy practices and behaviors that maintain or improve the health of self and others, *such as three activities from the plan to have 60 minutes of physical activity for five days.* (Joint Committee on National Health Education Standards, 2007, p. 35)	7.12.2 Students demonstrate *three* activities from the plan that helps the teen be physically active for 5 days with 60 minutes of physical activity each day.
SEL–Social-Awareness: Perspective-taking, empathy, recognize community resources. SEL–Social-Awareness: Perspective-taking SEL–Social-Awareness: Empathy SEL–Social-Awareness: Recognize community resources.	Students demonstrate taking perspective of a teen who is inactive, empathize with that teen, then help the teen design a daily 60-minute workout from a valid and reliable website.

Step 3 – Instruction
Design the instruction so that students learn the content, skill, and competency to be successful on the assessment. Ask yourself the question, "What do I need to teach so that the students will be successful when assessed?"

one barrier to exercising for 60 minutes on another. On the wall or white board, write Benefits of exercising for 60 minutes each day. Next to it, write the Barriers to exercising for 60 minutes each day. Invite the students up to place their ideas underneath the appropriate heading. Add any information or additional student input that may be missing.

b. Use **Worksheet 5.9 Benefits of and Barriers to Exercising for 60 Minutes Each Day** and the rationale on the board to role play. One teen explains the reasons why he/she cannot exercise and how miserable he/she feels. The other students put themselves in his/her shoes (perspective-taking) and empathize (share the feelings) then try to help by using the information on the worksheet and from the board to provide a rationale regarding the benefits of exercising 60 minutes each day. Conclude the role play with suggestions to overcome the barriers.

c. Benefits of being active for 60 minutes each day.
1) Improves heart and lung function
2) Boosts the immune system
3) Helps develop strong muscles, bones, and good posture
4) Helps to maintain weight and avoid being overweight.
5) Reduces the risk of high blood pressure, anxiety, depression and type 2 diabetes.
6) Breaks up long periods of sitting and studying
7) Helps to improve concentration and memory.
8) Provides the opportunity to learn new skills.
9) Increases self-confidence
10) Reduces stress
11) Improves sleep (raisingchildren.net.au, 2020)

d. Barriers to being active for 60 minutes each day.
1) No time to be physically active
2) Prefer screen time to active time
3) Do not have any energy
4) Not motivated
5) Afraid of injury
6) Not skilled in any physical activities
7) The weather makes being active difficult (too hot, too cool, etc.) (Centers for Disease Control and Prevention, 2020)

3. 3.12.1. Evaluate the validity of health information, products, and services *about physical activity.*
   a. Explain the SPAT method to evaluate a website (see Table 5.8).
   b. Use **Worksheet 5.10 Using SPAT to Evaluate a Website**.
4. 7.12.2 Demonstrate a variety of healthy practices and behaviors that maintain or improve the health of self and others, *such as three activities to have 60 minutes of physical activity for five days.*
   a. Use **Worksheet 5.11 Making a Plan to Become Physically Active** to design a physical activity plan
   b. Students demonstrate, through video, three of the physical activities completed during the five days.
5. Read the practice prompt. Students answer the reflection questions and discuss.

Practice Prompt: Lisseth

Lisseth is in the 10th grade. She used to be very active until she started working. As soon as school is over, she goes to the pizza shop and works until 7:00 PM. She snacks while she works and when she gets home, snacks again, spends time with her family, does her homework, checks social media, and goes to bed. She is putting on weight and getting very grumpy.

Manny and Melanie have seen a change in Lisseth. They used to hang out after school and bike, run, and do all sorts of fun things together. Although her friends invite her to join them on the weekend, Lisseth tells them, "I am too tired to do anything." As a result, she spends a lot of time on her phone or the computer.

Her friends have noticed that Lisseth is grumpy and asked why. "...because all I do is work! I stand in front of the register and take orders then, I get the orders off the shelf, call the person's number, and give them their order. The only exercise I get is in school, walking from class to class."

Mannie and Melanie feel bad for their friend and they know, if they were in the same position, they would be miserable too. They want to help. They made plans to meet on Saturday morning. They went for a walk and talked about getting active again. Lisseth said, "I don't see how I can get any physical activity in. I do not have any free time and, anyway, I am too tired. It is easier just to check social media and forget about being active!" Her friends reminded her that they were out walking now and walking is physical activity. "You are right, and I feel so much better being out with you and moving!"

They went back to Lisseth's house to check out openphysed.org for activities that teens can do at home. They evaluated the site in health class and know it is a valid and reliable place to get information about physical activity. They think walking, biking, and jumping rope will work best for them, which was the easy part. The challenge was to find the time to do it.

The friends decided to meet at school a half hour before the bell rings and walk around the building. That half hour, walking between classes, and throughout the day should give them the 60 minutes of activity they need. If they need more time, they will jump rope at home. On Saturday mornings, they plan to meet and go bike riding. There is a nice five-mile bike trail near their homes.

Lisseth thanked Manny and Melanie for helping her. They told her that they know she would do the same for them if they needed help. Lisseth is thankful for such good friends, feels so much better that she has more control over her life, and is confident she can be physically active, if she is mindful and follows through.

6. Use the review questions in **Table 5.11** to help the students understand how to demonstrate perspective-taking, empathy, and recognizing and using resources.
7. End of class review. Ask the students to put away their materials then ask review questions.
   a. What are three benefits of being physically active? (1.12.7)
   b. What are three barriers to being physically active? (1.12.7)
   c. Demonstrate how to evaluate a website using the SPAT method. (3.12.1)
   d. What are three physical activities busy teens can fit into their schedule? (7.12.2)
8. Exit ticket (Social-Awareness: Perspective-taking, empathy, and recognizing school resources)

   Use a sticky note to explain how taking perspective and being empathetic promotes and encourages positive friendships.

Table 5.11 How to Take Perspective of and Demonstrate Empathy for a Teen Who Needs Help Being Physically Active and Recognize Community Physical Activity Resources

Question	Answer
How did Lisseth <u>compare and contrast three benefits of</u> and three barriers to being active for 60 minutes each day. (1.12.7)	Benefits to Lisseth of being active for 60 minutes each day. • Spends time with friends • Doing fun activities • Feels more self-confident and in control of her life. Lisseth's Barriers to being active for 60 minutes each day. • Does not have time for physical activity because she works. • Is tired because she is in school all day and works until 7:00 PM. • It is easier just to check social media and forget about being physically active.
How did the friends <u>evaluate</u>, using the SPAT technique, the validity of Openpe.org website for information *about physical activity?* (3.12.1)	The friends knew openphysed.org was a valid and reliable site to find physical activity information because they used the SPAT method in health class to evaluate the site.
How did the friends demonstrate three activities from the plan that helps the teen be physically active for five days with 60 minutes of physical activity each day? (7.12.2)	The friends chose activities they did not have to learn. They knew they planned to find time to walk, bike, and jump rope.
SEL-Social-awareness: Perspective-taking, empathy, recognize community resources. SEL–Social-Awareness: Perspective-taking	Manny and Melanie took perspective of the situation and knew Lisseth was unhappy and that she would help them if they had the same problem.
SEL–Social-Awareness: Empathy	Lisseth's friends showed empathy when they felt badly when their friend was unhappy.
SEL–Social-Awareness: Recognize community resources	The friends used the SPAT method to evaluate openpe.org then use the information to find physical activities they could do at home.

Section 2. Appreciating Diversity/Respecting Others/Persevering in Addressing Challenges

Diversity is defined as a group of people from many cultures with different customs and habits.

From 2000 to 2017, the United States population increased by 15% from 282.2 million to 325.3 million. Adults 25 and older increased by 21% to 221.1 million. The college-age population (18–24) increased 13% to 30.8 million. School-age children aged 5–17 declined from 2010 to 2017 to 53.7 million (National Center for Education Statistics, 2020).

Because almost half of our school population represents minority groups, teachers take the perspective of the students and share their feelings (empathy). Being empathetic helps the teacher find and use appropriate instructional strategies. How teachers work with English Learners, students adapting to a new and different culture, and other groups, effects the relationship with all students. When teachers and students are respectful and positive, the classroom is more conducive to mutual understanding, respect, and sensitivity to a variety of cultures, ethnicities, races, and student needs. (Randy M. Page., 2015, p. 12)

Grades PreK–2: Social-Awareness: Appreciating Diversity/Respecting Others/Persevering in Addressing Challenges

Lesson Overview: Respecting Differences

Students explore their similarities and differences, how their physical, emotional, and social health is affected by not accepting differences, and who to talk to when there is a problem.

Resources:

- Online book: All Kinds of Children by Norma Simon. https://www.albertwhitman.com/book/all-kinds-of-children/

Materials needed:

- **Worksheet 5.12 Similarities and Differences**

Table 5.12 provides an overview of the lesson objectives, assessment, and instruction for this lesson.

Step 3 – Instruction

1. Define
   a. Identify: To recognize a particular person or an object.
   b. Recognize: To identify a person or thing because there is a history of having seen or

Table 5.12 Lesson Objectives, Assessment, and Instruction

Step 1 – Lesson Objectives	Step 2 – Assessment
The verb of the *infused* performance indicator and the SEL competency generate the assessment and instruction.	Design the assessment based on the objectives. Ask yourself the question, "What can my students do to show me they have met the standard?"
1.2.2 Recognize that the multiple dimensions of health *are affected when diversity is respected.* [Joint Committee on National Health Education Standards, 2007, p. 24]	1.2.2 Students recognize *one way* how not being respected for differences affects physical, emotional, and social health.
3.2.1 Identify trusted adults and professionals who help promote health *and diversity.* [Joint Committee on National Health Education Standards, 2007, p. 28]	3.2.1 Students identify *two* adults that help promote respecting diversity.
SEL-Social-awareness: Appreciating diversity, respecting others, persevering addressing challenges	Students demonstrate how to appreciate diversity, be respectful of differences, and keep trying when faced with a challenge.

Step 3 – Instruction
Design the instruction so that students learn the content, skill, and competency to be successful on the assessment. Ask yourself the question, "What do I need to teach so that the students will be successful when assessed?"

Table 5.13 Peer Similarities

Head	Body	Arms
Legs	Brain	Fingers
Toes	Hair	Other similarities

Table 5.15 Physical, Emotional, and Social Needs

Physical Needs	Emotional Needs	Social Needs
Food	Acceptance	Friends
Sleep	Respect	Kindness
Shelter		
Clothing		

interacted with that person or thing in the past.

   c. Diversity: A group of people from many cultures with different customs and habits.

2. 1.2.2 <u>Recognize</u> that the multiple dimensions of health *are affected when diversity is respected.*

   a. Distribute **Worksheet 5.12 Similarities and Differences, Page 1.** Students draw a picture of themselves with the details that make them unique. Students share their pictures with a peer and put a circle around features that are the same and a box around features that are different.

   b. To reflect, ask the children to stand if they have the items listed in **Table 5.13**.

   c. Reflect that the class has a lot of similarities. Now check the differences.

   d. To reflect, ask the children to stand if they have/are the items listed in **Table 5.14**.

   e. Reflect that even though there are lots of similar features, there are many things that make us different. Those differences make us a diverse classroom and an interesting place to be and to learn.

      Pages two and three of the worksheet are for the teacher.

   f. On page two, project or draw the graphic. Tell the students that we have many similarities and differences, but we all have physical, emotional, and social needs. Cut out

or project the needs (and any other that are appropriate for your students) and sort accordingly (**Table 5.15**).

3. 3.2.1 <u>Identify</u> trusted adults and professionals who help promote health *and diversity.*

   a. When finished sorting, reflect on who the students can turn to if they have problems in school or the community about accepting differences (diversity), respect, or when trying to overcome challenges related to diversity.

   b. Examples: teachers, parents, administrators, guidance counselors, clergy, community leaders, coaches, etc.

4. Read the practice prompt. Students answer the reflection questions and discuss.

Practice Prompt: Rashon

Rashon attends a school that has children from many cultures. The children get along most of the time but when a new student from a different culture comes to school, sometimes things do not go so smoothly.

The other day, Rashon heard his classmates talking about a new student, Rasheed, who is from another country and how different he looked and talked. He didn't look or sound different to Rashon because their families were from the same country.

The bus passes Rasheed's house and it is similar to everyone else's. His parents wait outside the house to make sure Rasheed gets on the bus safely and they looked nice. Rasheed's hair and skin color are different from his classmates but the same as his. Rasheed dresses like everyone else. Although the children were respectful, they weren't very accepting. Rashon invited Rasheed to sit with him during lunch. They got to know each other a little bit and realized they had a lot in common.

During afternoon recess, Rashon approached Rasheed. "How are you doing?" "I am OK, thanks, but many of our classmates stare at me and don't include

Table 5.14 Peer Differences

Boy	Girl	
Glasses	Skin is a beige/medium color	Hair is wavy
Do not have glasses	Skin is a dark color	Hair is curly
Skin is a light color	Hair is straight	Hair is light colored
Hair is a medium color	Hair is a dark color	*Other differences

*The children may be too young to ask about sexual orientation. Use your discretion.

(continues)

Practice Prompt: Rashon *(continued)*

me. They don't like me. I don't know what to do! You are my only friend! I don't think I will come to school tomorrow. I don't feel well." "Give them a little time," Rashon said. "You look different to them and they just need to get to know you. Then the differences won't matter." Rasheed thanked Rashon for being so kind and invited him to his house over the weekend. Both boys were pleased to have a new friend.

Meanwhile, the boys talked to their teacher about the situation and she thought it might be a good time to have their annual cultural celebration. She invited parents to the event and asked them to bring food and make a presentation about their background.

Community leaders also attended and brought gifts for the children that represented different cultures. Rasheed felt much better when he saw how different his classmates, their parents, and the community members were and realized he is not the only one who is different. He realizes he just needs to be himself and let his peers get to know him.

The celebration was a great success and Rasheed is looking forward to going to school tomorrow!

5. Use the review questions in **Table 5.16** to help the students understand how to accept differences, be respectful, and to keep trying when faced with a challenge.

6. End of class review. Ask the students to put away their materials then ask review questions.
   a. When peers do not accept differences in others, how does it affect physical, emotional, and social health? (1.2.2)
   b. When peers do accept differences in others, how does it affect physical, emotional, and social health? (1.2.2)
   c. Who is one adult who can help with accepting diversity, being respectful, and meeting the challenges of acceptance and respect? (3.2.1)

7. Exit ticket (Social-Awareness: Perspective-taking, empathy, and recognizing school resources)
   How does accepting differences, being respectful, and solving challenges help us to have a better learning environment?

Table 5.16 How to Appreciate Diversity/Respect Others/Persevering in Addressing Challenges

Question	Answer
What was one way that Rasheed's differences affected his physical, emotional, and social health? (1.2.2)	Physical health when differences were not accepted ■ Because of how the peers reacted to him, Rasheed felt sick and did not want to go to school the next day. Physical health when differences were accepted ■ Rasheed felt much better after the cultural festival and looked forward to going to school the next day. Emotional health when differences were not accepted ■ Rasheed did not feel accepted by his peers and that made him feel bad. Emotional health when differences were accepted ■ Rasheed realized after the cultural celebration that his peers are also very different and so are their parents and members of the community and that he just needs to be himself and let his peers get to know him. Social health when differences were not accepted Rasheed's classmates were respectful but not very accepting and that made him feel left out. ■ Rasheed felt that Rashon was his only friend. Social health when differences were not accepted ■ Rasheed realized after the cultural celebration that his peers are also very different and so are their parents and members of the community and that he just needs to be himself and let his peers get to know him.
Which two adults helped promote diversity, respect, and meeting challenges? (3.2.1)	The classroom teacher realized it was time to have the annual cultural celebration and invited the parents of her students and community members.

SEL-Social-Awareness: Appreciating diversity, respecting others, persevering in addressing challenges	
SEL-Social-Awareness: Appreciating diversity	The boys demonstrated how to appreciate diversity when they became friends and Rashon told Rasheed to give their classmates time. Rashon told Rasheed that when the classmates got to know him, the differences wouldn't matter.
SEL-Social-awareness: Respecting others	The peers in Rasheed's class were respectful of his differences.
SEL-Social-awareness: Persevering in addressing challenges	Rashon and Rasheed thought of a way to overcome the acceptance challenge. They spoke to their teacher and the teacher responded by organizing the annual cultural festival. This festival showed the children that each of them have differences and that the community and school support and accept them.

Grades 3–5: Social-Awareness: Appreciating Diversity/ Respecting Others/Persevering in Addressing Challenges

Lesson Overview: Accepting Differences

Students explore how their peers are different (diverse), how to accept those differences, and how to meet the challenges presented by being different.

Supportive background:

- Because the United States is becoming more diverse, students need to learn how to interact in a diverse learning environment.
- Cultural diversity enhances the school experience.
- Students who attend schools with a diverse population develop a different perspective about learning with children from different backgrounds.
- In the classroom,
  - use instructional strategies that include different perspectives.
  - Establish rules and norms for the classroom that encourage respect for and value differences. (Greatschoolstaff, 2012)
  - Model acceptance of others who have different attitudes and values.
  - Model respect and enthusiasm for learning about diversity.

- Use morning meetings to discuss how students in the same class may experience classroom and interpersonal events differently.
- Discuss how the behavior of one student affects all students.
- Acknowledge students who demonstrate respectful behavior.
- Ask students to explain how it feels when being respectful of others. (Collaborative for Academic Social Emotional Learning, 2020)

Resources:

- Simon, N. Reading book: Why am I different
- Corlis, M. Reading book: Same, Same But Different
- Teaching Tolerance Classroom Resources. https://www.tolerance.org/classroom-resources/teaching-strategies
- Teaching Tolerance: Mix it up: https://www.tolerance.org/mix-it-up
- Davis, M. Edutopia: Preparing for Cultural Diversity: Resources for Teachers. https://www.edutopia.org/blog/preparing-cultural-diversity-resources-teachers

Materials needed:

- **Worksheet 5.13 Appreciating Diversity**
- **Worksheet 5.14 Storybook to Identify Resources at Home, School, and the Community**

Table 5.17 provides an overview of the lesson objectives, assessment, and instruction for this lesson.

Table 5.17 Lesson Objectives, Assessment, and Instruction

Step 1 – Lesson Objectives	Step 2 – Assessment
The verb of the *infused* performance indicator and the SEL competency generate the assessment and instruction.	Design the assessment based on the objectives. Ask yourself the question, "What can my students do to show me they have met the standard?"

(continues)

Table 5.17 Lesson Objectives, Assessment, and Instruction *(continued)*

Step 1 – Lesson Objectives	Step 2 – Assessment
1.5.3 <u>Describe</u> ways a safe and healthy school and community environment *models acceptance of student differences, respect, and how to respond to the challenges of diversity.* (Joint Committee on National Health Education Standards, 2007, p. 24)	1.5.3 Students <u>describe</u> *three* ways the school and community models acceptance of student differences, respect, and how to respond to the challenges of diversity.
3.5.2 <u>Locate</u> resources from home, school, and community that provide valid health information about diversity, respecting differences, overcoming diversity challenges. (Joint Committee on National Health Education Standards, 2007, p. 28)	3.5.2 Students <u>locate</u> one resource from home, school, and the community that provide valid information about diversity, respecting differences, and meeting diversity challenges.
SEL–Social-Awareness: appreciating diversity, respecting others, and persevering in addressing challenges	Students demonstrate ways of appreciating the diversity of their peers, respecting the differences in their peers, and meeting diversity challenges.

Step 3 – Instruction

Design the instruction so that students learn the content, skill, and competency to be successful on the assessment. Ask yourself the question, "What do I need to teach so that the students will be successful when assessed?"

Step 3 – Instruction

1. Define
   a. Describe: To use words that help others envision the physical attributes of a person, place, or thing.
   b. Locate: To determine exactly where someone or something can be found.
   c. Diversity: A group of people from many cultures with different customs and habits.
   d. Strategy: The skill of making or carrying out plans to achieve a goal.
2. 1.5.3 Describe ways that a safe and healthy school and community environment *models acceptance of student differences, respect, and how to respond to the challenges of diversity*

   a. Read an online story to explain same and different such as Same, Same But Different by Megan Corlis. There are many book choices available. Find the one that best suits your students.
   b. On the board, write down Types of Diversity in Our School and ask the children to brainstorm the different ways students are different from each other. Examples are found in **Table 5.18** Diversity Examples: Peers. Add any additional group, as needed.
   c. On the board, write and explain.
      1) Strategies to help students accept peers who are different (diverse)/strategies to overcome the challenges of that diversity.

Table 5.18 Diversity Examples

From different countries	Who are visually impaired	Who have physical disabilities (wheelchair, etc.)
From different races	Who are hearing impaired	Who have speech and language disabilities
Who do not speak English	Who have learning disabilities (ADHD, writing, reading, etc.)	
From different cultural backgrounds	Who have medical disabilities (asthma, diabetes, allergies, etc.)	

2) Strategies to show respect to all peers but particularly to those who are different (diverse)/strategies to overcome the challenges of that diversity.

d. Ask students to write down their thoughts on sticky notes on how to meet the challenge of each and place them on the board under the appropriate category. The strategies listed below may contribute to the activity but should not limit the responses of the students.

e. Strategies to help students accept peers who are diverse/strategies to overcome the challenges of diversity.

1) Create a culture of acceptance in the classroom by providing opportunities for peers to get to know each other.

2) Spend time with another student and get to know him/her personally so they do not feel alone.

3) Buddy up for a day with a peer who is different to get to know and relate to him/her better. (Wiggs, 2014)

f. Strategies to show respect to all peers but particularly to those who are different/strategies to overcome the challenges of diversity.

1) Open the door for a person who has a physical disability.

2) Carry someone's book bag

3) Invite someone to sit with you at lunch.

4) Invite someone to play during recess.

5) Offer to interpret for an English learner.

6) Offer to be a tutor for a peer who is struggling in a subject or has a learning disability.

7) Plan a "Swap lunch" day where two peers from different cultures swap lunches. Note: Be mindful of food allergies.

g. Use **Worksheet 5.13 Appreciating Diversity** to reinforce how to appreciate diversity, be respectful, and meet the challenges of diversity.

3. 3.5.2 Locate resources from home, school, and community that provide valid health information about diversity, respecting differences, overcoming diversity challenges

a. Locate sources of valid information about diversity, respecting differences, and overcoming diversity challenges and distribute to the children.

b. Use **Worksheet 5.14 Storybook to Identify Resources at Home, School, and the Community** to identify, locate, and explain valid sources of information about diversity.

c. Resources (access local and community resources).

1) Home
   • Parents with high expectations: Keys to success in the family–school partnership. The Pacer Center, Champions for Children: https://www.pacer.org/pdf/ge/GE-1.pdf

2) School
   • Guidance
   • Special education liaison
   • English as a second language teacher
   • Disability coordinator

3) Community
   • Church
   • Boys/Girls Club
   • YMCA
   • Local government
   • Community centers

4. Read the practice prompt. Students answer the reflection questions and discuss.

Practice Prompt: Kaanta

Kaanta is one of many immigrants in his classroom. Many students do not speak English but are desperate to learn because they want to improve their lives. Kaanta's parents do not speak English and have a hard time communicating with the school. Kaanta interprets when his parents visit the school and receive mail in English.

Some of his classmates are friendly and some are not. Mrs. Elaina recognizes that the students are getting along well but decided to make a few changes in the classroom. One day, she asked the students to write down the characteristics that make them special. Students included what they look like, their culture, language, and what they like to do for fun.

The next day, pictures of each student were placed around the room. On the back of the picture was the description the student wrote. All the descriptions were placed into a large container and one by one, students took a description and tried to match it to the pictures. Mrs. Elaina walked from picture to picture to highlight the special qualities of each student. It helped Kaanta learn about his peers and realize he was not the only student who felt different.

(continues)

Practice Prompt: Kaanta
(continued)

Another day, Mrs. Elaina told the students they were going to "Buddy up" for a day. Kaanta and Joaquin were buddies. They didn't really know each other at the beginning of the day but by the end, realized they like the same food, go to the same church, and like to play soccer. It was fun to be together. It helped Kaanta feel less alone and more a part of the school.

Another day, Mrs. Elaina challenged the students to be mindful of showing respect to each other. It could be something as simple as holding the door or something harder like helping a peer with an assignment. Each time a peer helped another, he/she wrote down the kindness, put it in the jar, and rang the bell. Everyone stopped and said, "Excellent!" and Mrs. Elaina asked each student to explain his/her kindness. Kaanta helped clean up after activity time and helped another Spanish speaker complete an assignment. He got to ring the bell twice and felt great! He couldn't wait to tell his parents!

The principal loved Mrs. Elaina's work and asked her to include places where the children could find information about diversity at school, at home, and in the community, which was challenging. She asked a few parents and the English as a second language (ESL) teacher for ideas and they took pictures of people at school and community agencies that help children and their parents.

Kaanta is feeling much more at home in his new school and community. He enjoys being with his new friends and learning about them.

5. Use the review questions in **Table 5.19** to help the students understand how to accept differences, be respectful, and to keep trying when faced with a challenge.
6. End of class review. Ask the students to put away their materials then ask review questions.
    a. What is one strategy that helps us appreciate our differences (diversity)? (1.5.3)
    b. What is one strategy that demonstrates how to show respect for differences (diversity)? (1.5.3)
    c. What is one strategy that demonstrates how to overcome the challenges of being different (diversity)? (1.5.3)
    d. What is one resource from home, school, and the community that supports diversity? (3.5.2)

Table 5.19 How to Appreciate Diversity/Respect Others/Persevering in Addressing Challenges

Question	Answer
What were *three* ways the school and community modeled acceptance of student differences, respect, and how to respond to the challenges of diversity? (1.5.3)	Mrs. Elaina modeled how to accept the differences and diversity in others by designing three activities. 1. Photo matching 2. Buddy up day 3. The Kindness Jar
What is one resource from home, school, and the community that provided Kaanta with valid information about diversity, respecting differences, and meeting diversity challenges? (3.5.2)	Mrs. Elaina sought the advice of the ESL teacher and a few parents and together they took pictures and labeled people and places in the school and community where students and their families could get help.
SEL–Social-Awareness: Appreciating diversity, respecting others, persevering in addressing challenges	Mrs. Elaina placed pictures of the children around the room and peers matched a description to the picture. This activity helped the children appreciate their differences and their similarities.
SEL–Social-Awareness: Appreciating diversity	Mrs. Elaina also had a "Buddy Up" day where peers were paired for the day and had the opportunity to spend time with someone different.
SEL–Social-Awareness: Respecting others	Mrs. Elaina set up a Kindness Jar and students that showed respect or kindness toward another wrote down the kindness, put it in a jar, and rang a bell. The whole class said, "Excellent!"
SEL–Social-Awareness: Persevering in addressing challenges	Mrs. Elaina asked a few parents and the ESL teacher to identify community people and agencies that help children and their parents.

7. Exit ticket (Social-Awareness: Perspective taking, empathy, and recognizing school resources)

    How does accepting differences, being respectful, and solving challenges to help us with our social and emotional health?

Grades 6–8: Social-Awareness: Appreciating Diversity/ Respecting Others/ Persevering in Addressing Challenges

Lesson Overview: Accepting Differences

Students explore how their peers are different (diverse), how to accept those differences, and how to meet the challenges presented by being different.

More than half of school-aged children are ethnic minorities with Latinos as the largest minority and Asians as the fastest growing minority. Greater diversity in the middle school, with equal numbers of ethnic groups, results in less of a sense of social vulnerability for African American, Latino, Asian, and White youth.

Greater diversity in the student body both at the school and in the classroom is associated with less peer victimization and loneliness and a greater sense of safety. (Juvonen, 2018, pp. 1268, 1269, 1278)

Cross-ethnic peer relationships provide students with the opportunities to gain a new perspective of self and others. When ethnic minority students interact with students from other ethnicities, it is associated with increased academic performance. (Lewis, 2018)

Materials needed:

- **Worksheet 5.15 Respect**
- **Worksheet 5.16 Problems and Solutions to Accepting Differences**
- **Worksheet 5.17 Accessing Information about Diversity Clubs**
- **Worksheet 5.18 Making a Diversity Club Plan**

Table 5.20 provides an overview of the lesson objectives, assessment, and instruction for this lesson.

Step 3 – Instruction

1. Define
    a. Describe: To use words that help others envision the physical attributes of a person, place, or thing.
    b. Access: To be able to locate and use something.

Table 5.20 Lesson Objectives, Assessment, and Instruction

Step 1 – Lesson Objectives	Step 2 – Assessment
The verb of the *infused* performance indicator and the SEL competency generate the assessment and instruction.	Design the assessment based on the objectives. Ask yourself the question, "What can my students do to show me they have met the standard?"
1.8.5 <u>Describe</u> ways to reduce or prevent injuries and other adolescent health problems *by accepting and respecting diversity.* (Joint Committee on National Health Education Standards, 2007, p. 24)	1.8.5 Students <u>describe</u> *three* ways the school prevents adolescent health problems *related to accepting and respecting diversity.*
3.8.2 <u>Access</u> valid health information from home, school, and community *regarding school diversity groups.* (Joint Committee on National Health Education Standards, 2007, p. 28)	3.8.2 Students <u>access</u> valid health information *about three school diversity groups.*
7.8.2 <u>Demonstrate</u> healthy practices and behaviors to maintain or improve personal health. (Joint Committee on National Health Education Standards, 2007, p. 35)	7.8.2 Students <u>demonstrate</u> *a plan for a diversity school club.*
SEL–Social-Awareness: Appreciating diversity, respecting others, persevering in addressing challenges	Students appreciating diversity Respecting others Addressing challenges

Step 3 – Instruction
Design the instruction so that students learn the content, skill, and competency to be successful on the assessment. Ask yourself the question, "What do I need to teach so that the students will be successful when assessed?"

Table 5.21 Meanings of the Word Respect

Showing consideration for other people.	Caring for ourselves		Appreciating individual differences	Treating others the way you want to be treated
		© Orange Vectors/Shutterstock; Photo: © Matejknezevic/Shutterstock		
Showing consideration for the property of others including school accessories (book bag, pens, pencils, books, notebooks, etc.)	Caring for family	Caring for school relationships	Accepting individual differences	Caring for friends (Beverly Woods Elementary School, 2020)

c. Respect: A demonstration of reverence for a person or an object.

d. Demonstrate: To show how something is accomplished.

e. Prejudice: An unfounded negative feeling toward another person due to personal or cultural characteristics.

f. Discrimination: The act of treating people wrongly who are different.

g. Diversity: A group of people from many cultures with different customs and habits.

2. 1.8.5 Describe ways to reduce or prevent injuries and other adolescent health problems *by accepting and respecting diversity*.

a. Brainstorm the meaning of the word, "Respect." **Table 5.21**. Splash the sticky notes on the board and discuss.

b. Ask the students to look at the meanings on the board then write down on a sticky note, examples of ways to demonstrate respect for that meaning (**Table 5.22**). Place the sticky note on the board next to the meaning. Discuss.

c. To reinforce, use **Worksheet 5.15 Respect** to establishing the meaning of respect and how a teen demonstrates respect.

d. Discuss the meaning of prejudice and discrimination and the problems that may result.

Table 5.22 Examples of How to Demonstrate Respect

Use kind words when speaking to a peer.	Actively listen to what others have to say.	Appreciate the differences among peers.
Use good manners.	Value the opinion of others even if it differs from your own.	Value someone else's likes or dislikes.
Be sensitive to the feelings of others (empathy).	Follow the rules.	Take care of the property of others whether at school, home, or in the community.
Help others.	Do not mock, tease, or talk about someone.	Do not pressure someone into doing something he/she does not want to do. (Beverly Woods Elementary School, 2020)

Data from Beverly Woods Elementary School. (2020, May 30). Character Education: RESPECT. Retrieved from Beverly Woods Elementary School: https://schools.cms.k12.nc.us/beverlywoodsES/Documents/RespectSeptember2015.pdf.

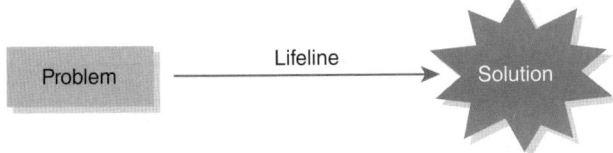

Figure 5.4 Providing a Solution and a Lifeline to Solve a Problem.

e. Use **Worksheet 5.16 Problems and Solutions to Accepting Differences** to explore the problems associated with being a student in a multiculture school.

1) Suggestion: Cut out the problems and distribute to the students. Distribute a "Solution Star" and when the solution suggestion is complete and approved, the student tapes the problem and the solution to the board, connected by a lifeline of string, yarn, paper, etc discuss (**Figure 5.4**).

2) Problems resulting from prejudice or discrimination. Possible responses may include but are not limited to the items shown in **Table 5.23**.

3) Strategies to overcome prejudice and discrimination and improve the acceptance of multicultural peers.
   - Accept the differences of the peer.
   - Respect the differences of the peer.
   - Get to know the peer.
   - Make the peer feel welcome.
   - Ask the peer to sit with you and your friends at lunch. (Lewis, 2018)
   - Speak up if bullying or harassment is observed.
   - Invite the peer to join a school club or athletic group.
   - Discover the things each of you have in common.

- Discuss how the media helps/does not help in solidifying differences instead of celebrating the differences.

3. 3.8.2 Access valid health information from home, school, and community *regarding school diversity groups*.

a. The web has an abundance of examples of diversity clubs. Below are just a few. By giving students valid and reliable websites, they access them rather than using the SPAT method to analyze the validity of websites.

b. As the students access the sites, use **Worksheet 5.17 Accessing Information about Diversity Clubs** as a tool to gather information about the different types of clubs.

1) Cultural Appreciation Clubs: https://blog.collegevine.com/cultural-appreciation-clubs-celebrating-your-heritage-educating-others-and-boosting-your-college-applications/

2) The World Culture Club: https://www.scarsdaleschools.k12.ny.us/Page/11905

3) Multicultural Club-Shawnee High School: www.lrhsd.org

4) Cultural Diversity Club Morton East High school: https://www.morton201.org/Page/516#calendar1534/20200529/month

4. 7.12.2 Demonstrate a variety of healthy practices and behaviors that maintain or improve the health of self and others *such as making a plan to establish school diversity groups*. (Joint Committee on National Health Education Standards, 2007, p. 35)

a. Use **Worksheet 5.18 Making a Diversity Club Plan** and the information on **Worksheet 5.16** to design a diversity club for your school.

5. Read the practice prompt. Students answer the reflection questions and discuss.

Table 5.23 Problems Resulting from Prejudice or Discrimination

Fear of someone who is different	Potential violence/bullying	Feeling alone/lonely	Irrational dislike of someone who is different
Uncertainty about being with someone who is different	Not feeling accepted by others.	Suspicion of peers who are different	Negative media depiction of peers who are different.
Discomfort in being with someone who is different.	Not feeling liked by peers	One group intolerant of another	(Meeks, 2020, p. 616)

Data from Meeks, L. H. (2020). *Comprehensive School Health Education*, (9th ed.). New York: McGraw Hill, p. 616.

Practice Prompt: George and Jose

George is in the 8th grade of a school where there are many different ethnicities. Each group stays together, however, and seldom hangs out with the other. Everyone is in different classes together and seem to get along but in the mornings before classes start, in the hall between classes, at lunch, and after school, there is a problem.

Mrs. Da'Shawni notices the problems during her duty times and wants to do something about it. As the students entered her health class, she gave them each a "Thought cloud" and asked them to finish the sentence: I can show respect to someone who is different from me by.... She taped the "clouds" to the board and asked the students to walk around and read them. The students were surprised that many of the comments were similar.

The teacher challenged the class to put themselves in the shoes of someone from a different ethnic group. She explained this exercise would help us gain perspective of people who are different from themselves. George decided to think about the Hispanic boy, Jose, who sits next to him. He likes Jose but because he looks and talks different, George only completes assignments with him and doesn't try to make friends. George realized that maybe his actions make Jose feel left out, unpopular, and uncomfortable. He decided to ask Jose if he wanted help with his writing and told him, "We can stay after school and go over the assignments and I'll help you." "Gracias," said Jose. At the afterschool homework club, the boys got to know each other. George helped Jose with his assignments and Jose was very happy to coach George for his Spanish class!

The boys looked for other ways to get to know each other but didn't find any. They approached Mrs. Da'Shawni and asked her if they could start a Multi-Cultural Club. She liked the idea but told them they would have to research other middle school diversity groups and come back with a plan. She gave them the websites of other schools in the nearby area that have those groups.

The boys researched and planned for two weeks. George asked a few of his friends to help and so did Jose. The group researched, put together ideas from several schools, and developed a plan. When they presented it, Mrs. Da'Shawni was very pleased and told the group that she would present it to the principal.

The principal loved the idea, met with the group and Mrs. Da'Shawni, and give her approval. They are very excited to start their club but know they have many obstacles to overcome to get the student body to join them. They plan to start with a Respect Campaign, conduct a survey to determine problems students experience, and then work together to develop a solution.

6. Use the review questions in **Table 5.24** to help the students understand how to accept differences, be respectful, and to keep trying when faced with a challenge.
7. End of class review. Ask the students to put away their materials then ask review questions.
   a. What is one way a school can help students with different ethnic backgrounds accept and celebrate their differences? (1.8.5)
   b. Why is it important to access valid information when researching? (3.8.2)
   c. Why is it important to demonstrate what is learned from accessing valid information? (7.8.2)
8. Exit ticket (Social-Awareness: Perspective-taking, empathy, and recognizing school resources)
   What is one way to show respect to a peer who is from a different cultural background?

Table 5.24 How to Appreciate Diversity/Respect Others/Persevering in Addressing Challenges

Question	Answer
What were three ways George's school prevented adolescent health problems related to accepting and respecting diversity? (1.8.5)	Mrs. Da'Shawni, the health teacher, observed that the different ethnic groups did not get along outside of class so she started class with a "Thought Cloud" activity where the students finished the sentence... I can show respect to someone who is different from me by.... Mrs. Da'Shawni challenged the class to gain perspective of a peer from a different culture by trying to put themselves in the shoes of a peer who is different from them. Mrs. Da'Shawni encouraged George and Jose to research diversity clubs. The principal supported starting a new multicultural club.

How did the students <u>access</u> valid health information *about three school diversity groups?* (3.8.2)	The teacher provided George and Jose with websites of *(continued)* different schools that have diversity clubs. The boys accessed them and researched the clubs.
How did George, Jose, and their friends <u>demonstrate</u> how to plan for a new multicultural club? (7.8.2)	George, Jose, and a few friends researched the diversity clubs of other schools and designed a plan for their school. The principal approved the idea and they planned a Respect Campaign and to use the results of a survey to develop programs.
SEL–Social-Awareness: Appreciating diversity, respecting others, persevering in addressing challenges	
SEL–Social-Awareness: Appreciating diversity	The school demonstrated it appreciates diversity by approving a new Multi-Cultural club.
SEL–Social-Awareness: Respecting others	Mrs. Da'Shawni demonstrated her concern about students respecting each other by starting class with a "Thought Cloud" activity.
SEL–Social-Awareness: Persevering in addressing challenges	The diversity challenges of the school were met by starting a new Multi-Cultural club.

Grades 9–12: Social-awareness: Appreciating Diversity/Respecting Others/Persevering in Addressing Challenges

Lesson Overview: Appreciating Diversity

Students explore discrimination and how to use the Whole School, Whole Community, Whole Child model to increase student connectedness.

A Pew Center survey found that 52% of U.S. Latina/os reported experiencing discrimination based on their race or ethnicity. Reducing discrimination in schools and enhancing school connectedness are protective factors for teens who are thinking of dropping out of school. (McWhirter, 2018)

Black students were 54% less likely than white students to be recommended for gifted-education programs, after adjusting for factors such as students'

standardized test scores. Solutions to reduce disparities are focused on social-emotional learning, better relationships, and building community. (Weir, 2016)

Resources:

- School connectedness: Strategies for increasing protective factors among youth, CDC: https://www.cdc.gov/healthyyouth/protective/pdf/connectedness.pdf

Materials needed:

- **Worksheet 5.19 Effects of Discrimination on the Components of Health**
- **Worksheet 5.20 Student Story of the Effects of Discrimination on the Components of Health**
- **Worksheet 5.21 School Connectedness**
- **Worksheet 5.22 Getting Connected!**

Table 5.25 provides an overview of the lesson objectives, assessment, and instruction for this lesson.

Table 5.25 Lesson Objectives, Assessment, and Instruction

Step 1 – Lesson Objectives	Step 2 – Assessment
The verb of the *infused* performance indicator and the SEL competency generate the assessment and instruction.	Design the assessment based on the objectives. Ask yourself the question, "What can my students do to show me they have met the standard?"
1.12.2 <u>Describe</u> *how discrimination affects* the interrelationships of emotional, intellectual, physical, and social health. (Joint Committee on National Health Education Standards, 2007, p. 25)	1.12.2 Students <u>describe</u> *one way discrimination affects* emotional, intellectual, physical, and social health.

(continues)

Table 5.25 Lesson Objectives, Assessment, and Instruction (continued)

Step 1 – Lesson Objectives	Step 2 – Assessment
3.12.2 <u>Use</u> resources from home, school, and community that provide valid health information *about how to increase school connectedness.* [Joint Committee on National Health Education Standards, 2007, p. 29]	3.12.2 Students <u>use</u> the resources from the Wellness Team to provide valid health information *about how to increase school connectedness.*
SEL–Social-Awareness: Appreciating diversity, respecting others, persevering in addressing challenges	Students appreciating diversity Respecting others Addressing challenges

Step 3 – Instruction
Design the instruction so that students learn the content, skill, and competency to be successful on the assessment. Ask yourself the question, "What do I need to teach so that the students will be successful when assessed?"

Step 3 – Instruction

1. Define
   a. Describe: To use words that help others envision the physical attributes of a person, place, or thing.
   b. Discrimination: The act of treating people wrongly who are different.
   c. Diversity: A group of people from many cultures with different customs and habits.
   d. Prejudice: An unfounded negative feeling toward another person due to personal or cultural characteristics.
   e. Protective factors: Individual or environmental characteristics, conditions, or behaviors that reduce the effects of stressful life events; increase an individual's ability to avoid risks or hazards; and promote social and emotional competence to thrive in all aspects of life now and in the future. (Centers for Disease Control and Prevention, 2009)
   f. Respect: A demonstration of reverence for a person or an object.
   g. Risk Factors: Individual or environmental characteristics, conditions, or behaviors that increase the likelihood that a negative outcome will occur. (Centers for Disease Control and Prevention, 2009)

   h. School connectedness: Belief by students that adults and peers in the school care about their learning as well as about them as individuals. (Centers for Disease Control and Prevention, 2009)
2. 1.12.2 Describe *how discrimination affects* the interrelationships of emotional, intellectual, physical, and social health.
   a. Ask students to brainstorm types of discrimination (**Table 5.26**).
   b. Use **Worksheet 5.20 Effects of Discrimination on the Components of Health** to analyze how discrimination affects emotional, intellectual, physical, and social health (**Table 5.27**).
   c. Once the students complete the graphic organizer and discuss the results, ask them to write a story about someone they know who has experienced discrimination. Include suggestions on how to decrease discrimination and improve personal health. Swap papers, make comments, and share.
3. 2.3.12.2 <u>Use</u> resources from home, school, and community that provide valid health information *about how to increase school connectedness.*
   a. Project, draw, or distribute the graphic organizer. (**Worksheet 5.21 School Connectedness**)

Table 5.26 Types of Discrimination

Racism	Immigrant status	Size (small, medium, large body)	Sexual orientation
Homophobia	Cultural/Ethnic background	Intellectual	Gender
Disability	Gender identity	Religion	

Table 5.27 The Effects of Discrimination on the Components of Health

Component of Health	Effect of Discrimination
Emotional Health	■ Depression ■ Distressed ■ Distracted ■ Anxiety
Intellectual Health	■ Difficulty achieving because expectations may be low. ■ Increased ADHD
Physical Health	■ Higher cortisol levels (evidence of stress) (Huynh, 2016) ■ Injured ■ Sleep problems ■ Bullied ■ Increased substance use
Social Health	■ Isolated from peers ■ Worried about social climate (Polakovic, 2018)

b. Ask the students to think of a definition for school connectedness. Write the definition in the graphic organizer circle. *Explain that school connectedness is important because students are more likely to engage in healthy behaviors and succeed academically when they are connected to school.* (Centers for Disease Control and Prevention, 2009, p. 5)

c. Read the statements in **Figure 5.5** and ask the students to align them to a connector. As an alternative, prepare the statements on stickies or clouds, and ask the students to place the statement next to the connector. (home, school, community).

d. Add additional connectors suggested by the students and discuss.

e. Use **Worksheet 5.22 Getting Connected!** To challenge the students to meet with the School Wellness Team and ask them what resources they provide to help teens connect to the school. Examples may include:

1) Health education: Peer leadership club
2) Physical Education & Physical Activity: Before and after school fitness clubs

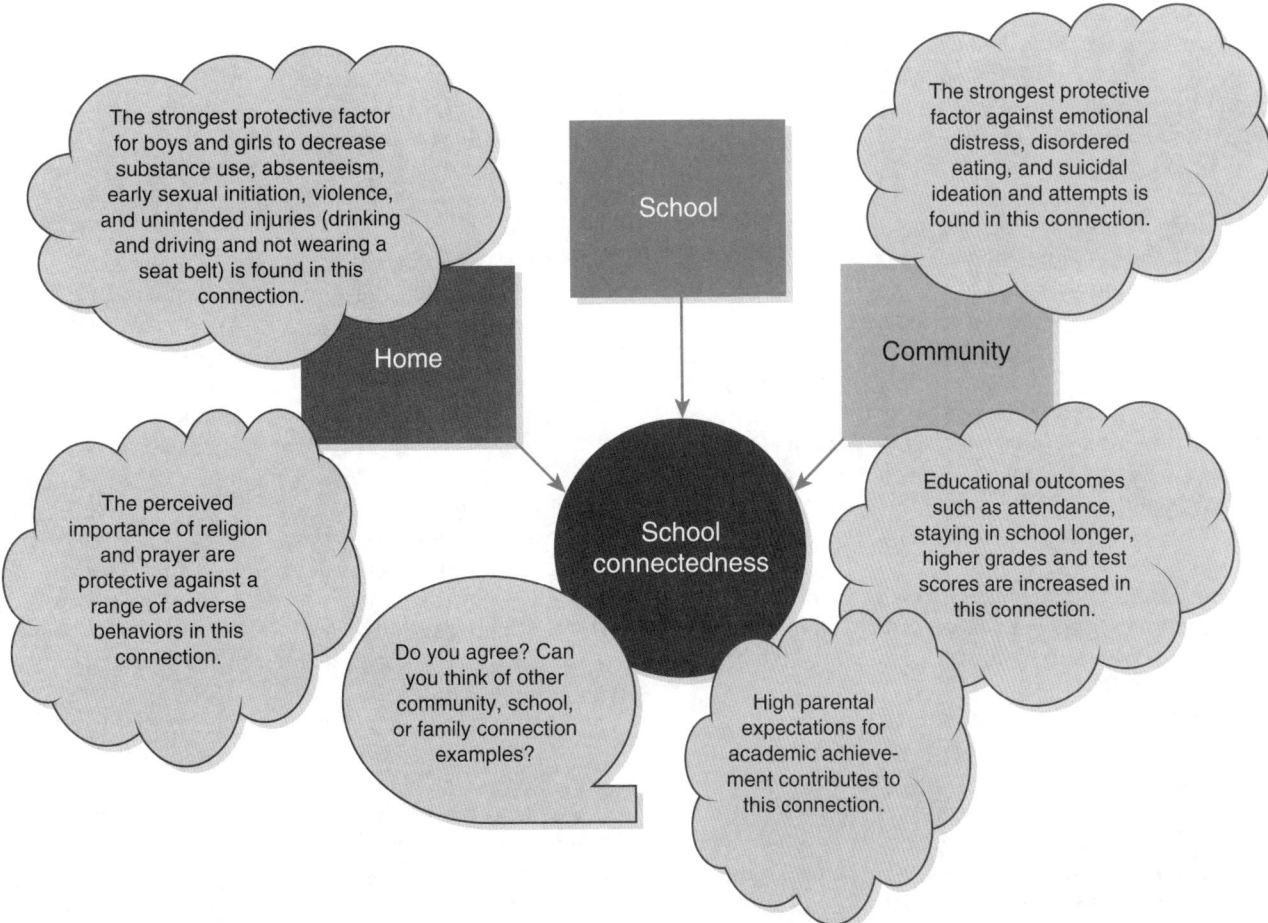

Figure 5.5 School Connectedness.

3) Nutrition Environment & Services: Executive lunch (students eat lunch in a special room set up for them to share ideas and ways to connect)

4) Health services: Future nurses club

5) Social & Emotional Climate: Pulse Club (Students survey to determine student needs then design programs to meet the needs)

6) Counseling, Psychological & Social Services: Public health club

7) Physical Environment: Custodial Connection (meet with the custodians and discuss ways the school environment can reflect the diversity of the school body.)

8) Employee Wellness: Make suggestions for professional development that helps teachers to work more effectively with diverse populations. (teacher expectations, classroom management, etc.)

9) Family Engagement: Attend parent-school meetings and provide suggestions about how the parents can connect better with the school to support students.

10) Community Involvement: Invite community members to school to brainstorm ways they can better connect with the school to provide support to students.

4. Read the practice prompt. Students answer the reflection questions and discuss.

Practice Prompt: Floyd

Floyd is in the 9th grade and thinking of quitting school. He doesn't feel connected to his teachers or to most of his peers. His courses are easy so sometimes he gets in trouble because he is bored and fidgety. He tried telling his teachers he can do more, but the message does not get through. His grades are not good so the teachers don't think he should be moved to a higher level. Floyd sees other peers moved up and wonders why he is being treated differently. He is very upset, has having trouble sleeping, and lost his appetite. He gets a headache as soon as he steps into the high school.

Floyd tried to make an appointment with his guidance counselor, but she was busy helping the students who were preparing their college applications. It is like he is invisible. He looks at his peers in the harder classes and he knows he can do the work. He does not understand why he is overlooked.

He enjoys wearing clothes that the other boys from the neighborhood wear but gets a lot of stares and comments from his peers when he walks by. Everyone seems to look at him with suspicion and it is stressing him out! Sometimes, he thinks the school is a very hostile place and doesn't want to be there.

His parents make him go to church every week and he enjoys the singing but questions the preaching. Why is everyone always trying to tell him what to do?

Floyd has a good voice and thought he would try out for the school play but no one he knows is interested in joining and he would look very different from everyone else there. He thought he would like to be a Peer Leader but does not know anyone in the club or how to join. He does not think he would be accepted, anyway.

His parents want him to do well in school but do not attend open house, parent conferences, or meetings of the parent parent-teacher group. They are different from the other parents and don't feel comfortable at school. Because they are not involved, it makes him feel alone and disconnected.

One day his guidance counselor, Mrs. Goodwill sent for him. He was surprised and wondered what he did wrong. She apologized for not being able to schedule him sooner but had plenty of time now. Floyd explained what was going on. She had several suggestions that really made him feel better. First, she will test him for a learning disability to rule out any problems then talk with his teachers. If he has no learning disability and if he is willing to work hard to catch up, she will try to schedule him in more challenging classes.

Next, she plans to call Floyd's parents and ask them to come to school. She will send the social worker to his home if his parents do not respond.

Then they talked about the school clubs. Mrs. Goodwill is the Chair of the Wellness Team and a friend of the health teacher. She thought that being a peer leader would be a great choice for him. He will have to bring up his grades to be accepted but Mrs. Goodwill thought the activities would increase his self-esteem and enable him to befriend other boys who are feeling disconnected.

"Taking on the drama club might be too much if you become a peer leader," said Mrs. Goodwill, "but joining the church teen choir would be excellent." She explained the more he got involved in things, the more connected he would feel.

Floyd felt great! He had a great day and told his parents all about it when he got home. They were very happy for him and agreed to attend the meeting with Mrs. Goodwill.

5. Use the review questions in **Table 5.28** to help the students understand how to accept differences, be respectful, and to keep trying when faced with a challenge.
6. End of class review. Ask the students to put away their materials then ask review questions.
   a. What is *one way discrimination affects* emotional, intellectual, physical, and social health? (1.12.2)

b. What is one way the Wellness team contributes to connecting students to school?
7. Exit ticket (Social-Awareness: Perspective-taking, empathy, and recognizing school resources)

What is one thing you can do to decrease discrimination in your school?

Table 5.28 How to Appreciate Diversity/Respect Others/Persevere in Addressing Challenges

Question	Answer
What is *one way discrimination affected* Floyd's emotional, intellectual, physical, and social health? (1.12.2)	Floyd's Emotional health ■ Is frustrated that he is in classes that are boring and do not challenge him. ■ Is easily distracted because he is bored. ■ Feels overlooked and not important. ■ Feels that everyone is trying to tell him what to do. ■ His parents do not attend any school meetings or events and that makes him feel alone and disconnected. ■ He feels invisible and lost. Floyd's Intellectual health ■ Is frustrated that he is in classes that are boring and do not challenge him. ■ Is easily distracted because he is bored. Floyd's Physical health ■ Is having trouble sleeping ■ Has lost his appetite ■ Gets headaches as soon as he enters the school. Floyd's Social health ■ Peers look at him with suspicion. ■ Cannot connect with clubs he is interested in joining.
How did Floyd <u>use</u> the resources from the Wellness Team to provide valid health information *about how to increase school connectedness?* (3.12.2)	Health education: Floyd will apply to become a peer leader. Counseling, Psychological, and Social Services: Mrs. Goodwill, the guidance counselor, helped Floyd with his courses and choosing a club. Family Engagement: Mrs. Goodwill will reach out to Floyd's parents to talk about what they can do together to help Jackson. Community Involvement: Floyd attends church with his parents and will try out for the choir.
SEL–Social-awareness: Appreciating diversity, respecting others, persevering in addressing challenges	
SEL–Social-Awareness: Appreciating diversity	The school demonstrated that they appreciate diversity by helping Floyd with his schoolwork and encouraging him to apply to peer leadership.
SEL–Social-Awareness: Respecting others	The guidance counselor demonstrated respect for Floyd by setting up an appointment with him, listening to him, having him tested for a learning disability, engaging his family, talking to his teachers about a different placement, and finding the appropriate club for his interests and skill.

(continues)

Table 5.28 How to Appreciate Diversity/Respect Others/Persevere in Addressing Challenges *(continued)*

Question	Answer
SEL–Social-awareness: Persevering in addressing challenges	The school demonstrated their willingness to meet diversity challenges by encouraging Floyd to apply to the Peer Leadership Club. Mrs. Goodwill told Floyd that becoming a member will be good for his self-esteem and he could help other boys who also experienced feeling alone and disconnected.

Sample Lesson Plan for Social Awareness

Unit: *State the unit of the lesson.*	Practicing Healthy Behaviors
Topic: *State the topic of the lesson.*	Coping with bullying by taking perspective, being empathetic, and accessing community resources.
Grade level: *State the grade level of the lesson.*	Grades 3–5
Time allotment: *State the time allotted for the lesson.*	40 minutes
Lesson summary: *Provide a summary of the lesson*	In this lesson, students intervene in bullying after taking perspective of the situation, being empathetic toward the victim, and accessing community resources
Risk behavior data: *Provide time rationale for this lesson by accessing the risk behavior the lesson reduces.*	38.6% (female: 44.8%; males: 32.6%) to 48.8% (females: 54.2%; males: 43.6%) of middle school students report ever being bullied on school property.
Standards and SEL Competency to reduce the risk factor(s): *List the Standard 1 and skills standards and the SEL competency/subcompetency.*	1.5.2. <u>Describe</u> the relationship between healthy behaviors and personal health. 3.5.2 <u>Locate</u> resources from home, school, and community that provide valid health information. SEL–Social-awareness: Perspective taking, empathy, community resources.
Objectives: *The objectives are the infused performance indicators and SEL competency.*	1.5.2. <u>Describe</u> the relationship between healthy behaviors, *such as being empathetic toward a bullying victim*, and personal health. 3.5.2 <u>Locate</u> resources from home, school, and community that provide valid health information *about bullying*. SEL–Social-awareness: Perspective taking, empathy, community resources.
Lesson assessment: *Design an assessment for each infused performance indicator and SEL competency.*	Students <u>describe</u> *three* effects on personal health of being empathetic to a bullying victim. Students <u>locate</u> school resources about bullying. SEL: Students take perspective of a child being bullied, show empathy, and recognize school resources.

Lesson instruction: *Provide a detailed description of how content, skill, and SEL competency are taught, "bell to bell."*	Review/Preview
	    Ask the children if they know anyone who has been bullied.
	    Ask what another child can do to help the victim of bullying.
	    Ask the children what empathy means to them. Explain.
	    Ask the children what taking perspective means. Explain.
	
	Lesson Objectives
	Students describe how being empathetic toward a victim affects their health and how to take perspective of a situation and locate school resources when someone is being bullied. Clarify definitions of vocabulary, if needed.

Lesson

1. 1. 1.5.1 Describe the relationship between healthy behaviors *such as being empathetic* and personal health
   a. Benefits of being empathetic
      1) Improves relationships
      2) Promotes understanding of self
      3) Improves the ability to take perspective of the experiences of others
   b. Model how to show empathy. Example: Set up a role play with a student. Approach the student and say,

      > "Melanie, it is OK. I understand that you are upset because you left your schoolwork at home. You are a responsible student and care about your work. (Empathy) Sometimes I forget things at home, and I know how upsetting it can be." (Perspective taking) Show me your work tomorrow and I'll grade you then. "Thank you," Melanie said with a smile on her face.

   c. Reflect
      1) Ask the children to explain what they observed.
      2) Explain that when we understand the feelings of another and try to help, we are showing empathy.
      3) Explain that when we put ourselves in another person's situation to understand better what is going on, that is taking perspective.
      4) How did the teacher show empathy to Melanie?
      5) How did the teacher take perspective of the situation?
      6) How did the student feel when the teacher told her she could pass in her work tomorrow?
   d. Use **Worksheet 5.3 Demonstrating How to Be Empathetic Toward a Bullying Victim and the Effect it Has on Personal Health.**

2. 3.5.2 Locate resources from home, school, and community that provide valid health information *about bullying*
   a. Ask the children where they can find information about bullying at school?
      1) Teacher
      2) Classroom/gymnasium
      3) Hallways
      4) Nurse's office
      5) Lunchroom
      6) Offices of the principal/assistant principle.
   b. Ask the children who are the trusted adults in the school they can go to if they are bullied or know someone who is bullied.

3. Read the practice prompt then ask the students the reenforcement questions.

Practice Prompt: Eloise

Eloise thought she had friends but all that has changed. The other day, the teacher was leading the class to the gymnasium when three girls behind her started making fun of her clothes. Eloise likes to dress a little differently, preferring colorful dresses to pants. Mrs. Dresser didn't hear the girls, but they were taunting her saying she looked like a cartoon character. They said, "Wait until we are in the gym, that dress won't be so colorful anymore!" They pointed at her and laughed. Eloise thought, "They didn't like what I was wearing last week either!" Eloise is upset but doesn't know what to do to make them stop.

Her line partner, Antoinette, heard the girls and looked back at them and told them to stop. In the gym, Antoinette told Eloise she heard the girls and didn't like what was happening. Eloise was relieved. She told Eloise that she would stay close by in case the girls started taunting her again.

Eloise and Antoinette felt empowered when they made a plan to tell the girls to stop and told them they were going to tell their teachers if they didn't. Once they reminded the girls that Mrs. Dresser taught their class about bullying, told the children that the school policy says bullying is not acceptable, and that bullies would be held accountable for their behavior, the bullying stopped.

Eloise and Antoinette became friends and have a lot of fun together. They sit together on the bus, are partners when they go to their specialist classes, eat lunch together, and invite each other to their homes. Together, they proudly told Eloise's parents about the bullying and how they got it to stop.

Eloise feels great that someone understood what she was going through and was willing to help her. Antoinette also feels great because she helped a peer and gained a friend!

(Stop Bullying, 2020)

4. Use the following review questions to help the children review healthy ways to cope with stress.

Question	Answer
What were three effects on Eloise's and Antoinette's personal health when Antoinette demonstrated empathy? (1.5.1)	Improved relationships ■ Eloise felt great because she gained a friend. ■ Antoinette felt great because she helped a peer and gained a friend. ■ Antoinette told the bullies to stop and if they didn't, she would tell the teacher. The bullies stopped. Promoted understanding of self ■ Eloise was relieved that Antoinette understood the situation and was willing to help her. ■ Eloise and Antoinette were proud to tell Eloise's parents about how they stopped the bullying. ■ Eloise and Antoinette felt empowered when they make a plan to tell their teacher if the bullying didn't stop. Helped to take perspective of the situations others experience ■ Antoinette told Eloise she heard the girls bullying her and didn't like it. Eloise was relieved. Antoinette told Eloise that she would stay close by in case the girls started taunting her again.
How did Eloise and Antoinette locate school resources about bullying? (3.5.2)	The girls knew Mrs. Dresser already taught their class about bullying, explained that the school policy says bullying is not acceptable, and that bullies would be held accountable for their behavior.
SEL–Social-awareness: Perspective taking, empathy, community resources.	
SEL–Social-awareness: Perspective taking	Antoinette knew that the words from the other peers couldn't make Eloise feel very good. (perspective-taking)

	SEL–Social-awareness: Empathy	Antoinette realized that Eloise was upset because the girls behind her were (empathy) taunting her.
	SEL–Social-awareness: Community resources.	Antoinette and Eloise developed a plan to tell the bullies to stop and if they didn't, Eloise and Antoinette would tell their teacher. (recognizing school resources)
Materials: *List the materials used to plan and implement the lesson, including formative assessments.*	**Worksheet 5.3 Demonstrating How to Be Empathetic toward a Bullying Victim and the Effect it Has on Personal Health.**	
Resources: *What resources were used to plan and implement the lesson?*	<ul><li>Arthur: So Funny I Forgot to Laugh (empathy): https://pbskids.org/arthur/friends/so-funny</li><li>Understood.org: How to show empathy to your students with compassionate curiosity: https://www.understood.org/en/school-learning/for-educators/empathy/using-compassionate-curiosity-to-drive-empathy?_ul=1*8pjd5t*domain_userid*YW1wLUdnNFdocGNScm9xUmlvQ1dXNmVRRVE</li><li>Understood.org: Teacher to Teacher: Use a Daily Warm-up to Build Empathy: https://www.understood.org/en/school-learning/for-educators/empathy/teacher-to-teacher-use-a-daily-warm-up-to-build-empathy?_ul=1*1ro98sf*domain_userid*YW1wLUdnNFdocGNScm9xUmlvQ1dXNmVRRVE</li><li>See additional resources in the chapter.</li></ul>	
Differentiated instruction: *What modifications are being made for students with disabilities and English Learners?*	Students work in groups specifically designed to support students with disabilities or English learners.	
Sample student products: *Provide exemplars of how other students successfully complete this assignment.*	Show previously completed worksheets.	
Collaboration: *Are the students completing the activity individually, in pairs, in groups, etc.?*	Students work in groups of four to pair up or work as a group.	
Teacher reflection: *What can I do to improve this lesson next time it is taught?*	Will vary.	

References

Morin, A. (2020). *The importance of teaching children impulse control*. Retrieved from verywellfamily https://www.verywellfamily.com/the-importance-of-teaching-children-impulse-control-1095019

Beverly Woods Elementary School. (2020). *Character education: RESPECT*. Retrieved from Beverly Woods Elementary School: https://schools.cms.k12.nc.us/beverlywoodsES/Documents/RespectSeptember2015.pdf

CASEL. (2019). *What is SEL?* Retrieved from CASEL: https://casel.org/what-is-sel/

Centers for Disease Control and Prevention. (2009). *School connectedness: Strategies for increasing protective factors among youth*. Atlanta, Georgia: U.S. Department of Health and Human Services.

Centers for Disease Control and Prevention. (2020). *2019 Middle School YRBS Ever Being Bullied on School Property*. Retrieved from Center for Disease Control and Prevention https://nccd.cdc.gov/youthonline/App/Results.aspx?TT=B&OUT=0&SID=MS&QID=M12&LID=LL&YID=RY&LID2=&YID2=&COL=&ROW1=&ROW2=&HT=&LCT=&FS=&FR=&FG=&FA=&FI=&FP=&FSL=&FRL=&FGL=&FAL=&FIL=&FPL=&PV=&TST=&C1=&C2=&QP=&DP=&VA=CI&CS=Y&SYID=&EYID=&SC=&SO=

Centers for Disease Control and Prevention. (2019). *2019 High School YRBS not physically active for all 7 days prior to the survey*. Retrieved from Centers for Disease Control and Prevention https://nccd.cdc.gov/youthonline/App/Results.aspx?TT=B&OUT=0&SID=HS&QID=QNPA7DAY&LID=LL&YID=RY&LID2=&YID2=&COL=&ROW1=&ROW2=&HT=&LCT=&FS=&FR=&FG=&FA=&FI=&FP=&FSL=&FRL=&FGL=&FAL=&FIL=&FPL=&PV=&TST=&C1=&C2=&QP=&DP=&VA=CI&CS=Y&SYID=&EYID=&SC=&SO=

Centers for Disease Control and Prevention. (2020). *Overcoming barriers to physical activity*. Retrieved from Centers for Disease Control and Prevention https://www.cdc.gov/physicalactivity/basics/adding-pa/barriers.html

Collaborative for Academic and Social Emotional Learning. (2020). *CASEL Competencies*. Retrieved from CASEL https://casel.org/wp-content/uploads/2019/12/CASEL-Competencies.pdf

Collaborative for Academic Social Emotional Learning. (2020). *www.casel.org/.../08/Sample-Teaching-Activities-to-Support-Core-Competencies-8-20-17.pdf*. Retrieved from CASEL.org www.casel.org/.../08/Sample-Teaching-Activities-to-Support-Core-Competencies-8-20-17.pdf[Au: This link is not working.]

Connolly, M. (2020). *Skills-based health education*, (2nd ed.). Burlington, MA: Jones and Bartlett.

Courtney Ward, J. R. (2020). *Lesson plans*. Retrieved from https://learningwardinstruction.wordpress.com/character-ed/self-control-bubbles/

de Brey, C. Musu, L., McFarland, J., Wilkinson-Flicker, S., Diliberti, M., Zhang, A., ...Wang, X. (2019). *Status and trends in the education of racial and ethnic groups 2018. NCES 2019-038*. Washington, DC: U.S. Department of Education. National Center for Education Statistics.

LaRue, E. M., Sereika, S., & Engberg, S. (2013). *Website evaluation tool*. Retrieved from SPAT http://www.spat.pitt.edu/research.php

Frey, N., Fisher, D., & Smith, D. (2019). *All learning is social and emotional: Helping students develop essential skills for the classroom and beyond*. Alexandria: ASCD.

Greatschools Staff. (2012). *How important is cultural diversity at your school?* Retrieved from greatschools.org https://www.greatschools.org/gk/articles/cultural-diversity-at-school/

Greytak, E. K., Kosciw, J. G., Villenas, C., & Giga, N. M. (2016). *From teasing to torment: School climate revisited a survey of U.S. Secondary School Students and Teachers*. Retrieved from GLSEN https://www.glsen.org/sites/default/files/2019-12/From_Teasing_to_Tormet_Revised_2016.pdf

GSA Network. (2020). *Resources: 10 Steps for starting a GSA*. Retrieved from GSA Network: https://gsanetwork.org/resources/10-steps-for-starting-a-gsa/

Huynh, V. (2016). Discrimination during teen years can have health repercussions later in life. *CSUN Today (California State University)*.

Joint Committee on National Health Education Standards. (2007). *National Health Education Standards*, (2nd ed.). American Cancer Society.

Jones, L. (2018). *If we're teaching social emotional skills, we need to assess them*. Retrieved from We Are Teachers https://www.weareteachers.com/assess-sel-skills/

Juvonen, J. K., Kogachi, K., & Graham, S. (2018). When and how do students benefit from ethnic diversity in middle school. *Child Development, 89*(4), 1268–1282.

Kenny, C. (2018). *LGBTQ youth share their stories, offer advice to adults to end bullying*. Retrieved from glaad—The Voice and Vision of a New Generation. https://www.glaad.org/amp/lgbtq-youth-share-stories-offer-advice-adults-to-end-bullying

Kenny, C. (2018, October 18). *lgbtq youth share their stories, offer advice to adults to end bullying*. Retrieved from GLAAD: https://www.glaad.org/amp/lgbtq-youth-share-stories-offer-advice-adults-to-end-bullying

Kidshealth from Nemours. (2015). *Stress*. Retrieved from Kidshealth from Nemours https://kidshealth.org/en/kids/stress.html

Kidshealth from Nemours. (2018). *Yoga for lowering stress*. Retrieved from https://kidshealth.org/en/kids/yoga-stress.html: https://kidshealth.org/en/kids/yoga-stress.html

Kidshealth from Nemours. (2020). *Yoga: Meditation and breathing*. Retrieved from Kidshealth from Nemours https://kidshealth.org/en/teens/meditation.html?WT.ac=ctg

Lewis, J. A., Nishina, A., Ramirez Hall, A., Cain, S., Bellmore, A., & Witkow, M. R. (2018). Early adolescents' peer experiences with ethnic diversity in middle school: Implications for academic outcomes. *Journal of Youth and Adolescence, 47*(1), 194–206.

McWhirter, E. H., Garcia, E. A., & Bines, D. (2018). Discrimination and other education barriers, school connectedness, and thoughts of dropping out among Latina/o students. *Journal of Career Development, 45*(4), 330–344.

Meeks, L. H. (2020). *Comprehensive School Health Education*, (9th ed.). New York: McGraw Hill.

Namaste Kid. (2020). *Downward Facing Dog*. Retrieved from Namaste Kid https://www.namastekid.com/teaching-tools/downward-facing-dog/

Namaste Kid. (2020). *Table Pose*. Retrieved from Namaste Kid https://www.namastekid.com/teaching-tools/table-pose/

Pico, I. (2019). *The Wheel of Emotion by Robert Plutchick*. Retrieved from PsicoPico https://psicopico.com/en/la-rueda-las-emociones-robert-plutchik/

Polakovic, G. (2018). Kids stress over public acts of discrimination, USC Study finds. *USC News (University of Southern California)*.

raisingchildren.net.au. (2020). *Why physical activity is important for pre-teens and teenagers*. Retrieved from raisingchildren.net.au: https://raisingchildren.net.au/teens/healthy-lifestyle/physical-activity/physical-activity-teens#why-physical-activity-is-important-for-pre-teens-and-teenagers-nav-title

Page., R. M., Page, T. S. (2015). *Promoting health and emotional well-being in your classroom*. Burlington, MA: Jones and Bartlett.

Ryan, C. P. (2009). *Helping Families Support Their Lesbian, Gay, Bisexual, and Transgender (LGBT) Children*. Retrieved from Edutopia https://nccc.georgetown.edu/documents/LGBT_Brief.pdf

Stop Bullying.gov. (2020). *What Kids Can Do*. Retrieved from stopbullying.gove https://www.stopbullying.gov/resources/kids

Teaching Tolerance. (2020). *Developing Empathy*. Retrieved from Teaching Tolerance https://www.tolerance.org/classroom-resources/tolerance-lessons/developing-empathy

Transforming Education. (2020). *Introduction to Social Awareness*. Retrieved from Transforming Education https://www.transformingeducation.org/wp-content/uploads/2019/04/Introduction-to-Social-Awareness.pdf

Weir, K. (2016). Inequality at school. What's behind the racial disparity in our education system? *American Psychological Association, 47*(10), 42.

Wiggs, B. (2014). *Rethinking Tolerance: Ensuring That All Students Belong*. Retrieved from George Lucas Educational Foundation, Edutopia https://www.edutopia.org/blog/rethinking-tolerance-ensuring-all-students-belong

Wilson, D. C., & Conyers, M. (2017). *4 Proven Strategies for Teaching Empathy*. Retrieved from George Lucas Educational Foundation, Edutopia https://www.edutopia.org/article/4-proven-strategies-teaching-empathy-donna-wilson-marcus-conyers

Wolpert-Gawrom, H. (2018). *Supporting a Gay-Straight Alliance in Middle School*. Retrieved from George Lucas Educational Foundation, Edutopia https://www.edutopia.org/article/supporting-gay-straight-alliance-middle-school

YTS Your Therapy Source. (April). *10 FUN Self Control Games to Practice Self Regulation Skills (No Equipment Needed) - Self Regulation*. Retrieved from YTS Your Therapy Source https://www.yourtherapysource.com/blog1/2017/05/16/games-practice-self-regulation-skills/

Chapter 5—Appendix A
Social Awareness: Scope, Sequence, Content, SEL Competency/Subcompetencies

<u>Note:</u> This page is organized by grade span, Standard 1, skill standards, the HECAT content areas, and SEL Competency/subcompetencies.

The HECAT content areas include: AOD – Alcohol and Other Drugs; HE – Healthy Eating; MEH – Mental/Emotional Health; PHW – Personal Health and Wellness; PA – Physical Activity; S – Safety; SH – Sexual Health; T – Tobacco; V – Violence Prevention

Impulse Control, Self-Discipline, Self-Motivation

Grade Span	Standard 1	Skill	HECAT Content Areas and Specific Content	SEL Competency and Subcompetencies
PreK–2	1.2.2. Recognize *empathy for a friend in each of the* multiple dimensions of health.	3.2.1 Identify trusted adults and professionals *in the school who* help promote health.	Mental/emotional health: Empathy for a friend and accessing community resources	SEL–Social-awareness: Perspective-taking, empathy, community resources.
3–5	1.5.2. Describe the relationship between healthy behaviors, *such as being empathetic toward a bullying victim,* and personal health.	3.5.2 Locate resources from home, school, and community that provide valid health information *about bullying*	Violence prevention: Bullying	SEL–Social-awareness: Perspective-taking, empathy, community resources.
6–8	1.8.5. <u>Describe</u> ways to reduce or prevent injuries and other adolescent health behaviors *by being empathetic toward LGBTQ*	3.8.1. <u>Analyze</u> the validity of health information, products, and services *about sexual orientation.*	Sexual health: LGBTQ	SEL–Social-awareness: Perspective-taking, empathy, community resources.
9–12	1.12.7 Compare and contrast the benefits of and barriers to practicing a variety of healthy behaviors *such as being active for 60 minutes each day*	3.12.1. <u>Evaluate</u> the validity of health information, products, and services *about physical activity.* 7.12.2 <u>Demonstrate</u> a variety of healthy practices and behaviors that maintain or improve the health of self and others, *such as three activities from the plan to have 60 minutes of physical activity for five days.*	Physical Activity	SEL–Social-awareness: Perspective-taking, empathy, recognize community resources.

(continues)

Impulse Control, Self-Discipline, Self-Motivation *(continued)*

Grade Span	Standard 1	Skill	HECAT Content Areas and Specific Content	SEL Competency and Subcompetencies
Appreciating Diversity/Respecting Others/Persevering in Addressing Challenges				
PreK–2	1.2.2 Recognize that the multiple dimensions of health *are affected when diversity is respected.*	3.2.1 Identify trusted adults and professionals who help promote health *and diversity.*	Mental Emotional Health: Embracing differences, respect, meeting the challenges of being different.	SEL–Social-awareness: Appreciating diversity, respecting others, persevering in addressing challenges
3–5	1.5.3 Describe ways that a safe and healthy school and community environment *model acceptance of student differences, respect, and how to respond to the challenges of diversity.*	3.5.2 Identify resources from home, school, and community that provide valid health information *about diversity, respecting differences, and overcoming diversity challenges.*	Mental Emotional Health: Embracing differences, respect, meeting the challenges of being different.	SEL–Social-awareness: Appreciating diversity, respecting others, persevering in addressing challenges
6–8	1.8.5 Describe ways to reduce or prevent injuries and other adolescent health problems *by accepting and respecting diversity.*	3.8.2 Access valid health information from home, school, and community *regarding school diversity groups.* 7.12.2 Demonstrate a variety of healthy practices and behaviors that maintain or improve the health of self and others *such as making a plan to establish school diversity groups*	Mental Emotional Health/Violence prevention: Embracing differences, respect, meeting the challenges of being different.	SEL–Social-awareness: Appreciating diversity, respecting others, persevering in addressing challenges
9–12	1.12.2 Describe *how discrimination affects* the interrelationships of emotional, intellectual, physical, and social health.	3.12.2 Use resources from home, school, and community that provide valid health information *about how to increase school connectedness.*	Mental Emotional Health: Embracing differences, respect, meeting the challenges of being different.– Discrimination	SEL–Social-awareness: Appreciating diversity, respecting others, persevering in addressing challenges

CHAPTER 6

Teaching Relationship Skills

LEARNING OBJECTIVES

Upon finishing this course, students will be able to:

- Plan skills-based health (SBH)/SEL lessons using backwards design and practice prompts.
- Incorporate the subcompetencies of relationship skills into assessment and instruction.

KEY TERMS

Communication
Relationship building

Social engagement
Teamwork

Social and Emotional Learning (SEL) Competencies*

- **RELATIONSHIP SKLLS Figure 6.1**
  - *The ability to establish and maintain healthy and rewarding relationships with diverse individuals and groups. The ability to communicate clearly, listen well, cooperate with others, resist inappropriate social pressure, negotiate conflict constructively, and seek and offer help when needed.* (CASEL, 2019)

Introduction

The CASEL competencies of social awareness and relationship skills are linked because they prepare youth to develop positive social skills. Social awareness challenges the student to examine personal social attitudes, norms, and family and community resources. Relationship skills challenge the student to use those skills to establish and maintain healthy relationships with others.

Social awareness and relationship skills are also considered an important factor in the workforce. The Partnership for 21st Century Skills surveyed a variety

---

*A scope and sequence document is included as an appendix at the end of this chapter.

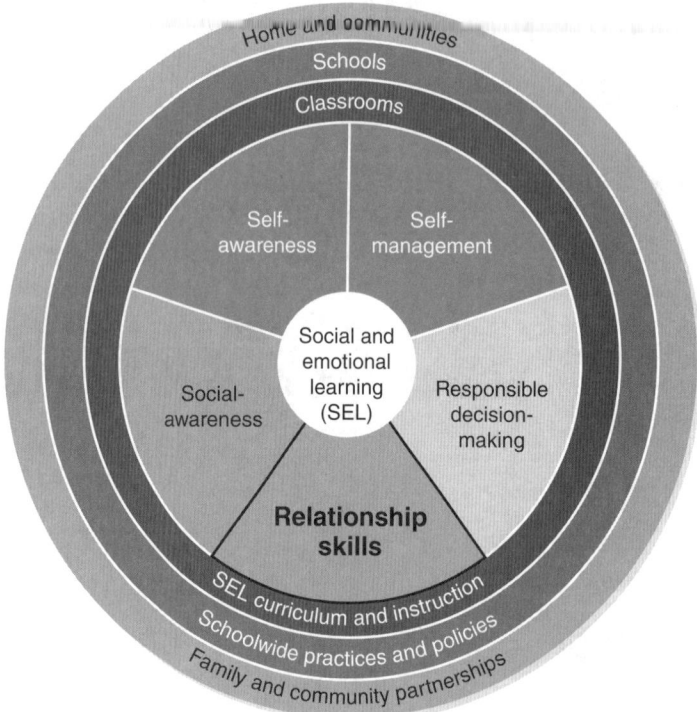

Figure 6.1 The CASEL Framework—Competency on Relationship Skills.

of employers. The results indicated that four of the five most important skills for high school students to acquire as they enter the work force are associated with social awareness and relationship skills: professionalism, collaboration, **communication**, and social responsibility. (Transforming Education, 2020)

When progressing through each chapter, it becomes evident that the skills and competencies from previous chapters are interwoven in the subsequent chapters. The richness of skills-based health/SEL is a result of multi-faceted, engaging, age-appropriate, and experiential assessment and instruction used to improve relationships and personal health in the school setting and the workplace.

Personal, family, and community health is enhanced by using effective communication skills. In Standard 4 of the National Health Education Standards, students learn to use verbal and nonverbal communication skills to establish and maintain healthy relationships. Advocacy, Standard 8, is an empowering skill that helps them promote healthy norms and behavior with their peers. Because advocacy, uses communication skills, it is included in this section. (Joint Committee on National Health Education Standards, 2007, pp. 30, 36)

Table 6.1 describes the alignment of relationship skills to Standard 4 of the National Health Education Standards: Students demonstrate the ability to use interpersonal communication skills to enhance health

and avoid or reduce health risks. (Joint Committee on National Health Education Standards, 2007, p. 30)

Preview

Unit Plan

In a skills-based/SEL unit, the planner accesses and analyzes data then selects a Standard 1 and skills performance indicator to reduce the risk factor and infuses them with content. The SEL competency and subcompetency are aligned with the infused performance indicators. Once established, the instructor plans the assessment and instruction. Once the content, skill, and competency are taught, the teacher distributes the performance task which consists of the unit prompt(s), the scoring rubric, back-up materials needed such as supplemental content, self-checks, and any other information the students need to show proficiency in the performance indicators and SEL competency. Students organize and practice for a few days and present their work to the class. This summative assessment is scored with an analytical rubric.

Skills-based Lesson Plan

The skills-based/SEL lesson plan contains an agenda, the lesson objectives (infused Standard 1 performance indicator and skills indicator and the SEL

Table 6.1 Alignment of Relationship Skills to Standard 4 of the NHES

Competency	Description	Subcompetencies
Relationship Skills	The ability to establish and maintain healthy and rewarding relationships with diverse individuals and groups. The ability to communicate clearly, listen well, cooperate with others, resist inappropriate social pressure, negotiate conflict constructively, and seek and offer help when needed. (Collaborative for Academic and Social Emotional Learning, 2020)	▪ Communication ▪ **Social Engagement** ▪ **Relationship Building** ▪ **Teamwork**

The relationship skills subcompetency, communication, is aligned with Standard 4—Demonstrate the ability to use interpersonal communication skills to enhance health and avoid or reduce health risks (Joint Committee on National Health Education Standards, 2007, p. 30) and Standard 8—Demonstrate the ability to advocate for personal, family, and community health. (Joint Committee on National Health Education Standards, 2007, p. 36)

Skills-based health/SEL educators use prompts, based on infused performance indicators, to develop relationship skills and demonstrate proficiency in content, skill, and SEL competency.

When students practice the Standard 4 skills of refusal and negotiation; assertive, passive, and aggressive communication; resolving conflict; and asking for and offering help; they are practice and gain proficiency in the competency, social awareness: communication.

Students who present public service announcements and design and distribute health-enhancing posters that advocate for personal, family, or community health, are practicing and gaining proficiency in social awareness: communication.

For example:

Infused performance indicators:

▪ 1.2.1 <u>Identify</u> that healthy behaviors, *such as resolving differences*, affect personal health (Joint Committee on National Health Education Standards, 2007, p. 24)
▪ 4.2.1 <u>Demonstrate</u> healthy ways to express needs, wants, and feelings *when experiencing a conflict*. (Joint Committee on National Health Education Standards, 2007, p. 30)
▪ SEL: Relationship skills—communication

Liam likes to keep his electronics in a certain place, so he always knows where they are. Dante, Liam's younger brother, found Liam's Xbox remote and hid it because Liam wouldn't play with him. Liam was upset but rather than getting angry with his little brother and threatening him, said, "When you take the remote, I think I have lost it, and I know mom and dad would get really upset if that happened. I really need for you to return the remote. I will play a game with you if you return it." Both boys were happy after resolving the conflict and had a good time playing the game together. (Connolly, 2020)

In this example, the lesson taught to PreK–2 students included communication skills. Liam was clear in expressing his needs, wants, and feelings, as was his little brother! (4.2.1) Both boys realized that resolving their differences was good for their emotional health because they both felt better and had a good time playing the game. (1.2.1)

competency/sub competency), a review/preview, the Standard 1 content, the skill, competency, a student engaging practice prompt, clarifying questions relating to the prompt and learning objectives, a lesson review, and an exit ticket.

Skills-based Lesson Infrastructure

The sections that follow present <u>infrastructure</u> for a <u>lesson</u>, not a unit. The infrastructure provides the teacher with guidance without interfering with individual creativity. Each begins with an overview, data (when available), and a list of resources. Following the overview, a table initiates backwards design,

which consists of the infused performance indicators and SEL competencies as the lesson objectives.

Assessments are designed for each of the performance indicators and SEL competency. The prompt and the review questions engage the learner and help the teacher determine if the students met the lesson objectives. An exit question concludes the lesson infrastructure and provides an opportunity for students to reflect on how to use the content, skill, and SEL competency taught.

When reading, let your imagination guide your planning. You may need more or fewer lessons to teach the material. You may like an idea and modify it to meet the needs of your students. You may find the worksheets valuable or may prefer to edit them.

Table 6.2 *Relationship Skills by Subcompetencies*

Communication	Relationship Building
Social Engagement	Teamwork

When modifying, maintain the integrity of the backwards design. Teach content, skill, and SEL each day. If the lesson infrastructure contains too much material, plan an additional day(s) but maintain the integrity of aligning SEL and teaching content through the infused performance indicators. Refer to the sample lessons at the end of each chapter to understand how to align SEL and teach content through the skill.

Organization

The learning activities for the core competency of social awareness are divided into two sections:

- Establishing and maintaining healthy and rewarding relationships/communicating clearly.
- Negotiating conflict constructively/seeking and offering help when needed.
- Resisting inappropriate social pressure/seeking and offering help when needed. (Collaborative for Academic Social Emotional Learning, 2020)

Each section that follows contains background information about the subcompetency followed by lesson suggestions and resources.

The National Health Education Standards are grouped according to the grade spans PreK–2, Grades 3–5, Grades 6–8, and Grades 9–12. The examples follow that structure. The classroom examples may require the teacher to be creative and adjust instruction to accommodate the age and abilities of the students.

The headings of each section represent a relationship skills subcompetency **Table 6.2**. The practice prompt is aligned with the competency and the infused performance indicators of the National Health Education Standards.

Section 1. Establishing and Maintaining Healthy and Rewarding Relationships/ Communicating Clearly

(Collaborative for Academic Social Emotional Learning, 2020)

Healthy relationships are fundamental to our well-being. In the classroom, we model and teach verbal, non-verbal communication and listening skills, interpersonal skills such as coping with peer pressure, refusal/negotiation skills, and where to find help when needed. We provide time for student practice and give effective feedback that helps youth develop, enhance, and maintain healthy relationships.

The following are specific strategies to help students develop healthy relationships:

- *Understanding the Individual.* (Randy M. Page., 2015, p. 64) Encourage students to discover what is important to a person (sports, music, art, etc.) and take an interest in it. One student may be interested in fishing and another while another knows nothing about it. To enhance or initiate a relationship with the fishing student, raise questions about fishing (fresh water, salt water, lures, bait, etc.), ask to accompany the student when he/she goes fishing, inquire about the success of the fishing day, etc.

- *Demonstrate courtesies and kindness.* (Randy M. Page., 2015, p. 64) Healthy relationships are respectful. In the classroom and throughout the school, to encourage students to demonstrate courtesy and kindness by saying, "Please," "Thank you," "Excuse me," "I am sorry," opening and holding the door for others, and offering to help.

- *Keep commitments.* (Randy M. Page., 2015, p. 64) In a healthy relationship, peers trust one another. To build trust, encourage students to follow through on what they say they are going to do. For example, if a student commits to completing a portion of an assignment, he/she should follow through. If the commitment cannot be met, encourage the student to communicate with his/her peer to explain the situation.

- *Clarify expectations.* (Randy M. Page., 2015, p. 64) To establish and reinforce healthy relationships, adults and peers need to clearly communicate expected behavior. Teachers clarify assignment expectations with clear directions and rubrics. Peers use their communication skills to assure they understand what is expected. For example, one student may tell another that they will get together afterschool but be speaking in general terms. Meanwhile, the other student may have interpreted the comment as occurring on that day and waits in anticipation. Clear communication is vital to avoiding misunderstandings.

- *Show personal integrity.* (Randy M. Page., 2015, p. 64) To help youths understand personal integrity, model positive character traits in actions and relationships with students and adults. To develop integrity, encourage peers to follow the school rules, work hard to complete assignments through effort, refuse to cheat, acknowledge mistakes, apologize when appropriate, and respect the opinions of others even when they disagree.

- *Apologize when needed.* (Randy M. Page., 2015, p. 65) To develop healthy relationships, it is important to encourage youth to acknowledge a mistake and apologize if they have done something wrong. (Randy M. Page., 2015, pp. 64-65)

PreK–2: Relationship Skills: Establishing and Maintaining Healthy and Rewarding Relationships/Communicating Clearly

The Robert Wood Johnson Foundation published in 2015, the results of a long-term study of the relationship between Kindergarten students and interpersonal skills. The results indicate that helping children develop social and emotional skills is crucial to preparing them for a healthy future.

The results show that Kindergarten students with interpersonal skills are

- Fifty-four percent more likely to attain a high school diploma.

- Twice as likely to attain a college degree in early adulthood.
- Forty-six percent more likely to have a full-time job by the age of 25. (Robert Wood Johnson Foundation, 2015)

Lesson Overview: Expressing Appreciation and Respect—Friendship

In this lesson, students learn the importance of using courteous words, "I" messages to express needs, wants, and feelings, and identifying respectful and disrespectful behaviors.

The lesson may be divided into three separate lessons: courteous words, "I" messages, and respectful behavior.

Resources:

- Michigan Model for Health, Kindergarten

Materials needed:

- **Worksheet 6.1 Respectful or Disrespectful Behaviors**

Table 6.3 provides an overview of the lesson objectives, assessment, and instruction for this lesson.

Table 6.3 Lesson Objectives, Assessment, and Instruction

Step 1 – Lesson Objectives	Step 2 – Assessment
The verb of the *infused* performance indicator and the SEL competency generate the assessment and instruction.	Design the assessment based on the objectives. Ask yourself the question, "What can my students do to show me they have met the standard?"
1.2.1 <u>Identify</u> that healthy behaviors, *such as expressing appreciation and demonstrating respect*, affect personal health. (Joint Committee on National Health Education Standards, 2007, p. 24)	1.2.1 Students <u>identify</u> two ways that healthy behaviors, *such as expressing appreciation and demonstrating respect*, affect personal health.
4.2.1 <u>Demonstrate</u> *one* healthy way to express needs, wants, and feelings by using "I" messages. (Joint Committee on National Health Education Standards, 2007, p. 30)	4.2.1 Students use "I" messages to <u>demonstrate</u> one way to express needs, one way to express wants, and one way to express feelings.
SEL-Relationship skills: Relationship Building, Communication	Relationship Building: Students use courteous words and demonstrate respectful behaviors, engage peers, and develop friendships. (4.2.1) Communication: Students use "I" messages to express wants, needs, and feelings. (4.2.1)

Step 3 – Instruction
Design the instruction so that students learn the content, skill, and competency to be successful on the assessment. Ask yourself the question, "What do I need to teach so that the students will be successful when assessed?"

Step 3 – Instruction

1. Define
   a. Identify: To recognize a particular person or an object.
   b. Demonstrate: To show how something is accomplished.
   c. Respect: A demonstration of reverence for a person or an object.
2. 1.2.1. <u>Identify</u> that healthy behaviors, *such as expressing appreciation, giving compliments, and demonstrating respect* (manners), affect personal health.
   a. Model how to give a compliment and ask the children to give an example of how to respond. Appropriate responses include saying, "Thank you."
   b. Model how to respond when someone says, "Thank you" by saying, "You are welcome."
   c. Model how to respectfully ask for something by saying, "Please," and when you receive the requested item, reply, "Thank you."
   d. Effects of *expressing appreciation and giving compliments* on personal health
      1) Being respectful is a skill that helps children develop and maintain positive relationships.
      2) Expressing appreciation, giving compliments, and demonstrating respect results in feelings of happiness.
      3) Giving compliments and showing appreciation are worthwhile because they helps us make new friends and keep current friends. (Michigan Model for Health, 2019, p. 58)
   e. Practice: Provide time for the children to practice responding to a compliment, using "Please" to ask for something, and responding with a "Thank you." Formatively assess and model complimenting the students.
   f. Ask the students how they felt when peers used appropriate language to compliment them. (appreciated and respected)
   g. Ask the students how manners affect whether you want to be friends with someone.
   h. Ask the children to provide the meaning of the word, respect and give an example of how to show it.
   i. Use **Worksheet 6.1 Respectful or Disrespectful Behaviors** to show pictures of situations and ask the children to circle the thumbs up, if the behavior is respectful, and thumbs down if it is not.

If the behavior is disrespectful, challenge the children to suggest how to improve it.

Numbers on each of the pictures on **Worksheet 6.1** correspond to the same below.
1) Take care of personal property and those of others. (respectful)
2) Use communication skills (say, "excuse me") (respectful)
3) Use manners (please, thank you, you are welcome) (respectful)
4) Sharing (disrespectful)
5) Being considerate (respectful)
6) Showing empathy (sharing feelings) (respectful)
7) Taking perspective (putting yourself in the place of another) (disrespectful)

3. 4.2.1 <u>Demonstrate</u> healthy ways to express needs, wants, and feelings by using "I" messages.
   a. Model using "I" messages
      1) <u>Expressing needs</u>: "Manny, I forgot my pencil. Could I please borrow one? Thank you."
      2) <u>Expressing wants</u>: "When I learned the Lego club was meeting before school, I really wanted to join. Thank you for telling me about the club."
      3) <u>Expressing feelings</u>: "I like it when you say, "Thank you" because I feel like you appreciate what I did for you.
      4) <u>Expressing feelings</u>: "I like it when you say, you're welcome because I feel respected." (Michigan Model for Health, 2019, p. 61)
   b. Provide scenarios for the children to practice using "I" messages to express wants, needs, and feelings.
4. Read the practice prompt. Students answer the reflection questions and discuss.

Practice Prompt: Breonna

Breonna is shy and does not have many friends. Her health teacher, Mrs. Bell, taught the class that using manners helps to make friends. Breonna always uses good manners but decided she would try harder. When Emily was leaving the classroom for lunch, Breonna offered to hold the door for her. When Emily walked by, she said, "Thank you" and gave Breonna a big smile. Breonna said, "You are welcome" and smiled back. It was like they had met for the first time.

When Breonna needed to sharpen her pencil, she raised her hand and asked the teacher if she could please sharpen her pencil. The teacher complimented her on her good manners and gave her permission to get out of her seat. As she walked to the sharpener, several students looked at her and smiled. Breonna smiled back.

During math, Breonna saw that Deena was having trouble with a problem. She offered to help. Together they solved the problem, and Deena was very thankful. She complimented Breonna on how she explained the steps of solving the math problem and told the other students that Breonna is really good in math! Breonna really liked the fancy pen Deena had on her desk and asked if she could use it during English. Deena said, "Sure." Breonna liked the way it had different colors and wrote so smooth. She was very careful with it and returned it right after she finished her assignment. Breonna said, "Thank you" to Deena and she said, "You are welcome!" Both girls felt good about trusting each other.

During the next health lesson, Mrs. Bell asked the class how they were doing with using courteous words and good manners. Deena told Mrs. Bell how helpful Breonna was when she needed help with math and that both girls used "Please," "Thank you," and "You're welcome" many times with each other. Mrs. Bell asked the girls how it felt to be courteous, and they said it made them feel happy and comfortable with each other.

Mrs. Bell told the class they were continuing their lesson on making friends. She asked the class, "What is one way to show respect to one another?" The students responded by saying, "Hold the door for someone, help someone if they dropped something, if you borrow something return it in the same condition, be willing to share, and just be nice! "Excellent!" said Mrs. Bell. Breonna felt great because she did all those things.

Mrs. Bell asked the children, "How do you ask for something you need or want?" "How do you express your feelings?" Most of the students responded that they just tell their parents that they want something. Mrs. Bell said she was going to teach them a special way of expressing needs, wants, and feelings that works really well.

When Breonna got home, she decided to try the new strategy. She said to her mother, "Mom, I really like to ride my bike, but I haven't been able to because it is broken. When we biked together, we had fun, and I really liked spending time together with the family. I would also like to ride bikes with my friends in the neighborhood. Do you think I could have a new bicycle?"

Breonna couldn't wait until the next health class to tell Mrs. Bell that she has a beautiful new bike and is having a great time with her family and her new and neighborhood friends!

5. Use the review questions in **Table 6.4** to help the children understand how to recognize empathy in each of the dimensions of wellness.
6. End of class review. Ask the students to put away their materials then ask review questions.
   a. What is one way to show appreciation when someone does something nice for you? (1.2.1)
   b. What is one way to show respect to someone? (1.2.1)
   c. Give an example of a courteous word. (1.2.1)
   d. Give an example of how to use "I" messages to express needs, wants, and feelings. (3.2.1)
7. Exit ticket

What should we say when someone says something nice to us? (thank you) (4.2.1)

What should we say when someone tells us they liked what we did for them? (you are welcome) (4.2.1) (Michigan Model for Health, 2019, p. 62)

Grades 3–5: Relationship Skills: Establishing and Maintaining Healthy and Rewarding Relationships/Communication

Lesson Overview: Coping with Grief

In this lesson, students learn to understand how grief affects the components of health and how to use verbal and nonverbal communication skills to help a friend.

Understanding how grief affects the components of health and how using communication skills strengthens a friendship during difficult times.

In light of the pandemic, this lesson may be helpful to students who lost a loved one. However, with minor adjustments, the lesson is appropriate for loss regardless of the cause.

Guidelines for teaching about loss, death, and grief

- Be honest and open when answering questions about death.
- Be as factual as possible when answering questions about death.
- Avoid personal values when discussing death. (Heaven, euthanasia, etc.)
- Be a good and supportive listener
- Ask reflecting and review questions at the end of lessons to check for understanding. (Telljohann, 2009, p. 410)

Table 6.4 Empathy, Perspective Taking, and Recognizing Community Resources

Question	Answer
How did Breonna <u>identify</u> two ways that healthy behaviors, *such as expressing appreciation and demonstrating respect*, affect her personal health? (1.2.1)	■ When Breonna held the door for Emily, Emily gave her a big smile and said, "Thank you." ■ When Breonna returned the pen to Deena as soon as she finished the assignment, she showed respect for Deena's possessions.
How did Breonna use "I" messages to express needs, one way to express wants, and one way to express feelings? (4.2.1)	"Mom, I really like to ride my bike, but I haven't been able to because it is broken. When we biked together, we had fun, and I really liked spending time together with the family. I would also like to ride bikes with my friends in the neighborhood. Do you think, I could have a new bicycle?"
SEL–Relationship skills: Relationship building, communication	
How did Breonna use her news skills to maintain healthy relationships?	Breonna made new friends with Emily and Deena by being courteous and respectful. She is much friendlier with her neighborhood friends, also, since she has a new bicycle and can go out and play.
How did Breonna use communication skills?	Breonna used "I" messages with her mother to express a need to exercise, a desire for a new bicycle, feelings of happiness when biking with family, and a desire to bike with neighborhood children and new friends.

Resources:

- American Academy of Child and Adolescent Psychiatry. (2018). Grief and Children: https://www.aacap.org/AACAP/Families_and_Youth/Facts_for_Families/FFF-Guide/Children-And-Grief-008.aspx

Materials needed:

- **Worksheet 6.2 Effects of Grief on Personal Health**

Table 6.5 provides an overview of the lesson objectives, assessment, and instruction for this lesson.

Table 6.5 Lesson Objectives, Assessment, and Instruction

Step 1 – Lesson Objectives	Step 2 – Assessment
The verb of the *infused* performance indicator and the SEL competency generate the assessment and instruction.	Design the assessment based on the objectives. Ask yourself the question, "What can my students do to show me they have met the standard?"
1.5.2 <u>Identify</u> examples of emotional, intellectual, physical, and social health *that occur when experiencing a loss.* (Joint Committee on National Health Education Standards, 2007, p. 24)	1.5.2 Students <u>identify</u> *one way experiencing a loss effects* emotional, intellectual, physical, and social health.
4.5.1 <u>Demonstrate</u> effective verbal and nonverbal communication skills to enhance *the* health *of a friend experiencing a loss.* (Joint Committee on National Health Education Standards, 2007, p. 30)	4.5.1 Characters in the role play <u>demonstrate</u> "I" messages, active listening, empathy, and perspective taking.
SEL–Relationship skills: Communication, social engagement, relationship building, teamwork	Characters in the story use verbal and nonverbal communication skills to support someone who has experienced a loss. (1.5.2) (4.5.1)
Step 3 – Instruction	

Design the instruction so that students learn the content, skill, and competency to be successful on the assessment. Ask yourself the question, "What do I need to teach so that the students will be successful when assessed?"

Step 3 – Instruction

1. Define
   a. Identify: To recognize a particular person or an object.
   b. Demonstrate: To show how something is accomplished.
   c. Grief: A feeling of deep sadness and loss.
2. 1.5.2 <u>Identify</u> examples of emotional, intellectual, physical, and social health *that occur when experiencing a loss.*
   a. Use **Worksheet 6.2 Effects of Grief on Personal Health** to discover the effects on the components of health when experiencing a loss.
3. 4.5.1 <u>Demonstrate</u> effective verbal and nonverbal communication skills to enhance *the* health *of a friend experiencing a loss.*
   a. To introduce grief, ask the children the following questions
      1) What happens when something dies? (Example: flower)
      2) Explain that death is a part of life by showing the Cycle of Life **Figure 6.2**. (Michigan Model for Health, 2019, p. 448)
      3) Who can tell me what grief is?
      4) When do people experience grief?
      5) What behaviors do you see when people are grieving? (anger, irritability, fear, anxiety, confusion, difficulty sleeping, physical complaints, stomach aches)
      6) To help cope with grief, it is normal to express sad feelings and helpful to talk with a trusted adult or friend.
   b. Model verbal skills ("I" messages) to help a friend cope with grief.
      1) "Monica, when I heard your dog died, I was very sad. I always loved Digger and

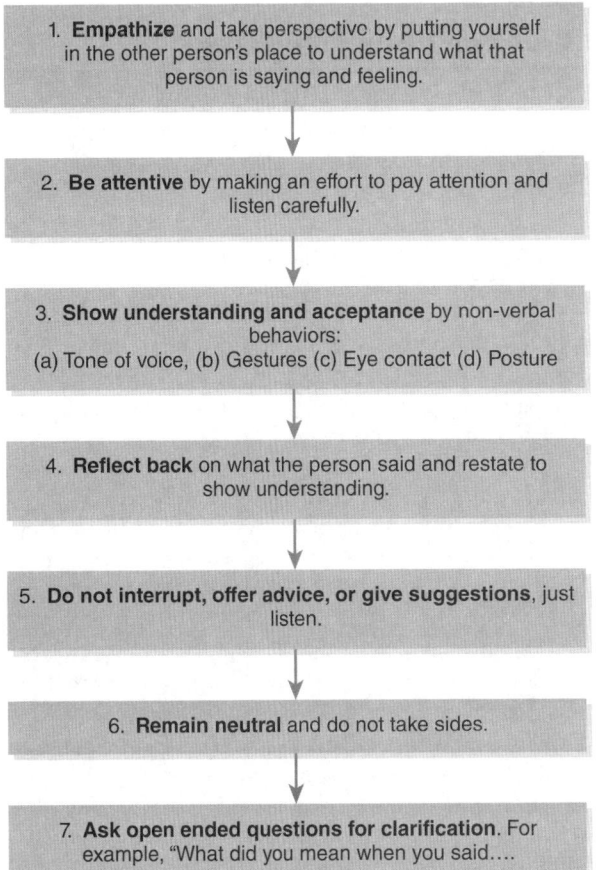

1. **Empathize** and take perspective by putting yourself in the other person's place to understand what that person is saying and feeling.

2. **Be attentive** by making an effort to pay attention and listen carefully.

3. **Show understanding and acceptance** by non-verbal behaviors:
(a) Tone of voice, (b) Gestures (c) Eye contact (d) Posture

4. **Reflect back** on what the person said and restate to show understanding.

5. **Do not interrupt, offer advice, or give suggestions**, just listen.

6. **Remain neutral** and do not take sides.

7. **Ask open ended questions for clarification**. For example, "What did you mean when you said…."

Figure 6.3 Active Listening Skills.

Reproduced from John W. Gardner Center. (2007). Youth Engaged in Leadership and Learning YELL A Handbook for Program Staff, Teachers, and Community Leaders. California: John W. Gardner Center for Youth and Their Communities 2nd Edition © 2007.

had lots of fun with him when I visited your house."
      2) "Danie, Mrs. Connolly told us that your grandmother died. I am so sorry. When my grandmother died, I was very sad for a long time. Talking to my friend helped. If you would like to talk, I would like to help."
   c. Active listening skills **Figure 6.3**
   d. Model active listening when helping a friend cope with grief.
   e. Provide simple practice prompts and time for the children to practice using "I" messages and active listening. Formatively assess and coach. Examples may include:
      1) Fatema's dog had to be put down.
      2) Marianne's grandfather passed away and she is just returning to school.
      3) Pedro rode his bicycle to school but did not lock it. Someone took his bicycle.
      4) Kenny's parents are separating, and his dad is moving to another city.
4. Read the practice prompt. Students answer the reflection questions and discuss.

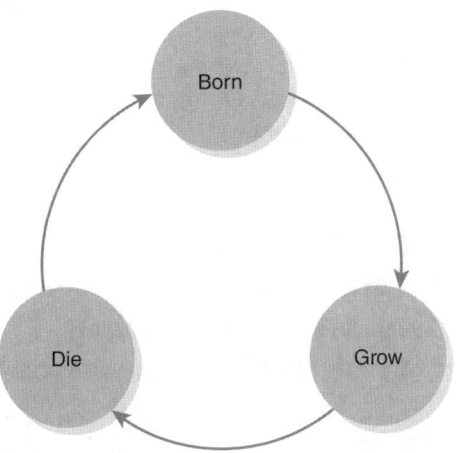

Figure 6.2 The Cycle of Life.

Practice Prompt: Annissa

Annissa loves her dog, Loki. When he was young, they played together, and had a great time. Annissa and her mom would take him for walks around the neighborhood and to the dog park. He had a great time playing with his dog friends. At home, he always found Annissa and snuggled up to her. They were great pals.

Lately, he has been sick, and her parents have spent a lot of time at the vet. Her mom and dad came home with Loki yesterday and Annissa could tell they both had been crying. Annissa asked, "What is wrong?"

Mom and dad explained that Loki was very sick and would not get better. Annissa insisted he would and that she would take care of him. She ran to Loki and gave him a big hug. Usually, Loki would lick her and wag his tail, but this time, he just sat down and looked sad and tired.

Dad explained that the vet said it was time to let Loki go. "What does that mean?" Annissa asked. Mom started to cry again and said that they would take Loki to the vet where he would get a shot that would make him very sleepy and eventually, he would stop breathing.

Annissa screamed, "NO! Don't kill Loki!" Her mom and dad explained that Loki is so sick and in pain that it is the right thing to do for him.

Annissa ran from the room and slammed her door shut. She cried and cried. Her mom tried to console her, but it did not help much. The next day, Loki was gone.

Annissa went to school but could not concentrate. She could not participate and often put her head down on her desk. Her teacher, Mrs. Neely, asked her what was wrong. Annissa broke into tears and told her that her dog went to the vet and was not coming back. Mrs. Neely understood immediately and brought her to the "Quiet Corner." Mrs. Neely

told Annissa how sorry she was. She explained that dying is a natural part of life but very difficult to experience when someone you love or a pet is no longer with you.

Mrs. Neely said, "When my dog died, it was terrible. I was upset for a very long time. Just looking at his toys made me cry." "You cried?" asked Annissa. "Yes," Mrs. Neely said. "Crying is a way of grieving and a perfectly normal reaction to such sadness." Annissa said she had a headache, so Mrs. Neely sent her to the nurse and then told the class about Annissa.

When Annissa returned, her classmates were very kind to her. They asked about Loki and listened carefully and attentively when she spoke. One classmate said, "When I am feeling sad, it helps when someone does something nice for me. Would you like me to help you with the work we did this morning? I noticed you had some trouble with it." "Yes," said Annissa. She felt better knowing that she was with people who cared about her and her feelings.

Mrs. Neely called Annissa's mom and told her that Annissa was emotionally upset about Loki but she improved as the day went on. Annissa's mom was grateful. She said, "I am so happy Annissa is a student at your school and has you for a teacher."

At the end of the day, Mrs. Neely said to her class, "I saw how you helped Annissa today and I wanted to compliment you on how you helped her, spoke, and listened to her. I am very proud of you."

Annissa is still sad but is getting better. She is completing her work and is able to sleep. She looks forward to going to school because she knows her teacher and classmates care about her.

Although it was difficult to cope with Loki's death, she now knows what to do to help others who experience the same loss.

5. Use the review questions in **Table 6.6** to help the children understand how to identify how grief affects the components of health and how to actively listen and use "I" messages to help a grieving friend.

6. End of class review. Ask the students to put away their materials then ask review questions.
   a. Name one component of health and how grieving affects it. (1.5.2)
   b. Give an example of how to use "I" messages when talking to a friend who is grieving. (4.5.1)
   c. Give an example of how to actively listen when a grieving friend talks to you. (4.5.1)

7. Exit ticket (Relationship skills: Maintaining healthy and rewarding relationships)

   What is one thing you can do to help a friend who is grieving?

Grades 6–8: Relationship Skills: Establishing and Maintaining Healthy and Rewarding Relationships/Communication

Learning how to listen and use communication skills to effectively communicate are essential skills. (Mendler, 2013)

Table 6.6 Empathy, Perspective Taking, and Recognizing Community Resources

Question	Answer
How did *experiencing Link's loss affect Annissa's* emotional, intellectual, physical, and social health. (1.5.2)	Annissa's Emotional health ■ Became upset when she learned Loki was sick and was going to die. ■ Cried when she told Mrs. Neely about Loki. ■ Felt better at the end of the day because she knew her teacher and her classmates care about her. ■ Knows it is normal to be sad when a pet dies and she feels confident she can help someone else who may experience the same kind of loss. ■ Looks forward to going to school. Annissa's Intellectual health ■ Could not concentrate at school ■ Could not complete her assignments Annissa's Physical health ■ Had a headache at school. Annissa's Social health ■ Felt better when her classmates were very kind and attentive to her. ■ Felt good to know that her teacher and her classmates care about her.
How did the characters in the story demonstrate verbal communication skills, active listening skills, empathy, and perspective taking with a friend who has experienced a loss? (4.5.1)	"I" messages ■ Mrs. Neely said, "When my dog died, it was terrible. I was upset for a very long time. Just looking at his toys made me cry." Active listening skills ■ Annissa's classmates listened carefully and attentively when she talked about Loki. Empathy (share feelings) ■ Annissa's parents shared her feelings (empathy) and tried to console her. ■ Annissa's teacher demonstrated empathy when she took Annissa to the Quiet Corner to talk. ■ Annissa's classmates demonstrated empathy when they were very kind. ■ A classmate said, "When I am feeling sad, it helps when someone does something nice for me. Would you like me to help you with the work we did this morning? I noticed you had some trouble with it." Perspective taking (put yourself in the position of the other person) ■ Mrs. Neely was able to take perspective because she also had a pet who died. ■ Annissa now knows she knows what to do to help a peer whose pet dies.
SEL–Relationship skills: Communication, social engagement, relationship building, teamwork Characters in the story use verbal and nonverbal communication skills to support someone who has experienced a loss.	"I" messages ■ Mrs. Neely said, "When my dog died, it was terrible. I was upset for a very long time. Just looking at his toys made me cry." Active listening skills ■ Annissa's classmates listened carefully and attentively when she talked about Loki.

Lesson Overview: Conversation Skills—Choosing Friends

Students discuss the effects of positive and negative friends on the components of health then use conversation skills to talk to a peer who is trying to make a friend and trying to end a friendship.

Materials needed:

- **Worksheet 6.3 Effects of Positive/Negative Friends on Components of Health**
- **Worksheet 6.4 Practice Conversation Skills**

Table 6.7 provides an overview of the lesson objectives, assessment, and instruction for this lesson.

Table 6.7 Lesson Objectives, Assessment, and Instruction

Step 1 – Lesson Objectives	Step 2 – Assessment
The verb of the *infused* performance indicator and the SEL competency generate the assessment and instruction.	Design the assessment based on the objectives. Ask yourself the question, "What can my students do to show me they have met the standard?"
1.8.2. <u>Describe</u> the interrelationships of emotional, intellectual, physical, and social health in adolescence *when communicating about whether or not to make a friend.* (Joint Committee on National Health Education Standards, 2007, p. 24)	1.8.2 Student <u>describes</u> the effect of a positive and negative friendship on the components of health.
4.8.1. <u>Apply</u> effective verbal and nonverbal communication skills to enhance health *when discussing positive and negative friendships.* (Joint Committee on National Health Education Standards, 2007, p. 30)	4.8.1 Student uses verbal and nonverbal communication skills to enhance health *when discussing positive and negative friendships.*
SEL–Relationship skills: Communication, social engagement, relationship building, teamwork	Use communication skills when discussing positive and negative friendships. (1.8.2) (4.8.1)

Step 3 – Instruction
Design the instruction so that students learn the content, skill, and competency to be successful on the assessment. Ask yourself the question, "What do I need to teach so that the students will be successful when assessed?"

Step 3 – Instruction

1. Define
   a. Describe: To use words that help others envision the physical attributes of a person, place, or thing.
   b. Apply: To use for an appropriate purpose.
2. 1.8.2. Describe the interrelationships of emotional, intellectual, physical, and social health in adolescence *when deciding to keep a friend.*
   a. Use **Worksheet 6.3 Effects of Positive/Negative Friends on Components of Health** to help the students organize their thoughts. Review by using the criteria below. Use the results when practicing communication skills.
   b. Effects of positive and negative friends on the components of health.
      1) Effects of having a positive friend on the components of health.
         a) Emotional: Shares feelings, encourages their friend to do their best, is fun to be with, trustworthy, honest, cares how others feel.
         b) Intellectual: Works hard in school to achieve and get good grades, encourages a friend to develop talents and reach their goals.
         c) Physical: Encourages a friend to do healthy activities, keeps him/herself clean and groomed.
         d) Social: Accepts that one person may have several friends, is friendly

toward others, is respectful to peers, willing to compromise.
      2) Effects of having a negative friend on the components of health.
         a) Emotional: Pushes a friend to do things they should not do, makes fun of people, does not show care or concern toward others.
         b) Intellectual: Does things that he/she knows are wrong but tries to convince others the behavior is fine, does not value school.
         c) Physical: Does dangerous things, uses physical force to get what he she wants, does not care about appearance or grooming.
         d) Social: Makes fun of others, gossips, spreads rumors, yells at others when angry, is disrespectful toward others, not willing to compromise, gets angry when a peer wants to be with other friends. (Michigan Model for Health, 2016, p. 197)
3. 4.8.1. Apply effective verbal and nonverbal communication skills to enhance health *when discussing positive and negative friendships.*
   a. Verbal and nonverbal communication skills: Conversation skills
      1) Share information about self and ask questions about the peer's interests. Show interest by responding, "Really," "Wow!" "That is interesting," etc.

2) Use the SLANT method to pay attention to physical cues (S-Sit up straight, L-Listen, A-Answer and ask questions, N- Nod to show interest, T-Track the speaker—keep track of what is being said)

3) Challenge put-downs or hurtful comments by asking, "How can you say that without being hurtful?"

4) Ask open-ended questions that stimulate discussion rather than a yes or no answer.

5) Rather than accepting "I don't know," as an answer, challenge your peer to wonder about the question and give the best thoughtful response.

6) Make eye contact when speaking and listening. (Adapted from Mendler, 2013)

b. Use **Worksheet 6.4 Practice Conversation Skills** to have a conversation about making a new friend or ending a friendship.

1) Students take turns talking using the information about the effect of positive and negative friends on the components of health.

2) Use "I" messages during the conversation (When you put down others, I don't like it and do not want to be with you.)

3) Use active listening skills during the conversation (see Figure 6.3)

4) Establish boundaries of proper language and being respectful.

5) At the conclusion, students evaluate how well they worked together to meet the criteria of the activity.

4. Read the practice prompt. Students answer the reflection questions and discuss.

Practice Prompt: Keto

Keto is very social and friendly with peers from many different groups. Some of his peers get themselves in trouble at school or the community but when he is with them, they just have fun.

The other day, there was a problem. Keto was hanging out with Jeremiah and Jedi when Keto's friends from soccer walked by. Jeremiah and Jedi made rude remarks and his teammates heard them. They looked at Keto then looked away. Jeremiah and Jedi laughed and told Keto not to worry. They were just jocks and they didn't matter. But it did matter to Keto; they are his teammates and friends. He is beginning to wonder if he should be hanging around with Jeremiah and Jedi.

A few hours later, Jeremiah, Jedi, and Keto went to the park. They headed to the children's section and Jeremiah and Jedi started misusing the equipment. Keto thought, "They are going to get hurt or damage the things the little kids play on." They told Keto to join them, but he didn't want to. They made fun of him and that made Keto realize that he didn't want to be with them any longer. He said, "I am going home." The boys got angry that he was leaving and had some very unkind things to say as he walked away.

Keto called his soccer teammates and said, "I am sorry for not speaking up when Jeremiah and Jedi were rude." His teammates came over his house and they started talking about Keto's choice of friends.

The boys went outside and got serious about the conversation. They sat so they could see each other and listened intently as they took turns talking. As each boy talked, the others kept eye contact and nodded when they agreed. They asked questions and paid attention, so they were right on track with whoever was talking.

They were glad that Keto realized the other boys were being rude but wondered why it took him so long to figure that out. Keto told them Jeremiah and Jedi are in his math class and are smart. Keto said, "When I am stuck on a math problem, they always help me." "We could have helped you, if you had asked!" said his teammate. Keto also explained, "They are clever and like to do different things that are exciting and fun. You know I like to be out and be physically active." His teammates reminded him that team practice includes lots of physical activity and that the three of them could always increase their training, which would be good for the team.

His teammates also pointed out, "They may help you in math and may be fun to be with, but we think they are rude and disrespectful not only to others but to you!" The boys continued, "Jeremiah and Jedi know some of the things they do are wrong, but they don't get caught and don't care. When you hang around with them, they convince you to do the same things and you could get hurt or in trouble. Is that kind of friendship good for you?"

Keto said, "No, that is not good for me. I guess I just enjoyed having different kinds of friends, but I realize now that the things I think are important in a friend are not the same as theirs." Keto felt good that his teammates cared enough about him to talk to him.

5. Use the review questions in **Table 6.8** to help the students understand the qualities of a good friend and the importance of using verbal and nonverbal communication skills with friends.

Table 6.8 Empathy, Perspective Taking, and Recognizing Community Resources

Question	Answer

What were the effects of positive and negative friends on the components of *Keto's* health? (1.8.2)	Emotional health
	■ Negative friends
	  • Keto was uncomfortable when Jeremiah and Jedi were rude to his teammates.
	  • Keto knew he didn't want to stay with Jeremiah and Jedi when he saw them disrespecting the children's play area.
	■ Positive friends
	  • Keto felt good that his friends cared enough about him to have a conversation about Jeremiah and Jedi.
	Intellectual health
	■ Keto liked that Jeremiah and Jedi helped him with the math problems he couldn't figure out.
	■ His teammates told Keto that they could have helped him with math.
	Physical health
	■ Keto liked that Jeremiah and Jedi liked to do physical things because he likes being active.
	■ His teammates reminded Keto that team practice provides a lot of activity and that the three of them could always increase their training.
	Social health
	■ Jeremiah and Jedi were a part of Keto's social network. He enjoyed having lots of friends from different groups.
	■ Keto did not like that Jeremiah and Jedi were rude to his teammates. He realized that his teammates were good friends and didn't like them being insulted.

What verbal and nonverbal communication skills did Keto and his teammates use *when discussing positive and negative friendships?* (4.8.1)	■ When the boys went outside to talk, they sat so they could see each other. ■ The boys listened intently as each took turns talking. ■ They kept eye contact when someone else was talking. ■ They nodded to show the speaker they were paying attention and keeping track of the conversation.
Relationship skills: Communication, social engagement, relationship building, teamwork	■ When the boys went outside to talk, they sat so they could see each other. ■ The boys listened intently as each took turns talking. ■ They kept eye contact when someone else was talking. ■ They nodded to show the speaker they were paying attention and keeping track of the conversation.

6. End of class review. Tell the students to put away their materials then ask the review questions.
   a. Name one component of health and describe how a good friend affects it. (1.8.2)
   b. Name one component of health and describe how a negative friend affects it. (1.8.2)
   c. Demonstrate how to use one of the conversation skills. (4.8.1)
   d. Demonstrate how to actively listen when someone is talking. (4.8.1)
7. Exit ticket (Relationship skills: Maintaining healthy and rewarding relationships)
   What is one thing you can do to improve your conversation skills?

Grades 9–12: Relationship skills: Establishing and Maintaining Healthy and Rewarding Relationships/Communication–Advocacy

Thirty-five percent of teens prefer to interact with friends by texting. Thirty-two percent of teens prefer to interact with their friends in person. Sixteen percent of teens prefer to interact with friends through social media. Ten percent of teens prefer to interact with friends through video chatting. (Victoria Rideout, 2018)

Lesson Overview: Value of Face-to-Face Conversation with a Friend Rather than Texting

Students examine the benefits of and barriers to communicating person-to-person and by texting. Students design and adapt health messages for a high school audience that encourages them to embrace the benefits of person-to-person communication.

Resources:

- 2018 SOCIAL MEDIA, SOCIAL LIFE: Teens Reveal Their Experienceshttps://www.common sensemedia.org/research/social-media-social-life-2018

Materials needed:

- **Worksheet 6.5 Pros and Cons of Communicating Face-to-Face or by Texting**
- **Worksheet 6.6 Public Service Announcements Encouraging Communicating Face-to-Face**

   Table 6.9 provides an overview of the lesson objectives, assessment, and instruction for this lesson.

Step 3 – Instruction

1. Define
   a. Compare and contrast: Analysis of what is similar and what is different about two situations or two people.
   b. Adapt: To modify something so that it functions more effectively.
2. 1.12.7 Compare and contrast the benefits of and barriers to practicing a variety of healthy behaviors *such as talking face to face rather than by texting*.
   a. Use **Worksheet 6.5 Pros and Cons of Communicating Face-to-Face or by Texting** to compare breaking up with a boy- or girlfriend by text or in person.
      1) Benefits of face-to-face communication
         a) Fifty-eight percent of communication is through body language.
         b) Thirty-eight percent of communication is through vocal tone, pitch, and emphasis.
         c) Four percent of communication is through the content of the message. (Kim Schneiderman, 2013)
      2) Barriers to resolving conflict in person
         a) Texting does not reveal emotions as much as a person-to-person conversation.
         b) Texting protects against hearing negative reactions.
         c) By texting, the person better controls the situation.
         d) Texting expends less energy. (Kim Schneiderman, 2013)

Table 6.9 Lesson Objectives, Assessment, and Instruction

Step 1 – Lesson Objectives	Step 2 – Assessment
The verb of the *infused* performance indicator and the SEL competency generate the assessment and instruction.	Design the assessment based on the objectives. Ask yourself the question, "What can my students do to show me they have met the standard?"
1.12.7 <u>Compare</u> and <u>contrast</u> the benefits of and barriers to practicing a variety of healthy behaviors *such as talking face to face rather than by texting*. (Joint Committee on National Health Education Standards, 2007, p. 25)	1.12.7 Students <u>compare</u> and <u>contrast</u> the three benefits of and three barriers to having a conversation by text or in person.
8.12.4. <u>Adapt</u> health messages and communication techniques *about the value of person to person communication rather than texting* to a specific target audience. (Joint Committee on National Health Education Standards, 2007, p. 36)	8.12.4 Students adapt a health message and a communication technique *about the value of person to person communication rather than texting* for high school students.
SEL–Relationship skills: Communication, social engagement, relationship building, teamwork	Use communication skills when discussing positive and negative friendships. (1.12.7) (8.12.4)
Step 3 – Instruction	
Design the instruction so that students learn the content, skill, and competency to be successful on the assessment. Ask yourself the question, "What do I need to teach so that the students will be successful when assessed?"	

h. Provide time for the students to complete the worksheet. Discuss. In the discussion, include the benefits of and barriers to face-to-face communication.

3. 8.12.4. Adapt health messages and communication techniques *about the value of person-to-person communication rather than texting* to a specific target audience.

   a. Active listening skills (see Figure 6.3)
   b. Face-to-face communication
      1) Gives the person your full attention
      2) Is more personal and intimate.
      3) Is showing a physical commitment to the conversation.
      4) Shows time was taken to be with the person.
      5) Provides time for questions and a discussion of the situation. (Contemporary Media Forum, 2010)
   c. Practice adapting messages
      a. Use **Worksheet 6.6 Public Service Announcements Encouraging Communicating Face-to-Face**
      b. Students present their public service announcement to the class.
      c. Discuss

4. Read the practice prompt. Students answer the reflection questions and discuss.

Practice Prompt: JaceLynne

One Saturday, JaceLynne and a few friends were hanging out at Harrison's house. It was good to see everyone. They watched a movie, enjoyed pizza, and had fun. While watching the movie, she looked around and noticed that a few of her friends were texting instead of watching the movie. She didn't say anything but thought it a little rude. Plus, they were there to spend time together, not to text others who were not there!

Before and after school, she noticed the same thing. Many peers were together but not talking to each other. It seemed weird.

JaceLynne also texts her friends but prefers talking to them face to face. She likes to hear their voice and see their expressions as they tell a story or share an experience. She knows texting is quicker and takes less energy, can protect against hearing negative reactions, and allows for more control in a situation, but she also realizes that those things are a normal part of relationships and that teens need to learn how to cope with those issues face to face.

During the next Wellness Club meeting, she presented the group with some texting research:

35% of teens prefer to interact with friends by texting; 32% of teens prefer to interact with their friends in person; 16% of teens prefer to interact with friends through social media; and 10% of teens prefer to interact with friends through video chatting. (Victoria Rideout, 2018)

The Wellness Team was shocked to hear that teens prefer to text rather than talk to friends. They decided to survey the student body to determine how often the students text instead of talking. The numbers were shocking! They decided to start a public service campaign to encourage the students to replace some of their texting with face-to-face conversations.

They role played different situations with diverse characters and used popular music to gain the attention of the audience. The video played in the morning and afternoon to raise awareness. They modeled how to give the person you are talking to your full attention, demonstrated that a personal conversation shows a commitment to the other person, and emphasized that it is important to set aside time to talk to one another. They modeled how to ask questions if something was not clear, keep eye contact when speaking, and demonstrate active listening.

The post campaign survey revealed the students had a hard time replacing texting with a face-to-face conversation but when they did, it was a much better way of really understanding what the person was saying.

The Wellness Team has their work cut out for them!

5. Use the review questions in **Table 6.10** to help the students understand the benefits of and barriers to having a conversation in person vs. texting and how to adapt advocacy message to a high school audience.

6. End of class review. Tell the students to put away their materials then ask review questions.
   a. What is one benefit of talking face to face? (1.12.7)
   b. What is one benefit of texting instead of talking? (1.12.7)
   c. What is one way to adapt a public service announcement to a high school audience? (4.12.4)
   d. How do you actively listen when someone is talking? (4.8.1)

7. Exit ticket (Relationship skills: Communication)

   What is one thing you can do to decrease your texting and increase your face-to-face conversations with friends?

Table 6.10 Benefits of Face-to-Face Communication Rather than Texting

Question	Answer
What three things did JaceLynne discover about the benefits of and three barriers to having a conversation in person rather than by text? (1.12.7)	Benefits of having a face-to-face conversation JaceLynne ■ Likes to hear the voice of her friends. ■ Likes to see the expressions on her friend's faces as they tell a story or share an experience. ■ Realizes that there are challenges in making conversation, but they are a normal part of relationships and that she thinks teens need to learn how to cope with those issues face to face. Barriers to having a face-to-face conversation JaceLynne understands texting ■ Is quicker and takes less energy. ■ Protects against hearing negative reactions. ■ Allows for more control in a situation.
How did the members of the Wellness Team adapt a health message and a communication technique *about the value of person-to-person communication rather than texting* for high school students? (8.12.4)	The Wellness Team ■ Role played different situations with diverse characters. ■ Used popular music to gain the attention of the audience. ■ Broadcasted the video in the morning and afternoon to raise awareness. ■ Modeled how to give a person your full attention, demonstrated that a personal conversation shows a commitment to the other person, and emphasized that it is important to set aside time to talk to one another. ■ Modeled how to ask questions if something was not clear, keep eye contact when speaking, and demonstrate active listening.
SEL–Relationship skills: Communication, social engagement, relationship building, teamwork Use communication skills when discussing the benefits of talking face to face.	The Wellness Team ■ Role played different situations with diverse characters. ■ Used popular music to gain the attention of the audience. ■ Broadcasted the video in the morning and afternoon to raise awareness. ■ Modeled how to give a person your full attention, demonstrated that a personal conversation shows a commitment to the other person, and emphasized that it is important to set aside time to talk to one another. ■ Modeled how to ask questions if something was not clear, keep eye contact when speaking, and demonstrate active listening.

Section 2. Negotiating Conflict Constructively/ Seeking and Offering Help When Needed

(Collaborative for Academic Social Emotional Learning, 2020)

Conflict is a normal part of our lives. Children experience conflict when they have different needs and wants from another child or they want the same thing that another child is using. Without conflict resolution skills, the conflict may result in arguing or physical aggression, or a passive response of backing away or avoiding the other child. (KidsMatter, Learning to Resolve Conflict, 2011)

Being able to resolve conflict seek and offer help when needed is enhanced with good communication skills. Teaching these skills to PreK–12 students prepares them to meet life's challenges with confidence. The key to adopting and using the skills with confidence is practice. Each grade span lesson infrastructure contains a practice prompt. Use it to review the information taught. Provide time for students to practice in the safe and supportive environment of the classroom. Elementary children may enjoy watching puppets resolve conflict before practicing the skills individually or in groups. Older students may enjoy writing their own prompts. However, the prompt must be written to the infused performance indicators and the SEL competencies in order to practice the content, skill, and SEL competency. (Randy M. Page., 2015)

Grades PreK–2: Relationship Skills: Negotiating Conflict Constructively/Seeking and Offering Help When Needed

To guide students to resolve their differences peacefully, teach the skill of conflict resolution. Begin by explaining that knowing how to resolve conflict is important for healthy relationships both in and out of the classroom. Model the skill so they know what it looks like, provide time for the children to practice, and formatively assess (coach) them as they demonstrate how to solve a problem in a practice prompt.

Lesson Overview: Resolving Conflict—Friendships

Students examine how to resolve conflict using healthy strategies.

Resources:

- 5 Strategies to Help Kids Resolve Conflict (Hurley, 2018)

Materials needed:

- **Red, yellow, and green circles**
- **Helps sign**
- **Hurts sign**

- **Worksheet 6.7 Healthy Ways to Resolve Conflict**

Table 6.11 provides an overview of the lesson objectives, assessment, and instruction for this lesson.

Step 3 – Instruction

1. Define
   a. Identify: To recognize a particular person or an object.
   b. Demonstrate: To show how something is accomplished.

   2.1.2.1 Understand that healthy behaviors, *such as being able to resolve conflict,* affect personal health.
   a. How resolving conflict affects personal social/emotional health.
      1) Learning how to handle conflict is an important social skill that they can use throughout their lives.
      2) Knowing how to resolve conflict helps children become more sensitive to the needs and feelings of others.
      3) Children develop self-confidence when they are successful at resolving conflict in a positive and assertive way.
      4) Problem solving helps children think creatively and evaluation solutions. (Childcare, 2019)

Table 6.11 Lesson Objectives, Assessment, and Instruction

Step 1 – Lesson Objectives	Step 2 – Assessment
The verb of the *infused* performance indicator and the SEL competency generate the assessment and instruction.	Design the assessment based on the objectives. Ask yourself the question, "What can my students do to show me they have met the standard?"
1.2 1 <u>Identify</u> that healthy behaviors, *such as being able to resolve conflict,* affects their personal *social/emotional* health. (Joint Committee on National Health Education Standards, 2007, p. 24)	1.2.1 <u>Identify</u> that children can experience conflict with a peer, resolve it, *maintain their relationship, and enhance their* personal *social/emotional* health.
4.2.1 <u>Demonstrate</u> healthy ways to express needs, wants, and feelings *when experiencing a conflict with a peer.* (Joint Committee on National Health Education Standards, 2007, p. 30)	4.2.1 Students <u>demonstrate</u> healthy ways to express needs, wants, and feelings *when resolving conflict with a peer.*
4.2.4 <u>Demonstrate</u> ways to tell a trusted adult if threatened or harmed *or need help resolving a conflict.* (Joint Committee on National Health Education Standards, 2007, p. 30)	4.2.4 Students <u>demonstrate</u> ways to tell an adult they need help *when resolving conflict.*
SEL–Relationship skills: Communication, social engagement, relationship building, teamwork	Students <u>demonstrate</u> healthy ways to express needs, wants, and feelings *when resolving conflict with a peer.*
Step 3 – Instruction	
Design the instruction so that students learn the content, skill, and competency to be successful on the assessment. Ask yourself the question, "What do I need to teach so that the students will be successful when assessed?"	

b. Place the signs "Helps" and "Hurts" on opposite sides of the classroom. Read the following situations and ask the children if the way it was resolved helped or hurt the relationship.

Below are two examples of conflicts. Add additional examples or adjust them to meet the needs of your students.

When the children decide if the example helps or hurts the relationship, ask why. Return to the second example after teaching the conflict resolution skills and challenge the children to use the steps to resolve the problem.

a) Rayshard and Kendi were playing with the Legos. Rayshard was building a space station and Kendi, a farmhouse. They were getting to the bottom of the Lego box. Rayshard wanted to make more docking stations and Kendi was finishing the barn. Rayshard said to Kendi, "You can have the rest of the Legos. I can stop building. I have enough docking stations, but you need more to finish the barn." "Thanks, Rayshard," Kendi said. "I would have been upset if I didn't have enough pieces to finish." They each gave an elbow bump and smiled. (Helps or Hurts?)

b) Marianne and Monica were looking forward to recess. They grabbed the jump ropes and started skipping around the playground. Dominique asked if she could play but the girls said, "No." Dominique got mad, called them names, and walked away. The girls skipped closer to Dominique and called her names. (Helps or Hurts?)

2. 4.2.1 Demonstrate healthy ways to express needs, wants, and feelings *when experiencing a conflict with a peer.* (Joint Committee on National Health Education Standards, 2007, p. 30)

3. 4.2.4 Demonstrate ways to tell a trusted adult if threatened or harmed. (Joint Committee on National Health Education Standards, 2007, p. 30)

Use the Marianne and Monica prompt above to model how to use the conflict resolution steps to resolve the problem.

a. Steps to resolving conflict

1) Step 1: STOP! Take three deep breaths to calm down.

2) Step 2: Help a friend by showing empathy
Say, "I can tell that you are upset. I am sorry. I get sad when I see you so upset."

3) Step 3: Use "I" messages to explain the problem.
Each person explains the problem from their point of view.
Say, "When you...........I felt........"
Be polite: No put-downs!
Listen

4) Step 4: Brainstorm 3 solutions
Agree to one solution that works for both people.
Ask an adult for help, if needed.
(Hurley, 2018)

b. Use **Worksheet 6.7 Healthy Ways to Resolve Conflict** to help the children practice conflict resolution skills

4. Read the practice prompt. Students answer the reflection questions and discuss.

Practice Prompt: Ronna

Ronna and Ryes are brothers. Both love riding their bike. The problem is, they share one bike.

Ronna's friend Reddy and his mother are coming over on Saturday. The plan is that the boys are going to set up an obstacle course in the driveway and have fun competing to see who can get through the fastest without hitting any of the obstacles.

Saturday was a beautiful day and Ronna was very excited to set up the course. Ryes asked if he could play. Ronna said, "No! Reddy is my friend and we have been looking forward to the challenge." "Can I ride the course?" asked Ryes. "No!" said Ronna. "You know we only have one bike and the course is for two riders!"

Ryes got really mad and pushed the bike over. It was scratched! Ronna went after his brother but he ran into the house and told his father what happened. "It was an accident, dad!" "No, it wasn't. I was right there and saw him push the bike over!"

"Alright boys, stop and calm yourselves down." Both boys did some deep belly breathing that they learned in health class. "I can tell you both are upset. Calm down and talk the problem through then see if you can solve it on your own."

Reyes said, "When you told me about setting up the obstacle course and riding through it, it sounded like a lot of fun and I wanted to play, too. I don't like it when you don't let me play when you have friends over."

Ronna explained that he likes playing with him, but he also likes to have time with his friends.

Their father came by and asked how they were doing. The boys told him they are working on it. Ronna said, "I know why Ryes got so mad." "Good. You are making progress. Have you figured out a solution?" Dad asked.

(continues)

Practice Prompt: Ronna *(continued)*

Ronna said, "How about you help me set up the course and try it out before Reddy comes over?" "Great! I would love that!" Reyes said, "I know you like to have time with your friend. I'll see if I can go visit my friend, Arno."

Dad checked in again and told the boys he was proud of them for solving the problem. He said, "Solving the problem should give you the confidence to know you can solve another problem if it comes up and also solve problems with your peers.

The solution worked! Reyes apologized for pushing the bike. "It's OK. I know you really wanted to play. You and I can set up a course any time and play together."

The boys felt good about solving the problem and gave each other a hug. Dad and mom were proud of them because they figured out how to resolve the conflict.

5. Use the review questions in **Table 6.12** to help the children understand how resolving conflict affects personal social/emotional health and a review of the steps of conflict resolution.
6. End of class review. Tell the students to put away their materials then ask review questions.

a. What is one way resolving conflict affects personal social/emotional health? (1.2.1)
b. What are the steps of conflict resolution? (4.2.1)
c. How can you tell when you need adult help or when you can handle conflict on your own? (4.2.4)

7. Exit ticket (Relationship skills: Relationship skills: Negotiating conflict constructively/seeking and offering help when needed)

Why is resolving conflict good for your social/emotional health?

Grades 3–5: Relationship Skills: Negotiating Conflict Constructively/Seeking and Offering Help When Needed

Lesson Overview: Resolving Conflict—Friendships

Students learn to resolve conflict and consequently, improve friendships and personal social-emotional health.

Resources:

- https://classroom.kidshealth.org/?WT.ac=ms_tab

Table 6.12 Identifying How Resolving Conflict Affects Personal Social/Emotional Health

Question	Answer
How did Ronna and Reyes <u>identify</u> why they were experiencing a conflict? How did they resolve it, *maintain their relationship, and enhance their personal social/emotional* health? (1.2.1)	■ Ronna and Reyes' dad told the boys he was proud of them and that being able to resolve conflict is a skill they will be able to use again. ■ The boys made suggestions to resolve the problem that demonstrated each understood the other's needs, feelings, and point of view. ■ The boys gained confidence when they were able to find a solution that worked for both of them. ■ The boys had to think creatively in order to find a solution that would work for both of them.
How did Ronna and Reyes <u>demonstrate</u> healthy ways to express needs, wants, and feelings *when resolving their conflict.* (4.2.1) How did the boys demonstrate how to tell a trusted adult when experiencing a conflict? (4.2.4)	■ **Step 1 – Stop!** Ronna and Reyes' dad told the boys to stop and calm down. The boys belly breathed to calm themselves. ■ **Step 2 – Show empathy:** Dad said, "I can tell you both are upset. Calm down and talk the problem through then see if you can solve it on your own." ■ **Step 3 – Use "I" messages to explain the problem:** Reyes said, "When you told me about setting up the obstacle course and riding through it, it sounded like a lot of fun and I wanted to play, too. I don't like it when you don't let me play when you have friends over." ■ **Step 4 – Brainstorm solutions:** Ronna suggested Reyes help set up the obstacle course and ride the bike through to test it and Reyes suggested he visit a friend while Reddy was at the house. Both boys agreed and the solution worked!
SEL–Relationship skills: Communication, social engagement, relationship building, teamwork	Same as above.

Materials needed:

- **Worksheet 6.8 Marysh's Tale**
- **Worksheet 6.9 Practice Resolving Conflict**

Table 6.13 provides an overview of the lesson objectives, assessment, and instruction for this lesson.

Step 3 – Instruction

1. Define
   a. Identify: To recognize a particular person or an object.
   b. Demonstrate: To show how something is accomplished.
2. 1.5.1 <u>Describe</u> the relationship between healthy behaviors *such as using a skill to resolve conflict* and personal health.
   a. Place the following statements around the room and cover them. Read the prompt. Uncover and discuss how the boys in the story accomplished each of the criteria below by resolving their conflict.
      1) Children improve their ability to get along with others. (social health)
      2) Children are happier knowing they have the skill to resolve conflict. (emotional health)
      3) Children have better friendships (social health)
      4) Children learn better. (intellectual health) (KidsMatter, Learning to Resolve Conflict, 2011)
   b. **Prompt**: Jay was using the computer but had to be excused to go to the bathroom. When he returned, Jondo was using his computer. "Hey, get up! I was using that computer," said Jay. "I didn't know you were using it; there was no one sitting here a few minutes ago," said Jondo. "That's because I had to go to the bathroom. Get up! I am working on my science assignment and I need to finish," said Jay. Mrs. Solveitall heard the boys arguing and asked, "What is the matter?" Jay explained that he was using the computer but had to get up to go to the bathroom and when he returned, Jondo was using his computer. "I didn't know that Jay was using the computer, Mrs. Solveitall, the screen was off, and the seat was empty, so I sat down and began my work," said Jondo.

      "Well, I need to finish my work," said Jondo, and "I need to finish my work," said Jay. "Boys, can you think of a way you can both get what you need and still be friends?" asked Mrs. Solveitall. Jay saved his work so he suggested he could use a different computer. Jondo suggested he could finish what he was doing and switch to another computer. The boys looked around and saw a few computers not being used and realized they were upset over nothing. They apologized and Jay went to a different computer, opened his assignment, and started working again. It was a good choice because they were both

Table 6.13 Lesson Objectives, Assessment, and Instruction

Step 1 – Lesson Objectives	Step 2 – Assessment
The verb of the *infused* performance indicator and the SEL competency generate the assessment and instruction.	Design the assessment based on the objectives. Ask yourself the question, "What can my students do to show me they have met the standard?"
1.5.1 <u>Describe</u> the relationship between healthy behaviors *such as using a skill to resolve conflict* and personal health. (Joint Committee on National Health Education Standards, 2007, p. 24)	1.5.1 Student <u>describes</u> *three* relationships between having the skill to resolve conflict and personal health.
4.5.3 <u>Demonstrate</u> nonviolent strategies to manage or resolve conflict *with a peer*. (Joint Committee on National Health Education Standards, 2007, p. 30)	4.5.3 Student <u>demonstrates</u> how to resolve conflict with a peer.
SEL–Relationship skills: Communication, social engagement, relationship building, teamwork	Student <u>demonstrates</u> how to negotiate conflict with a peer.(4.5.3)

Step 3 – Instruction	
Design the instruction so that students learn the content, skill, and competency to be successful on the assessment. Ask yourself the question, "What do I need to teach so that the students will be successful when assessed?"	

working on the same assignment and started helping each other.

c. Place the terms emotional health, intellectual health, and social health in a hat. Using calling sticks, ask a student to pull one of the pieces of paper out of the hat and read it. Point to each of the statements and ask the students to match the term with the statement.

3. 4.5.3 <u>Demonstrate</u> nonviolent strategies to manage or resolve conflict.

a. Use **Worksheet 6.8 Marysh's Tale** to learn the steps of conflict resolution.
   1) What is the conflict?
   2) Who are the characters having the conflict?
   3) How does each character feel about the conflict? (Use "I" messages)
   4) What are the wants and needs of each character?
   5) List three possible solutions. (The Nemours Foundation/KidsHealth, 2016)
   6) Select the solution that works for each person in the conflict.
   7) Reflect on the solution

b. Use **Worksheet 6.9 Practice Resolving Conflict** to provide time for students to practice and demonstrate resolving conflict.

4. Read the practice prompt. Students answer the reflection questions and discuss.

Practice Prompt: Keila

Keila and Kesey have been friends since second grade. Keila invited Kesey to her house on Wednesday to work on their COVID-19 health project. Kesey checked with her parents, got permission to get off the bus at a different stop, and was looking forward to going to Keila's house.

On Tuesday, Keila cancelled. She told Kesey that her parents had something to do. Kesey was disappointed but understood. Sometimes, her parents changed plans and she had to cancel things with her friends.

On Wednesday, Keila spent a lot of time talking and laughing with another friend, Lida. That afternoon, Kesey saw Keila and Lida get off the bus together and run into Lida's house laughing all the way.

Kesey was hurt and mad. Keila said she couldn't work on the project because of a change in plans at home. She lied!

The next day, Kesey confronted Keila who tried to explain but Kesey walked away said, "You lied to me and I don't want to be your friend anymore!" Keila was upset and couldn't concentrate on her work. Kesey had the same problem.

Keila went to the nurse and explained why she was so upset. Her grandmother is sick and her parents were going to visit her in another town and made arrangements for Keila to stay with Lida until they came back.

"Does Kesey know what happened?" asked the nurse. "No, she wouldn't let me explain" said Keila. "Well," said the nurse, "think of some ways to fix the situation." "I could say nothing and just try to be friends again. I could ask my parents to talk to her parents and explain the situation, or I could explain what happened, myself" said Keila. "Which solution do you think would be good for both of you?" asked the nurse. Keila told the nurse that she should talk to Kesey because they were good friends and she wants to be friends again.

The nurse called the teacher and asked her to send Kesey to her office. When she arrived, she saw Keila, glared at her, and ignored her. The nurse explained that she knows about the problem and Keila is upset and wants to fix the situation.

Keila said, "I had to go to Lida's house on Wednesday because my grandmother is sick, and my parents had to visit her. My parents and Lida's parents are friends and they made arrangements for me to stay there overnight."

"I didn't know that" said Kesey. "I thought you just didn't want to be with me" said Kesey.

"I am sorry that I hurt you," said Keila "I am sorry that I yelled at you instead of asking what happened. I was very hurt and then I hurt you" said Kesey. "Can we still be friends?" asked Keila. "Only if we agree to talk to each other when we have a problem" said Kesey. "That makes us better friends!" said Keila."

The girls felt good that they solved the problem and were eager to get back to class to work on their project. Now that they solved their problem, they could concentrate better.

5. Use the review questions in **Table 6.14** to help the children understand how resolving conflict affects their personal health.

6. End of class review. Ask the students to put away their materials then ask review questions.

a. What is one relationship between having the skill to resolve conflict and personal health? (1.5.1)

b. What is the first step in resolving conflict? (4.5.3)

c. What is the second step in resolving conflict? (4.5.3)

d. What is the third step in resolving conflict? (4.5.3)

e. What is the fourth step in resolving conflict? (4.5.3)

f. What is the fifth step in resolving conflict? (4.5.3)

Table 6.14 Identifying How Resolving Conflict Affects Personal Health

Question	Answer
What were *three* relationships between having the skill to resolve conflict and personal health? (1.5.1)	By resolving the conflict, the girls ■ Improved their ability to get along with each other. (emotional/social health) ■ Were happier that they learned how to resolve conflict. (emotional health) ■ Feel they have a better friendship. (social health) ■ Could concentrate better on their health project. (intellectual health)
How did the girls demonstrate the steps to resolving conflict? (4.5.3)	**What was the conflict?** ■ Keila explained that Kesey was upset with her because she thought she lied about cancelling their afterschool time together. **List the characters in the conflict.** ■ Keila explained who was involved to the nurse. (Kesey and Lida) **How did each character feel about the conflict?** ■ Keila and Kesey both felt very bad. ■ Lida didn't know there was a conflict, so she was just happy that Keila was staying over. **What were the needs and wants of each character?** ■ Keila values Kesey's friendship and wanted to resolve the conflict. ■ Kesey was angry until Keila explained what happened. When Kesey understood, she was sorry and wanted to be friends again. **What were three solutions Keila thought of?** ■ Keila could say nothing and just try to be friends again. ■ Keila could ask her parents to talk to Kesey's parents and explain the situation. ■ Keila could explain what happened herself.
SEL–Relationship skills: Communication, social engagement, relationship building, teamwork How did the girls negotiate conflict constructively and seek help, when needed?	Same conflict resolutions skills as above. The nurse and the teacher intervened to help the girls resolve their conflict.

g. What is the sixth step in resolving conflict? (4.5.3)

7. Exit ticket (Relationship skills: Relationship skills: Negotiating conflict constructively/seeking and offering help when needed)

   Why is it important to reflect on how a conflict was resolved?

Grades 6–8: Relationship Skills: Negotiating Conflict Constructively/Seeking and Offering Help When Needed

Between 38.6% and 47.2% of middle school teens report ever being in a physical fight. (Centers for Disease Control and Prevention, 2020)

Middle school teens need to understand that conflict is a natural and important part of our social life. In order to resolve conflict, teens must learn and practice the skill of conflict resolution. Once learned, practiced, and integral to how teens relate to one another, a teen may gain self-confidence and experience improved relationships.

Lesson Overview: Resolving Conflict: Friendships

Students examine the benefits of and barriers to maintaining a healthy relationship and demonstrate their conflict resolutions skills.

Resources:

- Michigan Model for Health

Materials needed:

- Sticky notes
- **Worksheet 6.10 Benefits of and Barriers to Maintaining a Healthy Relationship**
- **Worksheet 6.11 Resolving Conflict**

Table 6.15 provides an overview of the lesson objectives, assessment, and instruction for this lesson.

Table 6.15 Lesson Objectives, Assessment, and Instruction

Step 1 – Lesson Objectives	Step 2 – Assessment
The verb of the *infused* performance indicator and the SEL competency generate the assessment and instruction.	Design the assessment based on the objectives. Ask yourself the question, "What can my students do to show me they have met the standard?"
1.8.7 <u>Describe</u> the benefits of and barriers to practicing healthy behaviors *such as maintaining a healthy relationship*. (Joint Committee on National Health Education Standards, 2007, p. 24)	1.8.7 Student <u>describes</u> the three benefits of and three barriers to practicing healthy behaviors *such as maintaining a healthy relationship*.
4.8.3 <u>Demonstrate</u> effective conflict management or resolution strategies *with peers*. (Joint Committee on National Health Education Standards, 2007, p. 30)	4.8.3 Student <u>demonstrates</u> how to resolve conflict with a peer.
SEL–Relationship skills: Communication, social engagement, relationship building, teamwork	Students <u>demonstrate</u> how to negotiate conflict constructively and seek or offer help when needed.
Step 3 – Instruction	
Design the instruction so that students learn the content, skill, and competency to be successful on the assessment. Ask yourself the question, "What do I need to teach so that the students will be successful when assessed?"	

Step 3 – Instruction

1. Define
   a. Describe: To use words that help others envision the physical attributes of a person, place, or thing.
   b. Demonstrate: To show how something is accomplished.
   c. Healthy relationship: A relationship that includes honesty, good listening skills, able to trust one another, and mutual respect. (Office on Women's Health, Office of the Assistant Secretary for Health, Human Services, 2015)
2. 1.8.7 <u>Describe</u> the benefits of and barriers to practicing healthy behaviors *such as maintaining a healthy relationship*
   a. Ask the students to define "healthy relationship." Agree on the definition. Use the definition above as a guide.
   b. Ask the students to write down on a sticky note or on the board, the characteristics (benefits of) of a healthy relationship. Students place their comments on the board. As they are posted, place similar responses together to determine which characteristics are the most common.
   c. Once the benefits of a healthy relationship are established and discussed, distribute **Worksheet 6.10 Benefits of and Barriers to Maintaining a Healthy Relationship** to explore the barriers to establishing or maintaining a healthy relationship.

d. Benefits of maintaining a healthy relationship
   1) **Talk Honestly:** Able to talk honestly; share thoughts, feelings, and experiences. Each respects the privacy of the other. Able to talk through conflicts.
   2) **Good Listener:** Able to express care for what the other person is saying. Look at the other person and minimize distractions. If you don't agree, acknowledge you see the other person's point of view. (perspective taking)
   3) **Trust and Respect:** Each feels valued for who they are, not because of superficial things like clothes, phones, computers, other belongings.
3. 4.8.3 <u>Demonstrate</u> effective conflict management or resolution strategies *with peers*.
   a. Brainstorm common conflicts experienced between peers and place them on the board.
   b. Use **Worksheet 6.11 Resolving Conflict** to review the steps of conflict resolution and model one of the student conflict examples. Provide time for the students to select another example and resolve on their own. Ask for volunteers to role play the scenario, demonstrating how the conflict was resolved.
   c. Conflict resolution skills
      1) Take some time to calm down. Try belly breaths.
      2) Put yourself in the other person's shoes to better understand why they are upset.

3) Explain how you feel using "I" messages.
4) Use active listening skills to listen to the other person's point of view.
5) Consider solutions to the problem that work for everyone. (Michigan Model for Health, 2016)
6) Reflect on the solution and try another, if needed.
4. Read the practice prompt. Students answer the reflection questions and discuss.

Practice Prompt: Jackson

Jackson and Philip have been friends for a long time. Jackson loves skateboarding and has given Philip his old skateboard and helmet so they could go to the park together. Jackson taught Philip how to navigate the ramps at the skatepark and he is getting pretty good.

Now that they are in middle school, Philip is interested in playing for the school soccer team. He tried out and made it! Lately, he is spending more time with his soccer teammates than with Jackson and Jackson is not happy. He thought they would always be friends.

One day, Jackson said, "Hey, since we are not hanging out anymore, I want my old skateboard and helmet back." "Why? asked Philip. "We can still go to the park."

"When you spend all your time with your new soccer teammates, I feel that we are not friends anymore" said Jackson. Philip looked at Jackson while he was talking and listened carefully. He couldn't believe what he was hearing. To calm down, he took a couple of deep breaths before he spoke.

"Wait a minute, Jackson," Philip said. "I am just excited I made the team. I don't want to disappoint anyone so I practice a lot with the team. It doesn't mean I don't want to be your friend or skateboard with you anymore! I love going to the park and working out with you!" Philip said.

"Well, OK, you can keep the skateboard. Let's figure out how to make sure you have the time you need for soccer and still find the time to go boarding," said Jackson.

"I have an idea," Philip said, "Let's set time aside each week to go to the park." "That is a good idea, but the weekends don't always work for me. How about we wait to go boarding until the soccer season is over?" "Or, the days I don't have soccer practice, we go to the park?" said Philip. "I like that idea," said Jackson.

"I like working with the team, but I also like solo sports. The team is very competitive and with Boarding, I compete against myself" said Philip. "That's not entirely true," said Jackson. "You are pretty competitive with me, but you will need more practice to keep up!"

The boys laughed and walked to the bus together. Both felt great that they resolved the problem. They value their friendship and are glad they got through that problem.

5. Use the review questions in **Table 6.16** to help the students understand how resolving conflict affects their peer relationships.
6. End of class review. Tell the students to put away their materials then ask review questions.
   a. What is the benefit of being able to talk honestly with a friend? (1.8.7)
   b. How does being a good listener help to maintain a healthy relationship? (1.8.7)

Table 6.16 Identifying How Resolving Conflict Affects Personal Health

Question	Answer
What were three benefits of and three barriers to practicing healthy behaviors *such as maintaining a healthy relationship when there is a conflict?* (1.8.7)	Benefits of maintaining a healthy relationship when there is a conflict. ■ **Talk Honestly:** The boys talked honestly share thoughts, feelings, and experiences. They talked through conflicts. ■ **Good Listener:** Each boy expressed care for what the other one was saying. Look at the other person and minimize distractions. ■ **Trust and Respect:** Each boy felt valued for who they were, not for superficial reasons. Barriers to maintaining a healthy relationship when there is a conflict. ■ It was difficult for Jackson to confront Philip because he was angry and hurt. ■ It was difficult, at first, for Philip to understand why Jackson did not want to be his friend anymore. ■ It was challenging for the boys to find a way to spend time boarding because Philip made a commitment to the soccer team and that took a lot of his time.

(continues)

Table 6.16 Identifying How Resolving Conflict Affects Personal Health *(continued)*

Question	Answer

How did Jackson and Philip resolve their conflict? (4.8.3)	1. Calm down
	   • Philip took some deep breaths before he spoke to calm down.
	2. Put yourself in the other person's shoes to better understand why they are upset.
	   • Philip told Jackson that just because he made the soccer team, it didn't mean he didn't want to be his friend.
	3. Explain how you feel using "I" messages.
	   • Jackson: "When you spend all your time with your new soccer teammates, I feel that we are not friends anymore."
	   • Philip: "I am just excited I made the team. I don't want to disappoint anyone so I practice a lot with the team. It doesn't mean I don't want to be your friend or skateboard with you anymore!"
	4. Use active listening skills to listen to the other person's point of view.
	   • Philip looked at Jackson while he was talking listened carefully.
	5. Consider solutions to the problem that works for everyone.
	   • "Let's set time aside each week to go to the park."
	   • How about we wait to go boarding until the soccer season is over?"
	   • "The days I don't have soccer practice, we can go to the park?"
	6. Reflect on the solution and try another, if needed.
	   • The boys were pleased with setting aside the days there is no soccer practice to go to the skate park.

SEL–Relationship skills: Communication, social engagement, relationship building, teamwork How did the boys negotiate conflict constructively and seek or offer help, when needed.	Same as above.

c. How does trust and respect help to maintain a healthy relationship? (1.8.7)

d. Demonstrate the steps of resolving conflict. (4.8.3)

7. Exit ticket (Relationship skills: Negotiating conflict constructively/seeking and offering help when needed)

Why is it important to ask for help when having a problem with a friend?

Grades 9–12: Relationship skills: Negotiating Conflict Constructively/Seeking and Offering Help When Needed

A key to a healthy dating relationship is respect for self and the other person. An unhealthy dating relationship may be characterized by exerting power and control over the other either physically, sexually, and/or emotionally. (Youth.gov, 2020)

Since conflict is a part of social interactions, it is important for teens to understand how to resolve conflict to preserve the healthy dating relationship.

Lesson Overview: Resolving Conflict in a Dating Relationship

Students predict characteristics of a healthy dating relationship then use conflict resolution skills to resolve common dating problems.

Resources:

• https://youth.gov/youth-topics/teen-dating-violence/characteristics

Materials needed:

• **Worksheet 6.12 Predicting Characteristics that Support a Healthy Dating Relationship**
• **Worksheet 6.13 Resolving Conflict and Strengthening Relationships**

Table 6.17 provides an overview of the lesson objectives, assessment, and instruction for this lesson.

Table 6.17 Lesson Objectives, Assessment, and Instruction

Step 1 – Lesson Objectives	Step 2 – Assessment
The verb of the *infused* performance indicator and the SEL competency generate the assessment and instruction.	Design the assessment based on the objectives. Ask yourself the question, "What can my students do to show me they have met the standard?"
1.12.1 <u>Predict</u> how a *healthy dating relationship* affects health status. (Joint Committee on National Health Education Standards, 2007, p. 25)	1.12.1 Students <u>predict</u> three ways a *healthy dating relationship* affects health status.
4.12.3 <u>Demonstrate</u> strategies to prevent, manage, or resolve interpersonal *dating* conflicts without harming self or others. (Joint Committee on National Health Education Standards, 2007, p. 31)	4.12.3 Students <u>demonstrate</u> how to resolve conflict *when dating*.
SEL–Relationship skills: Communication, social engagement, relationship building, teamwork	Students negotiate conflict constructively/seek and offer help when needed.

Step 3 – Instruction
Design the instruction so that students learn the content, skill, and competency to be successful on the assessment. Ask yourself the question, "What do I need to teach so that the students will be successful when assessed?"

Step 3 – Instruction

1. Define
   a. Describe: To use words that help others envision the physical attributes of a person, place, or thing.
   b. Demonstrate: To show how something is accomplished.
   c. Healthy relationship: A relationship that includes honesty, good listening skills, the ability to trust one another, and mutual respect. (Office on Women's Health, Office of the Assistant Secretary for Health, Human Services, 2015)
2. 1.12.1 <u>Predict</u> how a *healthy dating relationship* affects health status.
   a. Ask the students to predict the characteristics of a healthy dating relationship on a piece of paper, fold it, and put it into a container.
   b. Characteristics of a healthy dating relationship
      1) **Mutual respect:** Value the other and understand the other person's boundaries.
      2) **Trust:** Trust the other and give each other the benefit of the doubt.
      3) **Honesty:** Demonstrate honesty, which builds trust and strengthens the relationship.
      4) **Compromise:** Acknowledge different points of view and be willing to give and take.

5) **Individuality:** Maintain personal identity. Continue to spend time with friends and participate in activities. Support one another and encourage each other to pursue new hobbies or friends.
6) **Good communication:** Speak openly and honestly. Give the other person time to think about what to say.
7) **Anger control:** Express anger in a healthy way by taking a deep breath, count to ten, or talk it out.
8) **Fighting fair:** Stick to the subject and avoid insults. Walk away for a while if the conflict escalates.
9) **Problem solving:** Break a problem into smaller parts and talk through the situation.
10) **Understanding:** Take the time to understand what the other person is feeling. (Youth.gov, 2020)
   c. Use **Worksheet 6.12 Predict Characteristics that Support a Healthy Dating Relationship** to expand or reinforce the written characteristics.
   d. Pull characteristics out of the container, one at a time, and see if they match those listed on the worksheet.
   e. Discuss

3. 4.12.3 ~~Demonstrate~~ strategies to prevent, manage, or resolve interpersonal conflicts without harming self or others.
   a. Brainstorm common dating conflicts and place them on the board.
   b. Use **Worksheet 6.13 Resolving Conflict and Strengthening Relationships** to review the steps of conflict resolution and model one of the student conflict examples. Provide time for the students to select another example and resolve on their own. Ask for volunteers to role play the scenario (do not role play violent examples), demonstrating how the conflict was resolved.
   c. Conflict resolution skills
      1) Take some time to calm down. Try belly breaths.
      2) Put yourself in the other person's shoes to better understand why they are upset.
      3) Explain how you feel using "I" messages.
      4) Use active listening skills to listen to the other person's point of view
      5) Consider solutions to the problem that works for everyone. (Michigan Model for Health, 2016)
      6) Reflect on the solution and try another, if needed.
4. Read the practice prompt. Students answer the reflection questions and discuss.

Practice Prompt: Davis

Davis and Lakeda have been dating a few months They look forward to being together and having fun alone or with their friends. They trust and respect each other and have always been honest.

Lakeda doesn't have as much confidence as Davis and becomes uneasy when she sees him with other girls. Before she dated Davis, Lakeda had a boyfriend who cheated on her and she was the last to know. It was humiliating. She is trying to get over that but is having trouble.

On Saturday, Lakeda thought they had plans to hang out, but Davis never showed up. She was angry and disappointed because she rented his favorite movie and asked her mom to buy his favorite snacks. She took some deep breaths to calm down then texted him. "I am sorry, Lakeda. I completely forgot. I made plans with the school Peer Leaders Friday afternoon. We are teaching a health lesson to the elementary students on Monday and we need to rehearse. Can we hang out tomorrow?" asked Davis. Lakeda was upset but said, "OK."

The next day, Davis was right on time but looked different. Lakeda assumed he was going to break up with her. They sat on the couch, facing each other and listened intently as each spoke. "I am sorry, Lakeda. I have been looking forward to being involved in Peer Leadership and when the group called the meeting, I just agreed and went," explained Davis.

"Is there another girl there that you like better than me?" asked Lakeda. "No, no! Nothing like that. We were just practicing our lesson. They are really nice, and I would like you to meet them."

"When you didn't show up at my house, I thought you were mad or decided to break up with me. I was hurt, afraid, and angry!" "I am sorry, Lakeda. I was thinking of myself and forgot," said Davis.

"Well, how can I fix this?" asked Davis.

"I care about you, Davis, and I want us to stay together," said Lakeda "but you have to remember when we have a date. How are you going to do that?" asked Lakeda.

"I have a schedule for peer leaders so I can check it when we are making a date; I can give you my schedule so you can make sure I don t make a mistake again; or I can ask the other peer leaders if you can come with me to practice and help out," said Davis.

"I like your last idea!" said Lakeda. That way we can be together, and you can practice!"

The next week, Lakeda went with Davis to practice. She met his new friends and really liked them. The group needed some help with props for another role play and Lakeda volunteered to help. Davis was pleased that Lakeda understood how important peer leadership was to him and Lakeda was pleased that Davis was comfortable asking her along.

5. Use the review questions in **Table 6.18** to help the students understand how to resolve conflict and maintain a healthy dating relationship.
6. End of class review. Ask the students to put away their materials then ask review questions.
   a. What is one characteristic of a healthy dating relationship? (1.12.1)
   b. What is one characteristic of an unhealthy dating relationship? (1.12.1)
   c. Demonstrate the steps of resolving conflict. (4.12.3)
7. Exit ticket (Relationship skills: Negotiating conflict constructively/seeking and offering help when needed)

   When would it be appropriate to ask for help when having a dating relationship conflict?

Table 6.18 Identifying How Resolving Conflict Affects Personal Health

Question	Answer
What are three predictions of how a *healthy dating relationship* affects health status. (1.12.1)	The relationship will withstand a conflict if both partners ■ Show mutual respect. ■ Trust each other. ■ Are honest with each other. ■ Compromise when there is a conflict. ■ Maintain their individuality. ■ Communicate well. ■ Control their anger. ■ Fight fairly. ■ Solve problems together. ■ Are understanding

How did Takeda and Davis resolve their conflict? (4.12.3)	1. Calm down
	  • Lakeda took deep breaths to calm down before texting Davis.
	2. Put yourself in the other person's shoes to better understand why they are upset.
	  • After talking to Lakeda, Davis understood why she was so upset.
	  • After talking to Davis, Lakeda understood how much peer leadership meant to him.
	3. Explain how you feel using "I" messages.
	  • Lakeda: "When you didn't show up at my house, I thought you were mad or decided to break up with me. I was hurt, afraid, and angry!"
	  • Davis: "I am sorry, Lakeda. I completely forgot."
	  • Davis: "I was thinking of myself and I forgot."
	4. Use active listening skills to listen to the other person's point of view.
	  • When Lakeda and Davis sat on the couch to talk, they faced each other and listened intently as each spoke.
	5. Consider solutions to the problem that works for everyone.
	  • "I have a schedule for peer leaders so I can check it when we are making a date."
	  • "I can give you my schedule so you can make sure I don't make a mistake again."
	  • "I can ask the other peer leaders if you can come with me to practice and help out."
	6. Reflect on the solution and try another, if needed.
	  • Lakeda liked the third solution and it worked out well because Davis could practice with the peer leaders and Takeda could go with him and help with the props.

SEL–Relationship skills: Communication, social engagement, relationship building, teamwork Students negotiate conflict constructively/seek and offer help when needed.	Same as above.

Section 3. Resisting Inappropriate Social Pressure/Seeking and Offering Help When Needed

Social pressure occurs when one person tries to influence the behavior of another. The pressure can be good, such as encouraging a peer to work hard on a project, eat healthy, being physically active, or joining a club; or negative, such as pressuring a peer to do something they know is wrong.

Some children and teens have difficulty resisting pressure because they want to be liked and fit in with the group. Resisting peer pressure is an interpersonal relationship skill that can be learned, with practice.

Grades PreK–2: Relationship Skills: Resisting Inappropriate Social Pressure/Seeking and Offering Help When Needed

Sixty percent of emergency-treated injuries occurred at recreation places or at schools.

Eighty-one percent of emergency-treated injuries involved falls or equipment failure; 42% involved falls from seesaws.

Seventy-two percent of emergency-treated injuries involved seesaws, swings, slides, or composite play structures. (Hanway, 2017, pp. 4-5)

Lesson Overview: Preventing Injuries on the Playground

Students examine how to resist the peer pressure to do something dangerous on the playground equipment.

Resources:

- Kidshealth, Playground Safety, https://kidshealth.org/en/parents/playground.html?view=ptr&WT.ac=p-ptr

Materials needed:

- Smiley face, face with a question mark, frowny face
- **Worksheet 6.14 PreK–2 Using Refusal Skills**

Table 6.19 provides an overview of the lesson objectives, assessment, and instruction for this lesson.

Step 3 – Instruction

1. Define
   a. List: A number of related elements that appear one after another in a group.
   b. Demonstrate: To show how something is accomplished
2. 1.2.4 List ways to prevent common childhood injuries *on the playground.*
   a. Playground safety rules to prevent injuries on the playground
      a) Never push or roughhouse while on the jungle gyms, slides, seesaws, swings, and other equipment.
      b) Use equipment properly (slide feet first, do not climb outside the guardrails, do not stand on the swing, etc.)
      c) Before jumping, check to see if no one is in the way. Land on two feet, with knees slightly bent.
      d) Leave bicycles, back packs, and bags away from the equipment to prevent tripping.
      e) Take off bicycle helmets while playing on the playground.
      f) Do not play on the equipment when it is wet because it will be slippery.
      g) If weather is very hot, check the equipment before going on it. The hot metal of the equipment may cause a burn.
      h) Do not play on the equipment if you are wearing clothes with a drawstring

Table 6.19 Lesson Objectives, Assessment, and Instruction

Step 1 – Lesson Objectives	Step 2 – Assessment
The verb of the *infused* performance indicator and the SEL competency generate the assessment and instruction.	Design the assessment based on the objectives. Ask yourself the question, "What can my students do to show me they have met the standard?"
1.2.4 List ways to prevent common childhood injuries *on the playground.* (Joint Committee on National Health Education Standards, 2007, p. 24)	1.2.4 Students list three ways to prevent injuries on the playground.
4.2.3 Demonstrate ways to respond to an unwanted, threatening, or dangerous situation *on the playground.* (Joint Committee on National Health Education Standards, 2007, p. 30)	4.2.3 Students demonstrate refusing to pressure a peer to get off the slide.
4.2.4 Demonstrate ways to tell a trusted adult if threatened or harmed. (Joint Committee on National Health Education Standards, 2007, p. 30)	4.2.4 Students demonstrate how to ask the teacher for help when there is a conflict on the playground.
SEL–Relationship skills: Communication, social engagement, relationship building, teamwork	Students demonstrate refusing to pressure a peer to climb higher on the jungle gym and telling a teacher about the incident. (4.2.3) (4.2.4)

Step 3 – Instruction
Design the instruction so that students learn the content, skill, and competency to be successful on the assessment. Ask yourself the question, "What do I need to teach so that the students will be successful when assessed?"

or cord because they can become entangled.

i) Wear sunscreen to avoid sunburn. (KidsHealth from Nemours, 2020)

b. Teach/review the playground rules in a creative, engaging manner. Example: Place a smiley face on one side of the room, a question mark face in the middle, and a frowny face on the other. Ask the children questions about the playground safety rules and direct them to stand by the smiley face if they agree, the question mark face if they are not sure of the answer, and the frowny face if they disagree.

a) 😊❓☹️ It is okay to push another peer if he or she is taking too long to go down the slide. Recess is very short, and you want your turn.

Answer: ☹️

b) 😊❓☹️ It is okay to slide head first. You have done that trick before and want to show your school friends how to do it.

Answer: ☹️

c) 😊❓☹️ When jumping off the equipment, check to make sure there is no one below.

Answer: 😊

d) 😊❓☹️ It is OK to keep your backpack close to where you are playing so you can keep an eye on it.

Answer: ☹️

e) 😊❓☹️ It is OK to keep your bicycle helmet on while you are playing in case you fall.

Answer: ☹️

f) 😊❓☹️ Do not play on the equipment if is wet; it might be slippery and dangerous.

Answer: 😊

g) 😊❓☹️ Stay off the metal equipment if it is sunny and hot. It may burn your skin.

Answer: 😊

h) 😊❓☹️ It is okay to play on the equipment if you tuck in the drawstring/cord of your clothes.

Answer: ☹️

i) 😊❓☹️ Wear sunscreen while playing to prevent sunburn.

Answer: 😊

3. 4.2.3 Demonstrate ways to respond when in an unwanted, threatening, or dangerous situation. (Joint Committee on National Health Education Standards, 2007, p. 30)

a. Refusal skill
   1) Say a direct, "No!"
   2) Say why you do not want to do the activity.
   3) Suggest another activity.
   4) Walk away.
   5) Tell an adult.

b. Use **Worksheet 6.14 PreK–2 Using Refusal Skills** to teach and model the skill. Use the safety examples above to provide prompts for the students to resist peer pressure to place a peer in a harmful situation on the playground.

c. Ask the children why it is important to tell the teacher when being pressured to place a peer in a dangerous situation on the playground.

4. Read the practice prompt. Students answer the reflection questions and discuss.

Practice Prompt: Aiden

Finally, it was time for recess!

Aiden and Jeremy ran to the slide and raced up the steps. Jeremy almost lost his grip on the ladder because Aiden pushed him to get by. "Hey, don't push! I almost fell!" Aiden laughed as he passed Jeremy, flew down the slide as fast as he could, and ran back up the ladder again. It was great fun until other children wanted to use the slide.

Dillon walked up and said, "Can I have a turn?" Aiden and Jeremy climbed over Dillon and kept on sliding. Dillon started to climb the ladder. Aiden knew he would slow down their fun so he said to Jeremy, "Climb up the slide so Dillon can't come down. That will make him go away." "No, I am not going to do that. I could get hurt. The slide is too hot to climb up and Dillon might slide into me and we will both get hurt!"

"Let's go on the swings" Aiden said. "There are two open. I bet I can go higher than you!" Aiden

(continues)

Practice Prompt: Aiden *(continued)*

didn't want to leave the slide and started calling him names.

Jeremy called to Dillon, "Hey, Dillon, do you want to go on the swings with me?" "Okay" said Dillon and off they went. They had a good time.

On the way back to the classroom, Jeremy told the recess teacher, Mrs. Modi, that Aiden wanted him to do something dangerous on the slide, but he didn't do it. Mrs. Modi thanked Jeremy and decided it was time to review the playground safety rules with the children so they would all be safe.

5. Use the review questions in **Table 6.20** to help the children understand why it is important to follow the playground safety rules and to refuse to do something dangerous or hurtful.
6. End of class review. Tell the students to put away their materials then ask review questions.
   a. It is okay to push another peer if he/she is taking too long to go down the slide. Recess is very short, and you want your turn.

   Answer:

   b. It is okay to slide head first. You have done that trick before and want to show your schoolfriends how to do it.

   Answer:

   c. When jumping off the equipment, check to make sure there is no one below.

   Answer:

   d. It is okay to keep your backpack close to where you are playing so you can keep an eye on it.

   Answer:

   e. It is okay to keep your bicycle helmet on while you are playing in case you fall.

   Answer:

   f. Do not play on the equipment if is wet; it might be slippery and dangerous.

   Answer:

   g. Stay off the metal equipment if it is sunny and hot. It may burn your skin.

   Answer:

Table 6.20 Using Refusal Skills on the Playground When Being Pressured to Do Something Dangerous

Question	Answer
How did Jeremy prevent injuries on the playground? (1.2.4)	■ Jeremy told Aiden not to push him when he went up the ladder. ■ Jeremy refused to climb up the ladder to stop Dillon from sliding. ■ Jeremy refused to climb up the ladder because it was very hot and he didn't want to burn himself.
How did Jeremy demonstrate refusal skills when being pressured to climb up the ladder so Dillon could not slide? (4.2.3)	■ **Say "No!"** When Aiden told Jeremy to climb up the ladder so Dillon could not slide, Jeremy said, "No, I am not going to do that." ■ **Say why.** Jeremy said, "I could get hurt. The slide is too hot to climb up and Dillon might slide into me and we will both get hurt!" ■ **Let's do something else.** Jeremy suggested that he and Aiden go on the swings instead of staying on the slide. ■ **Walk away.** When Aiden didn't want to leave the slide, Jeremy asked Dillon if he wanted to play on the swings with him. ■ **Tell an adult.** On the way back to the classroom, Jeremy told the recess teacher, Mrs. Modi, that Aiden wanted him to do something dangerous on the slide, but he didn't do it.
SEL–Relationship skills: Communication, social engagement, relationship building, teamwork How did Jeremy resist inappropriate social pressure and seek help, when needed?	**Tell an adult.** On the way back to the classroom, Jeremy told the recess teacher, Mrs. Modi, that Aiden wanted him to do something dangerous on the slide. When the children and Mrs. Modi returned to the classroom, she reviewed the playground safety rules and encouraged the children to follow them to be safe.

h. It is okay to play on the equipment if you tuck in the drawstring/cord of your clothes.

Answer:

i. Wear sunscreen while playing to prevent sunburn.

Answer:

7. Exit ticket (Relationship skills: Resisting inappropriate social pressure/seeking and offering help when needed).

Why is it important to tell an adult when you see one peer pressuring another to do something harmful or dangerous?

Grades 3–5: Relationship Skills: Resisting Inappropriate Social Pressure/Seeking and Offering Help When Needed

Lesson Overview: Using Refusal Skills to Reject Being Pressured to Be a Bully

Students learn to refuse inappropriate social pressure to bully, observe the effects that being a bully have on personal health, and how to seek help when needed.

Resources:

- Michigan Model for Health, Grade 5

Materials needed:

- **Worksheet 6.15 Effects of Bullying on the Bully**
- **Worksheet 6.16 Grades 3–5 Practicing Refusal Skills**

Table 6.21 provides an overview of the lesson objectives, assessment, and instruction for this lesson.

Step 3 – Instruction

1. Define
   a. Describe: To use words that help others envision the physical attributes of a person, place, or thing.
   b. Demonstrate: To show how something is accomplished.
2. 1.5.3. Identify examples of emotional, intellectual, physical, and social health when being pressured to bully.
   a. Effects of being pressured to be a bully on the components of health.
      1) Emotional health
         a) Feel uncomfortable
         b) Feel upset
         c) Feel guilty
         d) Lack of self-control
      2) Intellectual health
         a) Trouble doing their best at school.
         b) Makes the school feel uncomfortable or unsafe.

Table 6.21 Lesson Objectives, Assessment, and Instruction

Step 1 – Lesson Objectives	Step 2 – Assessment
The verb of the *infused* performance indicator and the SEL competency generate the assessment and instruction.	Design the assessment based on the objectives. Ask yourself the question, "What can my students do to show me they have met the standard?"
1.5.2 Identify examples of emotional, intellectual, physical, and social health *when being pressured to bully.* (Joint Committee on National Health Education Standards, 2007, p. 24)	1.5.2 Students describe *two* effects on each of the components of health when acting as a bully.
4.5.2 Demonstrate refusal skills that avoid or reduce health risks *when being pressured to bully.* (Joint Committee on National Health Education Standards, 2007, p. 30)	4.5.2 Students demonstrate refusal skills when being pressured to bully.
SEL–Relationship skills: Communication, social engagement, relationship building, teamwork	Students demonstrate refusal skills and how to seek help from an adult when needed. (4.5.2)

Step 3 – Instruction
Design the instruction so that students learn the content, skill, and competency to be successful on the assessment. Ask yourself the question, "What do I need to teach so that the students will be successful when assessed?"

3) Physical Health
   a) Stress
   b) Frequent fights
   c) Drink alcohol
   d) Smoke/vape
4) Social Health
   a) Feel they have to choose whether to be friends with the bullies and be safe from being bullied themselves or choose a more positive friend.
   b) Experience disrespect from some peers.
   c) Experience trouble at school or with the law. (Michigan Model for Health, 2016, p. 42)
   b. Use **Worksheet 6.15 Effects of Bullying on the Bully** to reinforce the content.
3. 4.5.2 <u>Demonstrate</u> refusal skills that avoid or reduce health risks *when being pressured to bully.*
   a. Refusal skill
   1) Say a direct, "No!"
   2) Suggest another activity.
   3) Repeat the same, "No!" message.
   4) Say why you do not want to do the activity by stating a fact or your feelings and opinions.
   5) Walk away (Michigan Model for Health, 2016)
   b. When refusing
   1) Maintain eye contact.
   2) Stand or sit tall.
   3) Face the person you are talking to.
   4) Use a firm, strong voice, but do not yell. (Michigan Model for Health, 2016)
   c. Use **Worksheet 6.16 Grades 3–5 Practicing Refusal Skills** to review and practice refusing.
4. Read the practice prompt. Students answer the reflection questions and discuss.

Practice Prompt: Kamya

Kamya and Cate are partners for their health project. They like to work together because they are friends and neighbors and it is easy to finish projects at home. They are also quite competitive. They work hard but Bianca and Trish always get higher grades and it is very annoying.

Kamya had an idea. "Let's text our friends that we saw Bianca and Trish copying and pasting from the Internet right onto their slides!" said Kamya. "No. I don't want to do that!" "Why not?"

asked Kamya. "Bianca and Trish didn't cheat. They work hard to get good grades. I don't like being pressured to do something I know is wrong," said Cate. "But we won't get caught and we will finally get a better grade than they will" said Kamya.

"No, Kamya. I am not going to spread a lie to get a better grade," said Cate. "Remember when Carlie was bullying Chase? Everyone turned on her for being a bully. No one wanted to work or play with her and she ended up going to another school. I do not want that to happen to me. I have been thinking. I don't want to be your partner or your friend anymore," said Cate as she walked away.

The next day, Mrs. Honestly asked Bianca and Trish to stay after class. At the bus stop, they were very upset. Cate asked, "What is the matter?" "Someone told the teacher that we cheated on our project and we didn't!" "That is awful," Cate said. Bianca explained, "Kamya texted to our friends that we copied from the Internet and then they told Mrs. Honestly. She asked to look at our slides and when she did, she could tell that we did not copy. We were relieved but very angry that Kamya would do that to us."

Cate told her mother what happened. Her mother told her, "Walking away and ending the friendship was the right thing to do. Kamya was not a true friend when she pressured you to text a lie."

Eventually, everyone learned that Kamya was the person who texted the lie and now no one trusts her, wants to be her friend, or work with her. Her grades are going down, she seldom speaks up in class, and always looks sad and lonely. She is a frequent flyer at the nurse's office and always seems to have a stomach ache or headache.

Cate feels bad for Kamya but is glad she did not take part in the bullying.

5. Use the review questions in **Table 6.22** to help the children understand the effects of being pressured to bully and how to refuse when being pressured to bully.
6. End of class review. Ask the students to put away their materials then ask review questions.
   a. What is one effect of being a bully on emotional health? (1.5.2)
   b. What is one effect of being a bully on intellectual health? (1.5.2)
   c. What is one effect of being a bully on physical health? (1.5.2)

Table 6.22 Using Communication Skills to Cope with a Bully

Question	Answer
What were two effects of Kamya's bullying on each of her components of health?	Kamya's emotional health ■ Looks sad ■ Looks lonely Kamya's Intellectual health ■ Her grades are going down. ■ She seldom speaks up in class. Kamya's physical health ■ Kamya always has a headache. ■ Kamya always has a stomach ache. Kamya's social health ■ No one trusts her. ■ No one wants to be her friend. ■ No one wants to work with her.
How did Cate demonstrate refusal skills when being pressured to bully?	Refusal skills 1) **Say "No."** – When first asked to text a lie, Cate said, "No. I don't want to do that!" 2) **Give a reason why you don't want to do the activity**. – Cate said, "Bianca and Trish didn't cheat. They work hard to get good grades. I don't like being pressured to do something I know is wrong." 3) **If necessary, say "No" again**. – Cate said, "No, Kamya. I am not going to spread a lie to get a better grade." 4) **Walk away**. – "I have been thinking. I don't want to be your partner or your friend anymore," Cate said as she walked away. **Tell a trusted adult**. – Cate told her mother what happened. Her mother told her that walking away and ending the friendship was the right thing to do. Kamya was not a true friend when she pressured you to text a lie.
SEL–Relationship skills: Communication, social engagement, relationship building, teamwork How did Cate demonstrate refusal skills and seeking help from an adult when being pressured to bully?	Refusal skills 5) **Say "No."** – When first asked to text a lie, Cate said, "No. I don't want to do that!" 6) **Give a reason why you don't want to do the activity**. – Cate said, "Bianca and Trish didn't cheat. They work hard to get good grades. I don't like being pressured to do something I know is wrong." 7) **If necessary, say "No" again**. – Cate said, "No, Kamya. I am not going to spread a lie to get a better grade." 8) **Walk away**. – "I have been thinking. I don't want to be your partner or your friend anymore," Cate said as she walked away. **Tell a trusted adult**. – Cate told her mother what happened. Her mother told her that walking away and ending the friendship was the right thing to do. Kamya was not a true friend when she pressured you to text a lie.

    d. What is one effect of being a bully on social health? (1.5.2)

    e. What are the steps to refuse? (4.5.2)

7. Exit ticket (Relationship skills: resisting inappropriate social pressure/seeking and offering help when needed)

    Why is it important to tell a trusted adult if you observe bullying?

Grades 6–8: Relationship Skills: Resisting Inappropriate Social Pressure/Seeking and Offering Help When Needed

Marijuana is the most commonly used illicit drug in the United States by teens as well as adults. Daily use of marijuana increased in 2019 among 8th grade and 10th grade students compared with 2018 rates. (National Institute of Drug Abuse, 2020)

Between 6.6% and 15% of middle school students have used marijuana. (Centers for Disease Control and Prevention, 2020)

21.7% of high school students currently use marijuana one or more times during the 30 days before the survey (Centers for Disease Control and Prevention, 2020).

Seven percent of 8th graders in 2017–2018 report vaping marijuana. (National Institute of Drug Abuse, 2019)

Lesson Overview: Using Refusal Skills to Avoid the Risks of Being Pressured to Smoke Marijuana

Students examine the benefits of and barriers of not smoking marijuana as well as practicing the skill of refusing to use marijuana.

Resources:

- NIDA for Teens
- Marijuana Facts for Teens (NIDA, National Institutes of Health)

Materials needed:

- **Worksheet 6.17 Reasons Not to Use Marijuana**
- **Worksheet 6.18 Grades 6–8 Using Refusal Skills**

Table 6.23 provides an overview of the lesson objectives, assessment, and instruction for this lesson.

Step 3 – Instruction

1. Define
   a. Describe: To use words that help others envision the physical attributes of a person, place, or thing.
   b. Demonstrate: To show how something is accomplished.
   c. THC: The active ingredient in marijuana
2. 1.8.9 Examine the potential seriousness of injury or illness if engaging in unhealthy behaviors *such as smoking marijuana.*
   a. Serious injury or illness related to using marijuana
      1) One in 11 users may become addicted to marijuana. If use begins during the teen years, the rate changes to one in six.
      2) Short-term effects include problems with learning and memory, distorted perceptions of sights, sounds, time, and touch, poor motor coordination, and increased heart rate.
      3) It is unsafe to use marijuana and drive. Marijuana is the most common illegal drug found in the blood of drivers who are in accidents. Marijuana affects alertness, concentration, coordination, and reaction time.

Table 6.23 Lesson Objectives, Assessment, and Instruction

Step 1 – Lesson Objectives	Step 2 – Assessment
The verb of the *infused* performance indicator and the SEL competency generate the assessment and instruction.	Design the assessment based on the objectives. Ask yourself the question, "What can my students do to show me they have met the standard?"
1.8.9 <u>Examine</u> the potential seriousness of injury or illness if engaging in unhealthy behaviors *such as smoking marijuana.* (Joint Committee on National Health Education Standards, 2007, p. 25)	1.8.9 Students <u>examine</u> *five* negative consequences of *smoking marijuana.*
4.8.2 <u>Demonstrate</u> refusal and negotiation skills that prevent or reduce health risks *from being pressured to smoke marijuana.* (Joint Committee on National Health Education Standards, 2007, p. 30)	4.8.2 Students <u>demonstrate</u> how to *refuse to smoke marijuana.*
SEL–Relationship skills: Communication, social engagement, relationship building, teamwork	Students <u>demonstrate</u> how to *refuse marijuana and seek help when needed.* (4.8.2)
Step 3 – Instruction	
Design the instruction so that students learn the content, skill, and competency to be successful on the assessment. Ask yourself the question, "What do I need to teach so that the students will be successful when assessed?"	

4) Marijuana use is associated with school failure. Users get lower grades and are more likely to drop out of school. Users experience negative effects on attention, memory, and learning that last for days after use. Long-time users report less satisfaction with their lives, having memory and relationship problems and poorer mental and physical health, lower salaries, and less career success.

5) High doses of marijuana can cause psychosis or panic when the person is high. (NIDA, National Institutes of Health, 2013)

b. Use **Worksheet 6.17 Reasons Not to Use Marijuana** to help the students understand the potential seriousness of injury or illness if choosing to smoke marijuana.

3. 4.8.2 <u>Demonstrate</u> refusal and negotiation skills that avoid or reduce health risks *from being pressured to smoke marijuana*.

a. Refusal skills

1) Step one: Verbal/nonverbal response

a) Say, "No!"

b) State your position simply but firmly.

c) Be sure your nonverbal body language is consistent with your spoken language: Stand tall and look the person in the eye.

2) Step two: Healthy alternative

a) Suggest an alternative healthy activity with which you are comfortable.

3) Step three: Clarify your position

a) Do not allow the other person to change your mind once you have refused.

b) Maintain eye contact and stand tall.

4) Step 4: Option to leave

a) If the pressure continues, leave. (Bronson, 2007)

b. Use **Worksheet 6.18 Grades 6–8 Using Refusal Skills** to practice skills building.

4. Read the practice prompt. Students answer the reflection questions and discuss.

Practice Prompt: Martin

Martin and Travis have been friends since elementary school. They are on the same sports team, are often paired for projects, and just enjoy hanging out on the weekends.

Lately, Travis started hanging out with other boys and behaving differently. Martin asked, "Where have you been, Travis? We haven't hung out together in a while." "Oh, I've been spending time with some guys who are friends with my brother. Do you want to join us?" Travis said.

"What do you do with them?" asked Martin. "Well, we go down to the river under the bridge. Some of the guys are into marijuana and I tried some," said Travis. "What? Are you crazy? You know what marijuana does to you! Your brother was hooked for a long time. Do you want the same thing to happen to you?" said Martin.

"I like it and I think you would like it, too. It is fun. The river and the clouds look so different when I am high. Nothing bothers me. I am happy," said Travis. "The fact that you like it makes marijuana even more dangerous for you!" said Martin.

"I'm not smoking weed and I won't be hanging out with your new friends," said Martin. "Oh, come on, remember you didn't like tacos and when you tried them you loved them!" said Travis. Martin reminded him that tacos and marijuana and not the same thing. "No. I am not interested," said Martin.

"Your grades have been going down this semester. Maybe smoking weed has something to do with it. Your attitude has changed. You are not the friend you used to be," said Martin. "Let's go to my house. I have a new video game I think you would like. We can have fun without getting high," said Martin.

"No, I am heading down to the river to meet up with the guys. I think you should come with me," said Travis.

"No. I am going home. I have things to do. Come by if you change your mind," said Martin.

At school, the next day, Martin went to the advisor of the Student Assistance Program (SAP) and asked what he could do to help a friend who was smoking weed. Mr. Helpman gave Martin a brochure about the SAP and told him to give it to his friend. "Your friend may not seek help right away but at least he will know there is help available. You are a good friend, Martin," said Mr. Helpman.

5. Use the review questions in **Table 6.24** to help the students understand the negative consequences of smoking marijuana, how to use refusal skills, and how to seek help.

6. End of class review. Ask the students to put away their materials then ask review questions.

a. What are three potential injuries or illnesses that may result from smoking marijuana? (1.8.9)

b. Using a scenario, demonstrate the refusal skills. (4.8.2)

Table 6.24 Identifying How Resolving Conflict Affects Personal Health

Question	Answer
What were the five negative consequences of smoking marijuana that Martin told Travis? (1.8.9)	<ul><li>Marijuana is addictive and Travis could be at risk because his brother was addicted.</li><li>Martin explained that because Travis liked the effects of marijuana, it makes it more dangerous for him to use.</li><li>Travis' grades are going down.</li><li>Travis' attitude has changed</li><li>Travis isn't the friend he used to be before he was smoking marijuana.</li></ul>
How did Martin refuse to go with Travis to smoke marijuana? (4.8.2)	**Step 1 – Say "No."** Martin said, "I'm not smoking weed and I won't be hanging out with your new friends." **Step 2 – Provide a healthy alternative.** Martin said, "Let's go to my house. I have a new video game I think you would like. We can have fun without getting high." **Step 3 – Clarify your position.** Martin said, "No. I am not interested." **Step 4 – If the pressure continues, leave.** Martin said, "I am going home. I have things to do. Come by if you change your mind." **Seeking help** – At school, the next day, Martin went to the advisor of the Student Assistance Program (SAP) and asked what he could do to help a friend who was smoking weed. Mr. Helpman gave Martin a brochure about the SAP and told him to give it to his friend. "Your friend may not seek help right away but at least he will know there is help available. You are a good friend, Martin," said Mr. Helpman.
SEL–Relationship skills: Communication, social engagement, relationship building, teamwork Students demonstrate how to refuse marijuana and seek help when needed.	**Step 1 – Say "No."** Martin said, "I'm not smoking weed and I won't be hanging out with your new friends." **Step 2 – Provide a healthy alternative.** Martin said, "Let's go to my house. I have a new video game I think you would like. We can have fun without getting high." **Step 3 – Clarify your position.** Martin said, "No. I am not interested." **Step 4 – If the pressure continues, leave.** Martin said, "I am going home. I have things to do. Come by if you change your mind." **Seeking help** – At school, the next day, Martin went to the advisor of the Student Assistance Program (SAP) and asked what he could do to help a friend who was smoking weed. Mr. Helpman gave Martin a brochure about the SAP and told him to give it to his friend. "Your friend may not seek help right away but at least he will know there is help available. You are a good friend, Martin," said Mr. Helpman.

7. Exit ticket (Relationship skills: Negotiating conflict constructively/seeking and offering help when needed).

Why is it important to seek help from a trusted adult, when needed?

Grades 9–12: Relationship Skills: Resisting Inappropriate Social Pressure/Seeking and Offering Help When Needed

- A single teen passenger increases a teen driver's crash risk by 44%. (National Safety Council, 2020)

Lesson Overview: Using Refusal Skills to Avoid the Risks of Driving with a Newly Licensed Driver

Students predict ways to get home safely from a party when offered a ride from a newly licensed driver and how to refuse when offered the ride.

Materials needed:

- **Worksheet 6.19 Grades 9–12 Practicing Refusal Skills**

Table 6.25 provides an overview of the lesson objectives, assessment, and instruction for this lesson.

Table 6.25 Lesson Objectives, Assessment, and Instruction

Step 1 – Lesson Objectives	Step 2 – Assessment
The verb of the *infused* performance indicator and the SEL competency generate the assessment and instruction.	Design the assessment based on the objectives. Ask yourself the question, "What can my students do to show me they have met the standard?"
1.12.5 <u>Propose</u> ways to reduce or prevent injuries and health problems *when being offered a ride by a newly licensed driver.* (Joint Committee on National Health Education Standards, 2007, p. 25)	1.12.5 Students <u>propose</u> *three* ways to get home safely from a party when being offered a ride by a newly licensed driver.
4.12.2 <u>Demonstrate</u> refusal, negotiation, and collaboration skills to enhance health and avoid or reduce health risks *associated with taking a ride from a newly licensed teen.* (Joint Committee on National Health Education Standards, 2007, p. 31)	4.12.2 Students <u>demonstrate</u> how to refuse a ride from a *newly licensed driver* and get home safely.
SEL–Relationship skills: Communication, social engagement, relationship building, teamwork	Students <u>demonstrate</u> how to resist inappropriate social pressure and seek help when needed. (1.12.5) (4.12.2)

Step 3 – Instruction

Design the instruction so that students learn the content, skill, and competency to be successful on the assessment. Ask yourself the question, "What do I need to teach so that the students will be successful when assessed?"

Step 3 – Instruction

1. Define
   a. Describe: To use words that help others envision the physical attributes of a person, place, or thing.
   b. Demonstrate: To show how something is accomplished.
2. 1.12.5 Propose ways to reduce or prevent injuries and health problems *when being offered a ride by a newly licensed driver.*
   a. To check for content knowledge, administer the true/false below before the instruction. Use Kahoot or another creative formative assessment to ask the true/false questions. The information in the pretest is also the rationale for refusing a ride from a newly licensed driver on **Worksheet 6.19 Grades 9–12 Practicing Refusal Skills.**
   b. True/False on teen driving.
      1) T F The number 2 killer of teens is car crashes. F—It is the number one cause of teen death.
      2) T F The safest way for a teen to build driving experience and skills is to ride with a parent and practice for one year after getting a license. T
      3) T F One of the most common teen driving errors is driving too slow for the conditions. F—Driving too fast.
      4) T F The radio is one of the biggest distractions teens experience when driving.

F—The biggest distraction is other teen passengers or brothers or sisters.
      5) T F Scanning the road constantly and knowing what to do in a variety of situations helps to keep the teen driver safe. T
      6) T F Driving in different weather conditions and traffic patterns is a risk for a new teen driver. T
      7) T F It is safer for new teen drivers to drive at night. F—16- and 17-year-old drivers are three times more likely to be in a fatal car crash at night than during the day.
      8) T F Teen drivers are the least likely to wear a seat belt. T
      9) T F If a teen has only six hours of sleep and drives, he or she is at greater risk to be in an accident. T—Teens need eight to 10 hours of sleep to function optimally.
      10) T F If a teen is tired because of a lack of sleep, busy school and work schedule, the safest thing to do is to call for a ride rather than driving. T
          https://www.nsc.org/driveithome/teen-driver-risks/drowsy-driving
   c. Brainstorm ways to get home safely from a party when the only person ready to leave is a newly licensed driver.
      1) Call an older sibling.
      2) Call a parent or other responsible adult.
      3) Order an Uber or Ride Share.

4) Check the other partygoers for a more experienced driver.

3. 4.12.2 <u>Demonstrate</u> refusal, negotiation, and collaboration skills to enhance health and avoid or reduce health risks *associated with taking a ride from a newly licensed teen*

a. Teach the steps of refusal skills or use **Worksheet 6.19 Grades 9–12 Practicing Refusal Skills** to teach and model the skill. Provide time for the students to brainstorm and practice other refusal situations.

   a) Step 1 – Calm down before speaking.

   b) Step 2 – Stand tall and look the person in the eye and simply but firmly say, "No!" Be sure your nonverbal body language is consistent with your spoken language. Repeat, if necessary.

   c) Step 3 – Give a reason why you do not want to do the activity.

   d) Step 4 – Suggest a healthy alternative or change the subject.

   e) Step 5 – Leave, if the pressure continues. (Michigan Model for Health, 2013, p. 97)

b. Use **Worksheet 6.19 Grades 9–12 Practicing Refusal Skills** to provide time for the students to practice refusing a ride with a newly licensed teen driver.

4. Read the practice prompt. Students answer the reflection questions and discuss.

Practice Prompt: Devin

Devin was at a party with his friends and it was getting late. He knew he should be going home soon so he called his parents but got no answer. Sometimes his parents do not take their phones with them when they go out and didn't expect to pick him up until much later.

One of his friends, Emily, just got her license and volunteered to take him home. She is very inexperienced, and Devin knows that inexperience is the #1 cause of teen crashes. Devin is worried because he saw Emily drive and she is not a good driver. She is easily distracted, plus state law says that she can only drive family members.

Devin was worried about his safety and anyone else who would get in the car, so he said, "Emily, you know you can't drive us! It's against the law." "I can do it! No one will know and I'll never get pulled over." Devin got mad because his older brother, when he just got his license, drove some friends home after a party and got in an accident. Some of his friends were seriously injured. Devin remembered that and doesn't want it to happen again.

Devin knew he had to step back and calm down before saying anything to Emily. He took a few deep breaths, faced her, looked her in the eye, and said, "No! My brother was in an accident as a new driver and he never got over it because people got hurt and I don't want that to happen to you!"

"I have an idea," Devin said. My friend Kaden has been driving for a while and is ready to go home. I'll ask him for a ride. If Kaden cannot drive me, I'll call an Uber."

"Devin, I told you, I can drive! Don't you trust me?" said Emily. "It has nothing to do with trust, Emily, I want us both to get home safe tonight. Thanks anyway. It is time for me to leave."

Right after talking to Emily, Devin texted his parents again and they responded saying they can pick him up whenever he is ready. Devin texted back that he is ready and will be waiting outside.

5. Use the review questions in **Table 6.26** to help the students understand how to get home safely from a party, refuse to drive with an inexperienced driver, and seek help when needed.

Table 6.26 Identifying How Resolving Conflict Affects Personal Health

Question	Answer
What were the *three* ways Devin proposed to get home safely from a party when being offered a ride by a newly licensed driver? (1.12.5)	<ul><li>Call his parents.</li><li>A more experienced driver, Kaden, was ready to go home. Devin will ask him for a ride.</li><li>If Kaden cannot drive Devin, he will call an Uber.</li></ul>
Students <u>demonstrate</u> how to refuse a ride from a newly licensed driver and get home safely. (4.12.2)	**Step 1 – Calm down before speaking**. Devin was angry because his brother was in an accident when he was a new driver and he didn't want the same thing to happen to Emily. He knew he had to step back and calm down before saying anything to Emily.

Step 2 – Stand tall and look the person in the eye and simply but firmly say, "No!" Devin took a few deep breaths, faced her, looked her in the eye, and said, "No! My brother was in an accident as a new driver and he never got over it because people got hurt and I don't want that to happen to you!"

Step 3 – Give a reason why you do not want to do the activity. Emily is very inexperienced, and Devin knows that inexperience is the #1 cause of teen crashes. Devin is worried because he saw Emily drive and she is not a good driver. She is easily distracted plus the state law says that she can only drive family members.

Step 4 – Suggest a healthy alternative or change the subject. "I have an idea," Devin said. My friend Kaden has been driving for a while and is ready to go home. I'll ask him for a ride. If Kaden cannot drive me, I'll call an Uber."

Step 5 – Leave, if the pressure continues. (Michigan Model for Health, 2013, p. 97) "It has nothing to do with trust, Emily, I want us both to get home safe tonight. Thanks anyway. It is time for me to leave."

Step 6 – Seek help when needed. Right after talking to Emily, Devin texted his parents again and they responded saying they can pick him up whenever he is ready. Devin texted back that he is ready and will be waiting outside.

SEL–Relationship skills: Communication, social engagement, relationship building, teamwork How did Devin demonstrate resisting inappropriate social pressure and seeking help when needed?	Same as above.

6. End of class review. Ask the students to put away their materials then ask review questions.
   a. Propose one way to get home safety when you do not want to drive with a newly licensed driver. (1.12.5)
   b. What is one reason to refuse to drive with a newly licensed driver?
   c. Demonstrate the steps of refusing. (4.12.2)

7. Exit ticket (Relationship skills: Negotiating conflict constructively/seeking and offering help when needed).

   Why is it important to seek or provide help when uncomfortable riding with a newly licensed driver?

Sample Lesson Plan for Relationship Skills

Unit: *State the unit of the lesson.*	Interpersonal Communication
Topic: *State the topic of the lesson.*	Relationship skills: Negotiating conflict constructively/seeking and offering help when needed
Grade level: *State the grade level of the lesson.*	Grades 3–5
Time allotment: *State the time allotted for the lesson.*	40 minutes
Lesson summary: *Provide a summary of the lesson.*	Students learn to resolve conflict and consequently improve friendships and personal social-emotional health.

Risk behavior data: *Provide time rationale for this lesson by accessing the risk behavior the lesson reduces.*	N/A
Standards and SEL Competency to reduce the risk factor(s): *List the Standard 1 and skills standards and the SEL competency/ subcompetency.*	1.5.1 <u>Describe</u> the relationship between healthy behaviors and personal health. 4.5.3 <u>Demonstrate</u> nonviolent strategies to manage or resolve conflict. SEL–Relationship skills: Communication, social engagement, relationship building, teamwork
Objectives: *The objectives are the infused performance indicators and SEL competency.*	1.5.1 <u>Describe</u> the relationship between healthy behaviors *such as using a skill to resolve conflict* and personal health. 4.5.3 <u>Demonstrate</u> nonviolent strategies to manage or resolve conflict *with a peer.* SEL–Relationship skills: Communication, social engagement, relationship building, teamwork
Lesson assessment: *Design an assessment for each infused performance indicator and SEL competency.*	1.5.1 Student <u>describes</u> *three* relationships between having the skill to resolve conflict and personal health. 4.5.3 Student <u>demonstrates</u> how to resolve conflict with a peer. SEL–Relationship skills: Communication, social engagement, relationship building, teamwork Student demonstrates how to negotiate conflict with a peer.
Lesson instruction: *Provide a detailed description of how content, skill, and SEL competency are taught, "bell to bell."*	Review/Preview Ask the students how they observe their peers resolving conflict. Is the strategy a healthy or unhealthy strategy? Why? What are some nonviolent ways to resolve conflict? Is that strategy healthy or unhealthy? Why? Lesson Objectives Students describe the relationship between using skills to resolve a conflict and personal health and how to use nonviolent strategies to resolve conflict. Define lesson vocabulary, if necessary.
	Lesson 1. 1.5.1 <u>Describe</u> the relationship between healthy behaviors *such as using a skill to resolve conflict* and personal health. a. Place the following statements around the room and cover them. Read the prompt. Uncover and discuss how the boys in the story accomplished each of the criteria below by resolving their conflict. 1) Children improve their ability to get along with others. (social health) 2) Children are happier knowing they have the skill to resolve conflict. (emotional health) 3) Children have better friendships (social health) 4) Children learn better. (intellectual health) (KidsMatter, Learning to Resolve Conflict, 2011) b. **Prompt**: Jay was using the computer but had to be excused to go to the bathroom. When he returned, Jondo was using his computer. "Hey, get up! I was using that computer," said Jay. "I didn't know you were using it, there was no one sitting here a few minutes ago," said Jondo. "That's because I had to go to the bathroom. Get up! I am working on my science assignment and I need to finish," said Jay. Mrs. Solveitall heard the boys arguing and asked, "What is the matter?" Jay explained that he was using the computer but had to get up to go to the bathroom and when he returned, Jondo was using his computer. "I didn't know Jondo was using the computer, Mrs. Solveitall, the screen was off, and the seat was empty, so I sat down and began my work," said Jondo

"Well, I need to finish my work," said Jondo, and "I need to finish my work," said Jay. "Boys, can you think of a way you can both get what you need and still be friends?" asked Mrs. Solveitall. Jay saved his work so he suggested he could use a different computer. Jondo suggested he could finish what he was doing and switch to another computer. The boys looked around and saw a few computers not being used and realized they were upset over nothing. They apologized and Jay went to a different computer, opened his assignment, and started working again. It was a good choice because they were both working on the same assignment and started helping each other.

   c. Place the terms emotional health, intellectual health, and social health in a hat. Using calling sticks, ask a student to pull one of the pieces of paper out of the hat and read it. Point to each of the statements and ask the students to match the term with the statement.

2. 4.5.3 <u>Demonstrate</u> nonviolent strategies to manage or resolve conflict.
   a. Use **Worksheet 6.8 Marysh's Tale** to learn the steps of conflict resolution.
      1) What is the conflict?
      2) Who are the characters having the conflict?
      3) How does each character feel about the conflict? (Use "I" messages)
      4) What are the wants and needs of each character?
      5) List three possible solutions. (The Nemours Foundation/KidsHealth, 2016)
      6) Select the solution that works for each person in the conflict.
      7) Reflect on the solution
   b. Use **Worksheet 6.9 Practice Resolving Conflict** to provide time for students to practice and demonstrate resolving conflict.

3. Read the practice prompt then ask the students the re-enforcement questions.

Practice Prompt: Keila

Keila and Kesey have been friends since second grade. Keila invited Kesey to her house on Wednesday to work on their COVID-19 health project. Kesey checked with her parents, got permission to get off the bus at a different stop, and was looking forward to going to Keila's house.

On Tuesday, Keila cancelled. She told Kesey that her parents had something to do. Kesey was disappointed but understood. Sometimes her parents changed plans and she had to cancel things with her friends.

On Wednesday, Keila spent a lot of time talking and laughing with another friend, Lida. That afternoon, Kesey saw Keila and Lida get off the bus together and run into Lida's house laughing all the way.

Kesey was hurt and mad. Keila said she couldn't work on the project because of a change in plans at home. She lied!

The next day, Kesey confronted Keila who tried to explain but Kesey walked away said, "You lied to me and I don't want to be your friend anymore!" Keila was upset and couldn't concentrate on her work. Kesey had the same problem.

Keila went to the nurse and explained why she was so upset. Her grandmother is sick and her parents were going to visit her in another town and made arrangements for Keila to stay with Lida until they came back.

"Does Kesey know what happened?" asked the nurse. "No, she wouldn't let me explain" said Keila. "Well," said the nurse, "think of some ways to fix the situation." "I could say nothing and just try to be friends again. I could ask my parents to talk to her parents and explain the situation, or I could explain what happened myself" said Keila. "Which solution do you think would be good for both of you?" asked the nurse. Keila told the nurse that she should talk to Kesey because they were good friends and she wants to be friends again.

The nurse called the teacher and asked her to send Kesey to her office. When she arrived, she saw Keila, glared at her, and ignored her. The nurse explained that she knows about the problem and Keila is upset and wants to fix the situation.

Keila said, "I had to go to Lida's house on Wednesday because my grandmother is sick, and my parents had to visit her. My parents and Lida's parents are friends and they made arrangements for me to stay there overnight."

"I didn't know that" said Kesey. "I thought you just didn't want to be with me" said Kesey.

"I am sorry that I hurt you," said Keila "I am sorry that I yelled at you instead of asking what happened. I was very hurt and then I hurt you" said Kesey. "Can we still be friends?" asked Keila. "Only if we agree to talk to each other when we have a problem" said Kesey. "That makes us better friends!" said Keila."

The girls felt good that they resolved the problem and were eager to get back to class to work on their project. Now that they solved their problem, they could concentrate better.

4. Use the following review questions to help the children understand how resolving conflict affects their personal health.

Question	Answer
Describe *three* ways the girls improved their personal health when they used refusal skills to resolve their differences (1.5.1)	By resolving the conflict, the girls ■ Improved their ability to get along with each other. (emotional/social health) ■ Were happier that they learned how to resolve conflict. (emotional health) ■ Feel that they have a better friendship. (social health) ■ Could concentrate better on their health project (intellectual health)
How did the girls demonstrate the steps to resolving conflict? (4.5.3)	**What was the conflict?** ■ Keila explained that Kesey was upset with her because she thought she lied about cancelling their afterschool time together. **List the Characters in the conflict.** ■ Keila explained who was involved to the nurse. (Kesey and Lida) **How did each character feel about the conflict?** ■ Keila and Kesey both felt very badly. ■ Lida didn't know there was a conflict, so she was just happy that Keila was staying over. **What were the needs and wants of each character?** ■ Keila values Kesey's friendship and wanted to resolve the conflict. ■ Kesey was angry until Keila explained what happened. When Kesey understood, she was sorry and wanted to be friends again. **What were three solutions Keila thought of?** ■ Keila could say nothing and just try to be friends again. ■ Keila could ask her parents to talk to Kesey's parents and explain the situation. ■ Keila could explain what happened herself.

	SEL–Relationship skills: Communication, social engagement, relationship building, teamwork	Same conflict resolution skills as above.
		The nurse and the teacher intervened to help the girls resolve their conflict.
	How did the girls negotiate conflict constructively and seek help, when needed?	

Materials: *List the materials used to plan and implement the lesson, including formative assessments.*	**Worksheet 6.8 Marysh's Tale** **Worksheet 6.9 Practice Resolving Conflict**
Resources: *What resources were used to plan and implement the lesson?*	https://classroom.kidshealth.org/?WT.ac=ms_tab
Differentiated instruction: *What modifications are being made for students with disabilities and English Learners?*	Students work in groups, specifically designed to support students with disabilities or English Learners.
Sample student products: *Provide exemplars of how other students successfully complete this assignment.*	Show previously completed worksheets.
Collaboration: *Are the students completing the activity individually, in pairs, in groups, etc.?*	Students work in groups of four in order to pair up or work as a group.
Teacher reflection: *What can I do to improve this lesson next time it is taught?*	Will vary.

References

Bronson, B. M. (2007). *Teen Health, Course 2.* New York: McGraw-Hill.

CASEL. (2019, September 21). *What is SEL?* Retrieved from CASEL https://casel.org/what-is-sel/

Centers for Disease Control and Prevention. (2020). *2019 Middle School YRBS Middle school students reporting ever smoking marijuana.* Retrieved from Centers for Disease Control and Prevention: https://nccd.cdc.gov/youthonline/App/Results .aspx?TT=B&OUT=0&SID=MS&QID=M28&LID=LL&YID =RY&LID2=&YID2=&COL=&ROW1=&ROW2 =&HT=&LCT=&FS=&FR=&FG=&FA=&FI=&FP=&FSL =&FRL=&FGL=&FAL=&FIL=&FPL=&PV=&TST =&C1=&C2=&QP=&DP=&VA=CI&CS=Y&SYID=&EYID =&SC=&SO=

Centers for Disease Control and Prevention. (2020). *High School YRBS 2019 Results-High school students currently used marijuana during the 30 days prior to the survey.* Retrieved from Centers for Disease Control and Prevention: https://nccd .cdc.gov/youthonline/App/Results.aspx?TT=B&OUT=0&SID =HS&QID=H47&LID=LL&YID=RY&LID2=&YID2=&COL =&ROW1=&ROW2=&HT=&LCT=&FS=&FR=&FG=&FA =&FI=&FP=&FSL=&FRL=&FGL=&FAL=&FIL=&FPL

=&PV=&TST=&C1=&C2=&QP=&DP=&VA=CI&CS=Y&SYID=&EYID=&SC=&SO=

Childcare. (2019). *Ways Child Care Providers Can Teach Young Children to Resolve Conflicts*. Retrieved from eXtension Alliance for Better Child Care https://childcare.extension.org/ways-child-care-providers-can-teach-young-children-to-resolve-conflicts/

Cohn-Vargas, B. & Adamson, C. (2020). *Helping Students Through a Period of Grief*. Retrieved from George Lucas Educational Foundation, Edutopia: https://www.edutopia.org/article/helping-students-through-period-grief

Collaborative for Academic and Social Emotional Learning. (2020). *CASEL Competencies*. Retrieved from CASEL https://casel.org/wp-content/uploads/2019/12/CASEL-Competencies.pdf

Collaborative for Academic Social Emotional Learning. (2020). *www.casel.org/.../08/Sample-Teaching-Activities-to-Support-Core-Competencies-8-20-17.pdf*. Retrieved from CASEL.org: www.casel.org/.../08/Sample-Teaching-Activities-to-Support-Core-Competencies-8-20-17.pdf

Connolly, M. (2020). *Skills-Based Health Education, Second Edition*. Burlington, MA: Jones and Bartlett.

Suler, J. (2010). Interpersonal guidelines for texting. *International Journal of Applied Psychoanalytic Studies*, 7(4), 358–361.

Dictionary.com. (2020). *Communication*. Retrieved from Dictionary.com: https://www.dictionary.com/browse/communication?s=t

Dictionary.com. (2020). *List*. Retrieved from Dictionary.com: https://www.dictionary.com/browse/list?s=t

Dictionary.com. (2020). *Teamwork*. Retrieved from Dictionary.com: https://www.dictionary.com/browse/teamwork?s=ts

Frey, N., Fisher, D., & Smith, D. (2019). *All learning is social and emotional: Helping students develop essential skills for the classroom and beyond*. Alexandria: ASCD.

Hanway, S. M. (2016). *Injuries and investigated deaths associated with playground equipment, 2009-2014*. Bethesda, MD: U.S. Consumer Product Safety Commission. Retrieved from https://www.cpsc.gov/s3fs-public/Injuries%20and%20Investigated%20Deaths%20Associated%20with%20Playground%20Equipment%202009%20to%202014_1.pdf?29GwYlhQ6fUwXskAQxLoGaHaE8aHZSsY

Hurley, K. (2018). *5 Strategies to Help Kids Resolve Conflict*. Retrieved from PBS for Parents https://www.pbs.org/parents/thrive/5-strategies-to-help-kids-resolve-conflict

John W. Gardner Center. (2007). *Youth Engaged in Leadership and Learning YELL A Handbook for Program Staff, Teachers, and Community Leaders*. California: John W. Gardner Center for Youth and Their Communities 2nd Edition © 2007. Retrieved from https://gardnercenter.stanford.edu/sites/g/files/sbiybj11216/f/YELL Handbook.pdf

Joint Committee on National Health Education Standards. (2007). *National Health Education Standards, Second Edition*. American Cancer Society.

KidsHealth from Nemours. (2020). *Playground Safety*. Retrieved from KidsHealth from Nemours: https://kidshealth.org/en/parents/playground.html?ref=search

KidsMatter, Learning to Resolve Conflict. (2011). *How Children Learn to Resolve Conflict*. Retrieved from KidsMatter www.kidsmatter.edu.au/resources/information-resources

Kim Schneiderman, L. M. (2013). *The Trouble with Texting*. Retrieved from Psychology Today https://www.psychologytoday.com/us/blog/the-novel-perspective/201301/the-trouble-texting

Krueger, K. R., Wilson, R. S., Kanenetsky, J. M., Barnes, L. L., Bienias, J. L., & Bennett, D. A. (2009). Social engagement and cognitive function in old age. *Experimental Aging Research*, 35(1), 45–60.

Lynch, A. E. (2012). *Choosing Health*. San Francisco: Pearson Education.

Meeks, L. H. (2020). *Comprehensive School Health Education, Ninth Edition*. New York: McGraw Hill.

Mendler, A. (2013). *Teaching Your Students How to Have a Conversation*. Retrieved from George Lucas Educational Foundation, Edutopia https://www.edutopia.org/blog/teaching-your-students-conversation-allen-mendler

Michigan Model for Health. (2013). *Michigan Model for Health, High School Edition, Skills for Health and Life*. Mt. Pleasant, Michigan: Michigan Model for Health Clearinghouse.

Michigan Model for Health. (2016). Lesson 9 Finding Ways to Resolve Conflict. *Michigan Model for Health, Grade 6 Curriculum*. Holt, Michigan, United States: Michigan Model for Health Clearinghouse.

Michigan Model for Health. (2016). *Michigan Model for Health, Grade 5*. Holt, Michigan: Michigan Model for Health Clearinghouse.

Michigan Model for Health. (2016). *Safe and Sound for Life, Middle School*. Michigan Model for Health Clearinghouse.

Michigan Model for Health. (2016). *Stay Drug Free for a Successful Tomorrow, Lesson 7*. Michigan Model for Health Clearinghouse.

Michigan Model for Health. (2019). *Michigan Model for Health, Grade 2*. Holt, MI: Michigan Model for Health Clearinghouse.

Michigan Model for Health. (2019). *Michigan Model for Health, Kindergarten*. Holt, MI: Michigan Model for Health Clearinghouse.

Michigan Model for Health Clearinghouse. (2016). Lesson 9, Finding Ways to Resolve Conflicts. *Michigan Model for Health, Grade 6 Curriculum*. Michigan, United States: Michigan Model for Health Clearinghouse.

National Institute on Drug Abuse. (2019). *Vaping of marijuana on the rise among teens*. Retrieved from National Institute on Drug Abuse https://www.drugabuse.gov/news-events/news-releases/2019/12/vaping-of-marijuana-on-the-rise-among-teens

National Institute on Drug Abuse. (2020). *Marijuana*. Retrieved from NIDA for Teens. https://teens.drugabuse.gov/drug-facts/marijuana#:~:text=Marijuana%20use%20has%20been%20linked%20with%20depression%20and,people%20with%20a%20genetic%20risk%20for%20developing%20schizophrenia.

National Safety Council. (2020). *How Many Teen Passengers Can Safely Ride with New Drivers?* Retrieved from National Safety Council https://www.nsc.org/driveithome/teen-driver-risks/passengers

National Safety Council. (2020). *Inexperience is the Leading Cause of Teen Crashes*. Retrieved from National Safety Council https://www.nsc.org/driveithome/teen-driver-risks/inexperience

NIDA, National Institutes of Health. (2013). *Marijuana Facts for Teens*. U.S. Department of Health and Human Services. Retrieved from file ///C:/Users/Mary's%20Surface%20Pro%206/OneDrive/Jones%20and%20Bartlett-Teaching%20SEL/Chapter%206-Teaching%20Relationship%20Skills/NIDA%20teens_brochure_2013.pdf. Sample-Teaching-Activities-to-Support-Core-Competencies-8-20-17.pdf (casel.org)

Office on Women's Health, Office of the Assistant Secretary for Health and Human Services. (2015). *Healthy Relationships*. Retrieved from Girls Health https://www.girlshealth.gov/relationships/healthy/index.html

Page, R. M., Page, T. S. (2015). *Promoting Health and Emotional Well-Being in Your Classroom, Sixth Edition*. Burlington, MA: Jones and Bartlett.

Robert Wood Johnson Foundation. (2015). *New Research: Children with Strong Social Skills in Kindergarten More Likely to Thrive as Adults*. Retrieved from Robert Wood Johnson Foundation: https://www.rwjf.org/en/library/articles-and-news/2015/07/new-research--children-with-strong-social-skills-in-kindergarten.html

Stop Bullying.gov. (2020). *What Kids Can Do*. Retrieved from stopbullying.gov https://www.stopbullying.gov/resources/kids

Telljohann, S. K., Symons, C. W., & Pateman, B. (2019). *Health Education, Elementary and Middle School Applications*. New York: McGraw-Hill. The year was 2009, 6th edition. The publisher is McGraw Hill.

The Nemours Foundation/KidsHealth. (2016). *Grades 3 to 5 • Personal Health Series, Conflict Resolution*. Retrieved from KidsHealth in the Classroom https://kidshealth.org/classroom/3to5/personal/growing/conflict_resolution.pdf

Transforming Education. (2014). *Introduction to Social Awareness*. Retrieved from Transforming Education https://www.transformingeducation.org/wp-content/uploads/2019/04/Introduction-to-Social-Awareness.pdf

Victoria Rideout, M. M., Robb, M. B. (2018). *Social Media, Social Life: Teens Reveal Their Experiences*. Retrieved from www.commonsense.org: https://www.commonsensemedia.org/sites/default/files/uploads/research/2018_cs_socialmedia sociallife_executivesummary-final-release_3_lowres.pdf

Wilson, D. C., Conyers, M. (2017). *4 Proven Strategies for Teaching Empathy*. Retrieved from George Lucas Educational Foundation, Edutopia https://www.edutopia.org/article/4-proven-strategies-teaching-empathy-donna-wilson-marcus-conyers

Youth.gov. (2020). *Characteristics of Healthy & Unhealthy Relationships*. Retrieved from Youth.gov https://youth.gov/youth-topics/teen-dating-violence/characteristics

Chapter 6—Appendix A

Relationship Skills: Scope, Sequence, Content, SEL Competency/Subcompetencies

<u>**Note:**</u> This page is organized by grade span, Standard 1, skill standards, the HECAT content areas, and SEL Competency/subcompetencies.

The HECAT content areas include: AOD – Alcohol and Other Drugs; HE – Healthy Eating; MEH – Mental/Emotional Health; PHW – Personal Health and Wellness; PA – Physical Activity; S – Safety; SH – Sexual Health; T – Tobacco; V – Violence Prevention

Establishing and Maintaining Healthy and Rewarding Relationships/Communicating Clearly

Grade Span	Standard 1	Skill	HECAT Content Areas and Specific Content	SEL Competency and Subcompetencies
PreK–2	1.2.1 <u>Identify</u> that healthy behaviors, *such as expressing appreciation and demonstrating respect,* affect personal health.	4.2.1 <u>Demonstrate</u> *one* healthy way to express needs, wants, and feelings by using "i" messages.	Mental/Emotional health- expressing appreciation and respect — Friendship	Relationship skills: Communication
3-5	1.5.2 <u>Identify</u> examples of emotional, intellectual, physical, and social health *that occur when experiencing a loss.*	4.5.1 <u>Demonstrate</u> effective verbal and nonverbal communication skills to enhance *the* health *of a friend experiencing a loss.*	Mental/Emotional health — Coping with grief.	Relationship skills: Communication, social engagement, relationship building, teamwork
6–8	1.8.2. <u>Describe</u> the interrelationships of emotional, intellectual, physical, and social health in adolescence *when communicating about whether or not to make a friend.*	4.8.1. <u>Apply</u> effective verbal and nonverbal communication skills to enhance health *when discussing positive and negative friendships.*	Mental/Emotional health: Conversation skills-choosing friends	Relationship skills: Communication, social engagement, relationship building, teamwork

(continues)

Establishing and Maintaining Healthy and Rewarding Relationships/Communicating Clearly *(continued)*

Grade Span	Standard 1	Skill	HECAT Content Areas and Specific Content	SEL Competency and Subcompetencies
9–12	1.12.7 <u>Compare</u> and <u>contrast</u> the benefits of and barriers to practicing a variety of healthy behaviors *such as talking face to face rather than by texting.*	8.12.4. <u>Adapt</u> health messages and communication techniques *about the value of person-to-person communication rather than texting* to a specific target audience.	Mental/Emotional health: value of face-to-face conversation with a friend rather than texting.	Relationship skills: Communication, social engagement, relationship building, teamwork

Negotiating Conflict Constructively/Seeking and Offering Help When Needed

Grade Span	Standard 1	Skill	HECAT Content Areas and Specific Content	SEL Competency and Subcompetencies
PreK–2	1.2 1 <u>Identify</u> that healthy behaviors, *such as being able to resolve conflict,* affect their personal *social/emotional* health	4.2.1 <u>Demonstrate</u> healthy ways to express needs, wants, and feelings *when experiencing a conflict with a peer.* 4.2.4 <u>Demonstrate</u> ways to tell a trusted adult if threatened or harmed.	Mental/Emotional Health-Resolving conflict. — Friendships	Relationship skills: Communication, social engagement, relationship building, teamwork
3–5	1.5.1 <u>Describe</u> the relationship between healthy behaviors *such as using a skill to resolve conflict* and personal health.	4.5.3 <u>Demonstrate</u> nonviolent strategies to manage or resolve conflict *with a peer.*	Mental/Emotional Health-Resolving conflict. Friendships	Relationship skills: Communication, social engagement, relationship building, teamwork
6–8	1.8.7 <u>Describe</u> the benefits of and barriers to practicing healthy behaviors *such as maintaining a healthy relationship.*	4.8.3 <u>Demonstrate</u> effective conflict management or resolution strategies *with peers.*	Mental/Emotional Health-Resolving conflict.— Friendships	Relationship skills: Communication, social engagement, relationship building, teamwork
9–12	1.12.1 <u>Predict</u> how a *healthy dating relationship* affects health status.	4.12.3 <u>Demonstrate</u> strategies to prevent, manage, or resolve interpersonal *dating* conflicts without harming self or others.	Mental/Emotional Health-Resolving conflict—Resolving conflict in a dating relationship.	Relationship skills: Communication, social engagement, relationship building, teamwork

Resisting Inappropriate Social Pressure/Seeking and Offering Help When Needed

Grade Span	Standard 1	Skill	HECAT Content Areas and Specific Content	SEL Competency and Subcompetencies
PreK–2	1.2.4 List ways to prevent common childhood injuries *on the playground.*	4.2.3 Demonstrate ways to respond to an unwanted, threatening, or dangerous situation *on the playground.* 4.2.4 Demonstrate ways to tell a trusted adult if threatened or harmed.	Safety: Preventing injuries on the playground— Responding to a dangerous situation on the playground and telling a trusted adult about the danger.	Relationship skills: Communication, social engagement, relationship building, teamwork

3–5	1.5.2 <u>Identify</u> examples of emotional, intellectual, physical, and social health *when being pressured to bully.*	4.5.2 <u>Demonstrate</u> refusal skills that avoid or reduce health risks *when being pressured to bully.*	Mental/Emotional Health – Effects on the components of health when acting as the bully and using refusal skills to reject being pressured to be a bully.	Relationship skills: Communication, social engagement, relationship building, teamwork
6–8	1.8.9 <u>Examine</u> the potential seriousness of injury or illness if engaging in unhealthy behaviors *such as smoking marijuana.*	4.8.2 <u>Demonstrate</u> refusal and negotiation skills that avoid or reduce health risks *from being pressured to smoke marijuana.*	Alcohol and other Drugs Negative effects of smoking marijuana and using refusal skills to avoid the risks of being pressured to smoke marijuana.	Relationship skills: Communication, social engagement, relationship building, teamwork
9–12	1.12.5 Propose ways to reduce or prevent injuries and health problems *when being offered a ride by a newly licensed driver.*	4.12.2 <u>Demonstrate</u> refusal, negotiation, and collaboration skills to enhance health and avoid or reduce health risks *associated with taking a ride from a newly licensed teen.*	Safety: Propose ways to get home safely when being offered a ride from a newly licensed driver and use refusal skills to avoid the risks of driving with a newly licensed driver.	Relationship skills: Communication, social engagement, relationship building, teamwork

CHAPTER 7

Teaching Responsible Decision Making

LEARNING OBJECTIVES

Upon finishing this course, students will be able to:

- Plan skills-based health (SBH)/SEL lessons using backwards design and practice prompts.
- Incorporate the subcompetencies of responsible decision-making skills into assessment and instruction.

KEY TERMS

Ethical responsibility
Ethical standards

Social and Emotional Learning (SEL) Competencies*

- **RESPONSIBLE DECISION-MAKING SKILLS**
  Figure 7.1
  - *The ability to make constructive choices about personal behavior and social interactions based on ethical standards, safety concerns, and social norms. The realistic evaluation of consequences of various actions, and a consideration of the well-being of oneself and others.* (CASEL, 2019)

Introduction

The CASEL competency of Responsible Decision Making is not paired like Self-Awareness/Self-Management and Social Awareness/Relationship Skills. However, proficiency in each of the other competencies contributes to proficiency in being able to make responsible decisions.

Being able to solve problems productively is a life skill that youth learn through skills-based health/SEL education. Problem solving is the first step in decision making because before a decision is made, we must identify the problem. For example, Mrs. Solver asks Merilee, "What is the matter?"

---

*A scope and sequence document is included as an appendix at the end of this chapter.

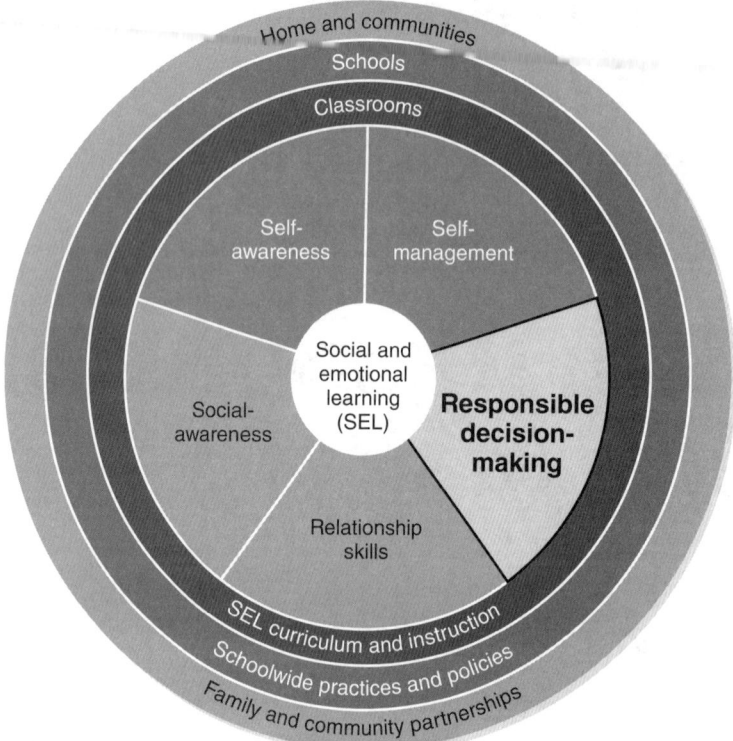

Figure 7.1 The CASEL Framework – Competency on Responsible Decision Making.

"Everything," Merilee replies. Mrs. Solver knows there is a problem, but the student's response is too general for her to help. "What part of everything is the problem?" asks Mrs. Solver. "I am mad at my mother," said Merilee. Now Mrs. Solver is getting somewhere but needs to help Merilee unfold more of the problem. "What is happening that you are mad at your mother?" she asks. "She will not let me go to the party on Saturday night!" Merilee exclaims. "Oh, did she tell you why?" asks Mrs. Solver. "Yes, she knows my friends and knows they won't social distance or wear a mask and she is afraid I will get sick with COVID-19," Marilee explains. "I see. How about we think of different solutions to the problem and see if any will help your cause," suggests Mrs. Solver. "OK" Merilee responds. "I'm not really mad at my mother but I get angry when she will not let me do something I really want to do and I think is safe," adds Merilee. Now the problem is clear, and Mrs. Solver can help Merilee use the responsible decision-making skill to find a solution.

An integral subcompetency of Responsible Decision Making is Ethical Responsibility. Ethics is defined as the principles of right and wrong that are accepted by an individual or social group. (Wordnet by Princeton University, Database: 3.0, 2020)

Because principles vary, using positive values as a compass may be the ethical standard that serves as

the foundation for responsible decision making. For example, honesty, integrity, truthfulness, reliability, and dedication to friends and family are examples of positive values. When decisions are based on these values, the outcomes reinforce positive personal standards. Basing decisions on positive rather than negative values (dishonesty, lack of integrity, lying, unreliable, not a supportive friend, or not a committed family member), may be a challenge to some whose norm includes negative values.

Before teaching decision making, challenge the students to examine the benefits of and barriers to making decisions according to positive and negative values (**Figure 7.2**). Discuss the results and the consequences. Help the students to understand that using positive values as an ethical foundation

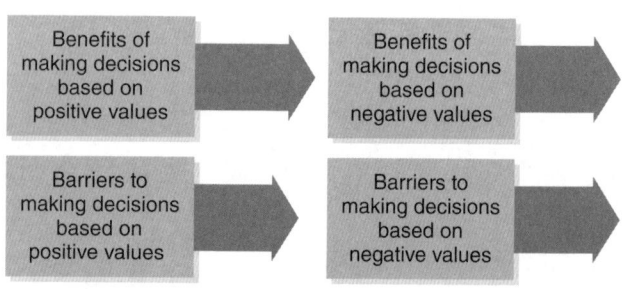

Figure 7.2 Benefits of and Barriers to Making Decisions Based on Positive and Negative Values.

for decision making may improve emotional, physical, intellectual, physical, and social health.

Teaching the Responsible Decision-Making competency and Standard 5, Decision Making, requires student practice. Students need time to understand the steps of the skill and practice using them. Over time, it may become natural for the student to target a particular problem, unpeel it to determine which part of the problem needs to be decided, weigh the pros and cons of each possible solution, and make a healthy choice based on positive values.

To assist and reinforce responsible decision making, provide opportunities for the students to make choices throughout the day. Students may choose which prompt they would like to tackle, write their own prompts, or organize a discussion about the pros and cons of health decisions made in the school, community, state, or even the nation. Comparing and contrasting is an excellent practice for making responsible decisions.

When progressing through each chapter, it becomes evident that the skills and competencies from previous chapters are interwoven in the subsequent chapters. The richness of skills-based health/SEL is a result of multi-faceted, engaging, age-appropriate, and experiential assessment and instruction used to improve relationships and personal health in school, community, and workplace.

Table 7.1 shows similarities in the NHES, DECIDE, and Responsible Decision-Making Model components.

The example below addresses the importance of family honesty (1.8.1) and demonstrates how to think through a problem and make a decision based on positive values (DECIDE-Identify your values; CASEL-Ethical Responsibility).

Decision-making example:

> Lisa wants to stay over Mari's house Friday night, but her mother doesn't want her to go. Lisa's mother does not trust Mari because she has been caught telling lies. She does not think the sleepover will be safe for her daughter so she said, "No." How can Lisa persuade her mother that it is safe to go to Mari's sleepover?

Standard 1 infused performance indicator:

- 1.8.1 <u>Analyze</u> the relationship between healthy behaviors, *such as being honest with parents*, and personal health.
- DECIDE Model **Table 7.2**

Table 7.1 NHES, DECIDE, and Responsible Decision-Making Model Component Similarities

Competency	Description	Subcompetencies
Responsible Decision Making	The ability to make constructive choices about personal behavior and social interactions based on **ethical standards**, safety concerns, and social norms. The ability to make a realistic evaluation of consequences of various actions as well as a consideration of the well-being of self and others. (Collaborative for Academic and Social Emotional Learning, 2020)	■ Identifying problems ■ Analyzing situations ■ Solving problems ■ Evaluating ■ Reflecting ■ **Ethical responsibility**

Responsible decision making directly aligns to Standard 5—Demonstrate the ability to use decision-making skills to enhance health (Joint Committee on National Health Education Standards, 2007, p. 32) and; therefore, it is not necessary to provide separate assessment or instruction.

Skills-based health/SEL educators use prompts, based on infused performance indicators, to develop decision-making skills and demonstrate proficiency in content, skill, and SEL competency. When students practice the Standard 5 skill of decision making, they are also practicing and gaining proficiency in the SEL competency, Responsible Decision Making.

There are a variety of decision-making models available. Skills-based Health/SEL educators use the performance indicators of the National Health Education Standards but may also use other models.

Many health educators use the DECIDE Model. Although the DECIDE and the CASEL models are closely aligned, DECIDE provides for more discrete thought and analysis. For example, exploring the options and consider the consequences are two steps, whereas CASEL combines the two into analyzing situations. Conversely, CASEL asks the students to separately evaluate and reflect whereas DECIDE only asks to evaluate. However, in order to evaluate, the student must reflect.

(continues)

Table 7.1 NHES, DECIDE, and Responsible Decision-Making Model Component Similarities *(continued)*

DECIDE is used in this chapter to teach responsible decision making. Because DECIDE and CASEL are so closely aligned, no additional instruction or assessment are required. Below are examples of PreK-2, 3-5, 6-8, and 9-12 alignment of the National Health Education Standards, the DECIDE and CASEL models. The same colored coded boxes, across models, show the component similarities.

PreK–2		
National Health Education Performance Indicators	**DECIDE Model**	**CASEL Responsible Decision Making**
5.2.1 Identify situations when a health-related decision is needed.	D – Define the decision to be made.	Identify the problem
5.2.2 Differentiate between situations when a health-related decision can be made individually or when assistance is needed.	E – Explore the options.	Analyze situations
	C – Consider the consequences.	Solve problems
	I – Identify your values.	Evaluate
	D – Decide and act.	Reflect
	E – Evaluate the results. (Kay, 2020)	Ethical responsibility (CASEL, 2019)
(Joint Committee on National Health Education Standards, 2007, p. 32)		

Grades 3–5		
National Health Education Performance Indicators	**DECIDE Model**	**CASEL Responsible Decision Making**
5.5.1 Identify health-related situations that might require a thoughtful decision.	D – Define the decision to be made.	Identify the problem
5.5.2 Analyze when assistance is needed in making a health-related decision.	E – Explore the options.	Analyze situations
5.5.3 List healthy options to health-related issues or problems.	C – Consider the consequences.	Solve problems
5.5.4 Predict the potential outcomes of each option when making a health-related decision.	I – Identify your values.	Evaluate
5.5.5 Choose a healthy option when making a decision.	D – Decide and act.	Reflect
5.5.6 Describe the outcomes of a health-related decision.	E – Evaluate the results. (Kay, 2020)	Ethical Responsibility (CASEL, 2019)
(Joint Committee on National Health Education Standards, 2007, p. 32)		

Grades 6–8		
National Health Education Performance Indicators	**DECIDE Model**	**CASEL Responsible Decision Making**
5.8.1 Identify circumstances that help or hinder healthy decision making.	D – Define the decision to be made.	Identify the problem
5.8.2 Determine when health-related situations require the application of a thoughtful decision-making process.	E – Explore the options	Analyze situations

5.8.3 Distinguish when individual or collaborative decision making is appropriate.	C – Consider the consequences.	Solve problems
5.8.4 Distinguish between healthy and unhealthy alternative to health-related issues or problems.	I – Identify your values.	Evaluate
5.8.5 Predict the potential short-term impact of each alternative on self and others.	D – Decide and act.	Reflect
5.8.6 Choose healthy alternatives over unhealthy alternatives when making a decision.	E – Evaluate the results. (Kay, 2020)	Ethical Responsibility (CASEL, 2019)
5.8.7 Analyze the outcomes of a health-related decision. (Joint Committee on National Health Education Standards, 2007, pp. 32-33)		
Grades 9–12		
National Health Education Performance Indicators	**DECIDE Model**	**CASEL Responsible Decision Making**
5.12.1 Examine barriers that hinder healthy decision making.	D - Define the decision to be made.	Identify the problem
5.12.2 Determine the value of applying a thoughtful decision-making process in health-related situations.	E – Explore the options.	Analyze situations
5.12.3 Justify when individual or collaborative decision making is appropriate.	C – Consider the consequences.	Solve problems
5.12.4 Generate alternatives to health-related issues or problems.	I – Identify your values.	Evaluate
5.12.5 Predict the potential short-term and long-term impact of each alternative on self and others.	D – Decide and act.	Reflect
5.12.6 Defend the healthy choice when making decisions.	E – Evaluate the results. (Kay, 2020)	Ethical Responsibility (CASEL, 2019)
5.12.7 Evaluate the effectiveness of health-related decisions. (Joint Committee on National Health Education Standards, 2007, p. 33)		

Reproduced from Joint Committee on National Health Education Standards. (2007). National Health Education Standards, Second Edition. SHAPE America.

Table 7.2 The DECIDE Model

DECIDE Model	Response
D – Define the decision to be made.	How can Lisa persuade her mother that it is safe to go to Mari's sleepover party?
E – Explore the options.	■ Lisa could lie and say she is sleeping over someone else's house. ■ She could tell her mother that if she feels unsafe, she will call her and go home. ■ She could go to Mari's house for the party and leave for the sleepover.
C – Consider the consequences.	■ If Lisa lies, her mother will not trust her. ■ If she tells her mother that she will call her if she feels unsafe, she will gain trust, but her mother will still be very worried. ■ If she goes to Mari's house for the party and leaves for the sleepover, Lisa will still have fun, her mother will worry, but she may miss out on a lot of fun.

(continues)

Table 7.2 The DECIDE Model *(continued)*

DECIDE Model	Response
I – Identify your values.	<ul><li>Honesty</li><li>Family</li><li>Friendship</li></ul>
D – Decide and act.	<ul><li>Although Lisa really wants to sleep over Mari's house, she does not want her mother to worry. She also wants her mother to have confidence in her ability to make a good decision and trust her. She has decided to go to the party and not stay for the sleepover.</li></ul>
E – Evaluate the results. (Kay, 2020)	<ul><li>Lisa made a good choice. Her mom was not the only worried parent. Other parents refused to allow their children to sleep over and Mari decided to just have a party, not a sleep over.</li></ul>

Data from Kay, J. (2020). The D.E.C.I.D.E. Model, A Tool For Teaching Students How To Make Healthy Decisions. Retrieved from Project School Wellness: https://www.projectschoolwellness.com/the-d-e-c-i-d-e-model-a-tool-for-teaching-students-how-to-making-healthy-decisions/

Preview

Unit Plan

In a skills-based/SEL unit, the planner accesses and analyzes data then selects a Standard 1 and skills performance indicator to reduce the risk factor and infuses them with content. The SEL competency and subcompetency are aligned with the infused performance indicators. Once established, the instructor plans the assessment and instruction. Once the content, skill, and competency are taught, the teacher distributes the performance task, which consists of the unit prompt(s), the scoring rubric, back-up materials needed such as supplemental content, self-checks, and any other information needed to show proficiency in the performance indicators and SEL competency. Students organize and practice for a few days and present their work to the class. This summative assessment is scored with an analytical rubric.

Skills-Based Lesson Plan

The skills-based/SEL lesson plan contains an agenda, the lesson objectives (infused Standard 1 performance indicator and skills indicator, and the SEL competency/subcompetency), a review/preview, the Standard 1 content, the skill, competency, a student-engaging practice prompt, clarifying questions relating to the prompt and learning objectives, a lesson review, and an exit ticket.

Skills-Based Lesson Infrastructure

The sections that follow present infrastructure for a lesson, not a unit. The infrastructure guides the teacher without impacting individual creativity. Each begins with an overview, data (when available), and a list of resources. Following the overview, a table initiates backwards design, which consists of the infused performance indicators and SEL competencies as the lesson objectives.

Assessments are designed for the Standard 1 performance indicator, The DECIDE model/SEL Responsible Decision-Making competency. The prompt and the review questions engage the student and help the teacher determine if the students met the lesson objectives. An exit question concludes the lesson infrastructure and gives the students the opportunity to reflect on how to use the content, skill, and SEL competency.

When reading, let your imagination guide your planning. You may need more or fewer lessons to teach the material. You may like an idea and modify it to meet the needs of your students. You may find the worksheets valuable, or you may prefer to edit them.

When modifying, maintain the integrity of the backwards design. Teach content, skill, and SEL each day. If the lesson infrastructure contains too much material, plan an additional day(s) but maintain the integrity of aligning SEL and teaching content through the infused performance indicators. Refer to the sample lessons at the end of each chapter to understand how to align SEL and teach content through the skill.

Organization

This chapter has only one section, Making Constructive Choices. The learning activities for the core competency of Responsible Decision Making are found here. (Collaborative for Academic Social Emotional Learning, 2020)

The National Health Education Standards are grouped according to the grade spans PreK–2, grades 3–5, grades 6–8, and grades 9–12. The examples

Table 7.3 Responsible Decision Making by Subcompetencies

Identifying problems
Analyzing situations
Solving problems
Evaluating
Reflecting
Ethical responsibility
(CASEL, 2019)

Data from CASEL. (2019, September 21). What is SEL? Retrieved from CASEL: https://casel.org/what-is-sel/

presented follow that structure. The classroom examples may require the teacher to be creative and adjust instruction to accommodate the age and abilities of the students.

Table 7.3 illustrates the subcompetencies of the Responsible Decision-Making Competency. In the section that follows, the practice prompt is aligned with the competency and the infused performance indicators of the NHES.

Making Constructive Choices

(Collaborative for Academic Social Emotional Learning, 2020)

The skill of responsible decision making helps youths make constructive and respectful choices about personal behavior and social interactions based on ethical standards, safety concerns, social norms, the evaluation of the pros and cons of various solutions, and the well-being of self and others. (Minnesota Department of Education, 2019)

To reinforce the responsible decision-making skill, provide time for student practice and give effective feedback as the students demonstrate the skill. Practice helps youth become more self-confident in the skill, increases their self-efficacy in using the skill outside the classroom and school, as well as achieving the long-term goal of developing, enhancing, and maintaining healthy behaviors.

PreK–2 Making Constructive Choices

Lesson Overview: Taking Medicine Safely

Students learn to make responsible decisions about taking medicine.

Resources:

- Minnesota Department of Education, SEL Implementation Guidance Document, Responsible Decision Making

Materials needed:

- **Cut out large letters: DECIDE**
- **Worksheet 7.1 A Story about the Benefits of Taking Medicine**
- **Worksheet 7.2 Medicine Safety Rules**

Table 7.4 provides an overview of the lesson objectives, assessment, and instruction for this lesson.

Table 7.4 Lesson Objectives, Assessment, and Instruction

Step 1 – Lesson Objectives	Step 2 – Assessment
The verb of the *infused* performance indicator and the SEL competency generate the assessment and instruction.	Design the assessment based on the objectives. Ask yourself the question, "What can my students do to show me they have met the standard?"
1.2.1 <u>Recognize</u> that healthy behaviors, *such as taking medicine safely*, affect personal health. (Joint Committee on National Health Education Standards, 2007, p. 24)	1.2.1 Students <u>recognize</u> two ways that healthy behaviors, *such as taking medicine safely*, affect personal health.
5.2.1–5.2.2 　　D – Define the decision to be made. 　　E – Explore the Options. 　　C – Consider the consequences. 　　I – Identify your values. 　　D – Decide and act. 　　E – Evaluate the results.	5.2.1–5.2.2 DECIDE Students <u>demonstrate</u> the skills to make a decision about taking medicine when sick.

(continues)

Table 7.4 Lesson Objectives, Assessment, and Instruction   *(continued)*

Step 1 – Lesson Objectives	Step 2 – Assessment
SEL – Responsible Decision Making	Students use the skills to make a decision about taking medicine when sick.

Step 3 – Instruction	
Design the instruction so that students learn the content, skill, and competency to be successful on the assessment. Ask yourself the question, "What do I need to teach so that the students will be successful when assessed?"	

Step 3 – Instruction

1. Define
   a. Identify: To recognize a particular person or an object.
   b. Analyze: To scrutinize something or someone in order to understand how it or they work(s).
   c. Solve: To find the solution to a problem or question. (Wordnet by Princeton University, Database: 3.0, 2020)
   d. Evaluate: To judge a person or thing after methodically examining the situation.
   e. Reflect: To think deeply about a subject. (Wordnet by Princeton University, Database: 3.0, 2020)
   f. Ethical responsibility: The obligation to behave according to the principles of right and wrong that are accepted by an individual or social group. Adapted from: (Wordnet by Princeton University, Database: 3.0, 2020)

2. 1.2.1 Recognize that healthy behaviors, *such as taking medicine when sick*, affects personal health.
   a. Use **Worksheet 7.1 A Story about the Benefits of Taking Medicine** to help students understand the benefits of taking medicine.
   b. Benefits of taking medicine
      1) Keeps us from getting sick. (immunizations)
      2) Helps us get better if we are sick or do not feel well. (antibiotics, pain reliever, cough syrup, etc.)
      3) Keeps us healthy when a body part needs help. (insulin, blood pressure medicine, etc.)
      4) Helps us be more comfortable when we are sick. (pain reliever)
   c. Use **Worksheet 7.2 Medicine Safety Rules** to help the children understand medicine safety rules.
      1) Know if you are allergic to any medicines

2) Do not
   a) Share medicine with other people.
   b) Take more medicine than parents or trusted adults give you.
   c) Take medicine prescribed by a doctor for someone else.
   d) Give medicine to other children. (Michigan Model for Health, 2016, p. 12)

3. **DECIDE Model/Responsible Decision Making**
   a. Explain that is important to learn the steps of making responsible decision making because they help children think before acting, weigh their values, and to make decisions based on positive values.
      1) On one side of the room, place a sign that says, "Helps" and on the other, "Does not help." For nonreaders, use symbols or emojis.
      2) Show a picture or describe a child who
         a) Is returning a pencil and explain this behavior is an example of being honest. (positive value)
         b) Is sneezing into his/her sleeve and explain this practice is an example of valuing your health and being respectful of others. (positive value)
         c) Is lying to another child, parent, or teacher and explain this deception is an example of dishonesty. (negative value)
         d) Is bullying another person. Explain that this aggressiveness is an example of disrespectful behavior. (negative value).
      3) Ask the children which type of value
         a) Makes us feel good about ourselves? (positive)
         b) Helps us have good relationships with family and friends? (positive)
         c) Is a good foundation for making a decision? (positive)

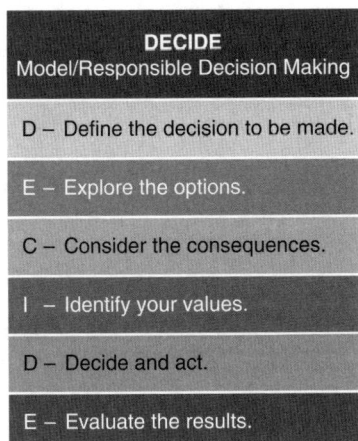

Figure 7.3 Decision-making Models.

b. Model decision making by reading the prompt below then explaining the acronym, DECIDE. Post the DECIDE letters/description in the classroom for easy reference when talking about making decisions **Figure 7.3**.

It was a long ride home on the bus and Carlos needed to run off some energy. His mom was talking to another parent and he wanted to run across the street on his own. His mom expects him to hold her hand while crossing the street.

What should Carlos do? **(D)** Should he wait for his mom, run across the street on his own, or cross with a friend and his parent?

If Carlos waits for his mom, she would be happy and proud of him for having patience. If he runs across the street on his own, his mother will be angry. If he crosses with a friend, his mother will not be happy because she believes it is her responsibility to make sure her child crosses the street safely. **(C)**

Carlos loves his mom and their family believes in being respectful. **(I)**

So, he decided to hop on one foot then the other to wear off some energy. His mother saw that Carlos needed to move so she finished the conversation, took Carlos' hand, and walked across the street. **(D)**

Carlos said, "Mom, I really wanted to run across the street on my own because I needed to move after the long bus ride but I knew you wouldn't like that so I decided to hop in place and wait for you." "You made a good choice, son. I am proud of you that you could show such patience when you really wanted to run." **(E)**

c. Provide time for the children to practice making another decision. Design a prompt that describes a situation where a child needs to make a decision. Guide the children through the process by bringing their attention to each of the components of the Responsible Decision-Making Model.

4. Read the practice prompt. Students answer the reflection questions and discuss.

Practice Prompt: Phillip

Phillip was feeling awful. His head hurt, he started sneezing, and he could not breathe. He went to the nurse for a little while and rested. The nurse called his mom. He wanted to go home but no one was home to watch him. He had to stay in school.

It was Wednesday, and Nonnie was picking him up and spending the afternoon with him and his brothers. Mom called her and asked her to stop at the pharmacy and pick up some cold medicine. Nonnie picked up the medicine before going to the school so they could go right home, take the medicine, and rest.

While driving home, Nonnie chatted with Phillip about his day. She knew he did not feel well and was trying to help him get his mind off feeling sick.

Phillip spied the pharmacy bag and knew it had medicine for him. He really wanted to open the bag and take the medicine. He knew how much to take and thought it would be safe. It would also be sneaky and knew Nonnie would not like it.

He thought he could ask Nonnie if he could open the package and take one of the pills. If she only knew how sick he was, she would say, "Okay." He realized she would never agree. She would have to pull over, open the package, find water in his backpack, then watch him safely take the pill.

They were getting close to home. He could decide to wait and have a nice cold glass of water with the pill. Nonnie would be there with him and it would feel good to have her next to him when he was feeling so sick. He loves Nonnie very much and would not do anything to upset her.

Before he knew it, they were home. His decision to wait was a good one. Nonnie fussed over him, made sure he safely took his medicine, wrapped him up in his favorite blanket, and read him a funny story. He felt much better and was glad he waited until he got home to take the medicine.

Later, Phillip was feeling a little guilty, so he told his mother he thought about taking the medicine in the car without telling Nonnie. "Well," mom said, "you thought about it but decided not to take the medicine because you knew it was not the right thing to do. I am proud of you, Phillip."

Now Phillip was really feeling better!

5. Use the review questions in **Table 7.5** to help the children understand how to make a responsible decision about taking medicine.
6. End of class review. Instruct the students to put away their materials then ask the review questions.
   a. How does taking medicine safely affect personal health? (1.2.1)
   b. What steps would you take to make a responsible decision about another health decision such as healthy snacking when you really want an unhealthy snack?

7. Exit ticket (responsible decision making)
   a. Why is it a good idea to base your decisions on positive values?

Grades 3–5: Responsible Decision Making

The practice prompt for this grade span includes a mask-making party. Post-COVID, the sample may still be appropriate or require alterations.

Table 7.5 PreK–2 Responsible Decision Making

Question	Answer
What are two ways taking the cold medicine safely affected Phillip's personal health? (1.2.1)	■ Phillip was glad that he waited because Nonnie was there with him when he took the medicine and it felt good to have her next to him when he was feeling so sick. ■ Phillip told his mother that he was thinking of taking the medicine in the car but decided not to. His mother said, "You decided not to take the medicine because you knew it was not the right thing to do. I am proud of you, Philip." After telling his mother, he really began to feel better.
How did Philip make a responsible decision about taking medicine when sick?	**D – Define the decision to be made.** Phillip was feeling very sick. In the car, he wanted to take the cold medicine Nonnie bought without telling her. **E – Explore the options.** Phillip could 1. Take the medicine and not tell Nonnie. 2. Ask Nonnie if he could take the medicine. 3. Wait until they got home to take the medicine. **C – Consider the consequences.** Phillip could 1. Take the medicine and not tell Nonnie but Nonnie would be very upset because that is not a safe way to take medicine. 2. Ask Nonnie if he could take the medicine but she would have to pull over, open the package, find water in his backpack, then watch him safely take the pill. 3. Wait until they got home to take the medicine and take it safely with Nonnie. **I – Identify your values.** Phillip's values include honesty, safety, and family. **D – Decide and act.** Phillip waited until he got home to take the medicine with Nonnie. **E – Evaluate the results.** Phillip's decision to wait was a good one. Nonnie fussed over him, made sure he safely took his medicine, wrapped him up in his favorite blanket, and read him a funny story. He felt much better and was glad he waited until he got home to take the medicine. Later, Philip was feeling a little guilty, so he told his mother he thought about taking the medicine in the car without telling Nonnie. "Well," mom said, "you thought about it but decided not to because you knew it was not the right thing to do. I am proud of you, Phillip." After telling his mother and knowing she was proud of him made him feel better.

SEL–Responsible Decision Making: Identifying the problem, analyzing the situation, solving the problem, evaluating the results, reflecting on the results, and demonstrating ethical responsibility.	See above.
How did Phillip use decision-making skills to make a good decision about taking medicine?	

Lesson Overview: Making Responsible Decisions about Getting Together with Friends

Students learn to make a responsible decision when there is a conflict in schedules.

Materials needed:

- **Worksheet 7.3 Effects of Making a Responsible Decision on the Components of Health**
- **Worksheet 7.4 Grades 3–5 Making Responsible Decisions**
- **Worksheet 7.5 Grades 3–5 Responsible Decision-Making Template**

Table 7.6 provides an overview of the lesson objectives, assessment, and instruction for this lesson.

Step 3 – Instruction

1. Define
   a. Identify: To recognize a particular person or an object.
   b. Analyze: To scrutinize something or someone in order to understand how it or they work(s).
   c. Solve: To find the solution to a problem or question. (Wordnet by Princeton University, Database: 3.0, 2020)

Table 7.6 Lesson Objectives, Assessment, and Instruction

Step 1 – Lesson Objectives	Step 2 – Assessment
The verb of the *infused* performance indicator and the SEL competency generate the assessment and instruction.	Design the assessment based on the objectives. Ask yourself the question, "What can my students do to show me they have met the standard?"
1.5.2 <u>Identify</u> examples of emotional, intellectual, physical, and social health *when making a responsible decision about getting together with friends*. (Joint Committee on National Health Education Standards, 2007, p. 24)	1.5.2 Students <u>identify</u> *two* ways emotional, intellectual, physical, and social health are affected when making a responsible decision about getting together with friends.

5.5.1–5.5.6
   D – Define the decision to be made.
   E – Explore the Options.
   C – Consider the consequences.
   I – Identify your values.
   D – Decide and act.
   E – Evaluate the results.
	5.5.1–5.5.6 DECIDE Students <u>demonstrate</u> the responsible decision-making model when making a decision about a conflict in a schedule.

SEL–Responsible Decision Making: Identifying the problem, analyzing the situation, solving the problem, evaluating the results, reflecting on the results, and demonstrating ethical responsibility.	Same as above.
Step 3 – Instruction	
Design the instruction so that students learn the content, skill, and competency to be successful on the assessment. Ask yourself the question, "What do I need to teach so that the students will be successful when assessed?"	

d. Evaluate: To judge a person or thing after methodically examining the situation.

e. Reflect: To think deeply about a subject. (Wordnet by Princeton University, Database: 3.0, 2020)

f. Ethical responsibility: The obligation to behave according to the principles of right and wrong that are accepted by an individual or social group. Adapted from: (Wordnet by Princeton University, Database: 3.0, 2020)

2. 1.5.2 Identify examples of emotional, intellectual, physical, and social health *when making a responsible decision* about a conflict in schedule.

a. Explain the components of health

b. Use **Worksheet 7.3 Effects of Making a Responsible Decision on the Components of Health** to help the children understand the impact of making responsible decisions on their emotional, intellectual, physical, and social health.

3. **DECIDE Model/Responsible Decision Making**

a. Explain the importance of learning the steps of responsible decision making is to help children think before they act. The steps also challenge children to think about their values and make decisions based on positive values.

   1) On one side of the room, place a sign that says, "Helps" and on the other, "Does not help."

   2) Show a picture of or describe a child who
      a) Cleans his/her room as expected by the parents/guardians. Explain this willingness is an example of integrity. (positive value)
      b) Helps an elderly person by opening a door and spending time chatting. Explain that this courtesy is an example of being a caring person. (positive value)
      c) Is lying to a teacher about completing an assignment. Explain this deceit is an example of dishonesty. (negative value)
      d) Posting lies about a peer. Explain that this behavior is disrespectful. (negative value)

   3) Ask the children which type of value
      a) Makes us feel good about ourselves? (positive)
      b) Helps us have good relationships with family and friends? (positive)
      c) Is a good foundation for making a decision? (positive)

b. Post the DECIDE Model in the classroom for easy reference when speaking about making decisions.

c. Explain the acronym DECIDE, why it is important to know how to make responsible decisions, and the steps to responsible decision making.

d. Use **Worksheet 7.4 Grades 3–5 Making Responsible Decisions** to model the decision-making process or to allow the children to read and parse the DECIDE steps on their own.

Tiffany's friend, Melanie, is having an outdoor party on Saturday and inviting a few classmates.

This time is the first since the pandemic started that her parents are allowing her to visit friends.

Her parents will only give permission if Tiffany promises to keep her mask on for the afternoon.

She hopes she can do it because she knows her friends don't wear a mask when they are outside. **(D)**

She really wants to be friends with this group and does not want to look silly. "What should I do?" I could wear my mask until my parents drop me off **(E)** *but she knows her parents would be very disappointed and upset that she placed her health at risk.* **(C)** If I leave the mask on for a while and take it off if no one else is wearing one **(E)**, *I would be disrespecting my parents and I do not want to lie to them when they ask about wearing the mask* **(C)**. If I leave the mask on for the afternoon **(E)**, *I may look silly if no one else is wearing a mask* **(C)**. If I stay six feet away from my friends **(E)**, *it would show my parents that I respect their rule and it would be similar to when the family goes for a walk and they take off their masks as long as they keep six feet away from others* **(C)**.

Her family values are important to Tiffany. She wants to be honest with her parents, but also wants to be with her friends. **(I)**

Tiffany decided to ask her mom, "If I stay six feet away from her friends, is it okay to take off the mask? It would be the same as when we go for our family walks and we keep six feet away from others!" **(D)**

Tiffany's parents agreed to let Tiffany go to the party and take off the mask as long as she keeps six feet away from her friends. Tiffany was happy! She wore the mask to the party and so did everyone else. Melanie's mom is also concerned about keeping the group safe so she set up rings in the backyard so each friend would have their own space, be safe, and have fun. It was a different party, but everyone had a great time! (**E**)

e. Use the blank **Worksheet 7.5 Grades 3–5 Responsible Decision-Making Template** to provide additional decision-making practice.

4. Read the practice prompt. Students answer the reflection questions and discuss.

Practice Prompt: Zavion

Zavion is very excited to go to Donnell's mask party on Saturday! Donnell's mom set up four stations, six feet apart, and bought all the ingredients to make a mask. The best decorated mask, which fits the best, gets a prize! He has a few ideas and has been sketching for a few days. He thinks he can win!

When Zavion told his parents about the party, his mother had a funny look on her face. That was never good news. "Zavion, I am so sorry, but your brother's 6th birthday party is Saturday. I forgot to tell you! We had to change the date because Auntie Marie is not available next week." "Mom! No! I already told Zavion I would go to his party! He is my best friend and he is counting on me to be there!" said Zavion.

Zavion ran to his room and shut the door. He was upset. His head hurt and he was stressed. He couldn't think clearly.

He could sneak out of the house and walk to Donnell's house but his family, especially his little brother, would be very upset if he wasn't at the birthday party. He could stay at home for the birthday party and miss Donnell's party, but Donnell will be very disappointed because they are best friends and have had the date for a few weeks. They even checked the date with his parents. He had

an idea. His brother's party starts at 1:00 P.M. and Donnell's party starts at 3:00 P.M. He could go to his brother's party and after the Happy Birthday song and the opening of presents, he can walk over to Donnell's house for his party. He will miss a little of both parties, but he thinks everyone will understand.

Zavion knows that plans change. He just didn't know the date for his brother's party was changed and wants to be a good brother, son, and friend.

He talked over his idea with his parents and little brother. They agreed that if Zavion stays for his brother's party, spends time with the family, stays for Happy Birthday and the opening of gifts, he can leave for Donnell's party.

Zavion was relieved and Donnell understood. He had a similar problem not long ago. Sometimes, parents forget to tell their kids that plans have changed.

Zavion had a great time at Donnell's party. Everyone was happy to see him and told him similar stories that happened in their families.

He researched different ways to decorate masks but the masks he found online did not cover the mouth and nose. The research was interesting but didn't help. Zavion colored his mask with bright colors. It was very creative. He didn't win the prize but had a great time trying.

Both parties were great fun and at the end of the day, Zavion felt good that he made the right decision for his family and his friend.

5. Use the review questions in **Table 7.7** to help the children understand how to make a responsible decision when there is a conflict in a schedule.

6. End of class review. Instruct the students to put away their materials then ask review questions.

a. Name one component of health and how making a responsible decision affects it. (1.5.2)

b. Think of a situation that requires a decision and work through the DECIDE model.

Table 7.7 Grades 3–5: Making a Responsible Decision

Question	Answer
What were two effects on Zavion's emotional, intellectual, physical, and social health as a result of making a responsible decision about getting together with his friend, Donnell? (1.5.2)	Emotional health Zavion <ul><li>Wants to be a good brother, son, and friend.</li><li>Received permission to leave the birthday party after the Happy Birthday song and the opening of the gifts. He was relieved and happy.</li><li>Had a great time decorating his mask.</li><li>Felt good that he made the right decision for his family and his friends.</li></ul>

(continues)

Table 7.7 Grades 3–5: Making a Responsible Decision _(continued)_

Question	Answer
	Intellectual health Zavion - Couldn't think clearly when he learned he had to attend his brother's birthday party and couldn't go to Donnell's party. - Was very creative in making his mask. - Researched different ways to decorate masks but the masks he found online did not cover the mouth and nose. The research was interesting but didn't help. Physical health Zavion - Had a headache when he learned he had to attend his brother's birthday party and couldn't go to Donnell's party. - Had a belly ache when he learned he had to attend his brother's birthday party and couldn't go to Donnell's party. Social health - Donnell understood that Zavion had to stay for his brother's birthday party. - Everyone was happy to see Zavion and told similar stories that happened in their families.
How did Zavion demonstrate how to use the responsible decision-making model when making a decision about a conflict in a schedule?	**D – Define the decision to be made.** The problem is Zavion accepted an invitation to a friend's party but then his brother's birthday was rescheduled to the same day. **E – Explore the options.** **Zavion** 1. Could sneak out of the house and walk to Donnell's house and skip his brother's party. 2. Could stay at home for the birthday party and miss Donnell's party. 3. Could go to his brother's party and after the Happy Birthday song and opening of presents, he would walk over to Donnell's party. **C – Consider the consequences.** **Zavion** 1. Could sneak out of the house and walk to Donnell's house and skip his brother's party but his family, especially his little brother, would be very upset if he was not at the birthday party. 2. Could stay at home for the birthday party and miss Donnell's party but Donnell would be very disappointed because they are best friends and have had the date for a few weeks. 3. Could go to his brother's party and after the Happy Birthday song and opening of presents, he would walk over to Donnell's party. He would miss a little of each party but he thinks everyone will understand. **I – Identify your values.** Zavion's values include honesty, family, friends, and keeping commitments. **D – Decide and act.** Zavion decided, with his brother's and parents' approval, to attend his brother's party and after the Happy Birthday song and opening of presents, he would walk over to Donnell's party. **E – Evaluate the results.** Zavion knows he made the right decision. Both parties were great fun and at the end of the day, Zavion felt good that he made the right decision for his family and his friend.

SEL–Responsible Decision Making: Identifying the problem, analyzing the situation, solving the problem, evaluating the results, reflecting on the results, and demonstrating ethical responsibility.	Same as above.

7. Exit ticket (responsible decision making)

Why is it important to base your responsible decision making on positive values?

Grades 6–8: Responsible Decision Making

When teaching responsible decision making, explain that knowing how the teenage brain works helps teens better understand why they make certain choices and how they can make better choices.

Although the brain reaches maximum size between the ages of 12 and 14, brain development continues. When a teen makes a rushed decision, it is a result of the influence of feelings and emotions from the limbic, or more developed, part of the brain. Whereas, taking time and thinking through a problem and solution is dependent on logic, thinking ahead, and assessing the pros and cons of behavior, which is rooted in the part of the brain, pre-frontal cortex, that is still developing.

Neural pathways are strengthened and reinforced with repeated use. Therefore, a teen who makes consistently good decisions, finds it easier to continue that behavior because the pathway is established and well used. The brain strengthens circuits that are well used and removes any that are not. (Scholastic and the Scientists of the National Institute of Drug Abuse, 2020)

It is curious why some teens behave one way in private and another when with peers. In studying teen brain circuitry, Jason Chein, et al., discovered that when peers are present, teens are more inclined to make risky decisions. (Jason Chein, 2011)

All of these factors are important when teaching responsible decision making. Helping teens understand the biology of their brain may help them take a step back and think before they act. The responsible decision-making model provides the foundation for this skill building.

Lesson Overview: Alcohol

Students learn to make a responsible decision when being influenced by friends.

Between 15.5% and 30.4 % of middle school students report ever drinking alcohol. (Centers for Disease Control and Prevention, 2020)

Between 5.6% and 13.6 % of middle school students report drinking alcohol for the first time before age 11. (Centers for Disease Control and Prevention, 2020)

Resources:

- CDC Middle School Youthonline
- Teens and Decision Making: What Brain Science Reveals. www.scholastic.com/headsup

Materials needed:

- **Worksheet 7.6 Grades 6–8 Making a Responsible Decision**
- **Worksheet 7.7 Grades 6–8 Responsible Decision-Making Template**

Table 7.8 provides an overview of the lesson objectives, assessment, and instruction for this lesson.

Table 7.8 Lesson Objectives, Assessment, and Instruction

Step 1 – Lesson Objectives	Step 2 – Assessment
The verb of the *infused* performance indicator and the SEL competency generate the assessment and instruction.	Design the assessment based on the objectives. Ask yourself the question, "What can my students do to show me they have met the standard?"

(continues)

Table 7.8 Lesson Objectives, Assessment, and Instruction   *(continued)*

Step 1 – Lesson Objectives	Step 2 – Assessment
1.8.7 <u>Describe</u> the benefits of and barriers to practicing healthy behaviors such as *making a healthy decision about alcohol when influenced by peers.* (Joint Committee on National Health Education Standards, 2007, p. 25)	1.8.7 Students <u>describe</u> *three* benefits of making a decision about alcohol when positively influenced by peers and *three* barriers to making a decision about alcohol when negatively influenced by peers.

5.8.1–5.8.7
    D – Define the decision to be made.
    E – Explore the Options.
    C – Consider the consequences.
    I – Identify your values.
    D – Decide and act.
    E – Evaluate the results.
	Students <u>demonstrate</u> the responsible decision-making model to make a good decision about drinking alcohol.

SEL–Responsible Decision Making: Identifying the problem, analyzing the situation, solving the problem, evaluating the results, reflecting on the results, and demonstrating ethical responsibility.	Students demonstrate the responsible decision-making model to make a good decision about drinking alcohol.

Step 3 – Instruction
Design the instruction so that students learn the content, skill, and competency to be successful on the assessment. Ask yourself the question, "What do I need to teach so that the students will be successful when assessed?"

Step 3 – Instruction

1. Define
   a. Identify: To recognize a particular person or an object.
   b. Analyze: To scrutinize something or someone in order to understand how it or they work(s).
   c. Solve: To find the solution to a problem or question. (Wordnet by Princeton University, Database: 3.0, 2020)
   d. Evaluate: To judge a person or thing after methodically examining the situation.
   e. Reflect: To think deeply about a subject. (Wordnet by Princeton University, Database: 3.0, 2020)
   f. Ethical responsibility: The obligation to behave according to the principles of right and wrong that are accepted by an individual or social group. Adapted from: (Wordnet by Princeton University, Database: 3.0, 2020)
2. 1.8.7 <u>Describe</u> the benefits of and barriers to practicing healthy behaviors such as *making a healthy decision about alcohol when influenced by peers.*
   a. In groups, direct the students to list the benefits of and barriers to making a healthy decision about alcohol. Discuss.
   b. Benefits of practicing healthy behaviors such as *making a healthy decision about alcohol when influenced by peers.*
      1) Peers can be a positive influence not to drink alcohol. (Scholastic, 2020)
      2) When a teen has nondrinking friends, it is easier to make a decision not to drink. (Pontz, 2020)
      3) Positive friends encourage each other to do what is healthy. (Michigan Model for Health, 2016, p. 31)
   c. Barriers to practicing healthy behaviors such as *making a healthy decision about alcohol when influenced by peers.*
      1) Instead of speaking out about not using alcohol, a teen may not say anything.
      2) A teen may be attracted to the step-by-step process of making a decision about alcohol and not think about the risks of drinking alcohol.
      3) Teens are still learning to control impulses and resist pressure from peers.
      4) Teens are more likely to engage in risky behavior when other peers are watching than when making behavior decisions alone. (Scholastic, 2020)

3. Explain that is important to learn the steps of making responsible decision making because they help teens think before they act. They also cause teens to think about their values and to make decisions based on positive values.

   a. To explore positive values as a foundation of decision making, place the following words and definitions on large post-its and place around the classroom. Direct the students to walk from one to the other and comment on how that positive value helps teens make positive decisions about alcohol. Discuss

     1) Honesty: Being truthful; acting or speaking without deception.

     2) Compassion: A feeling of caring and wanting to help someone who is less fortunate.

     3) Sincerity: A quality of a person who is genuine, open, and not deceitful.

     4) Integrity: A code of positive principles including honesty, morality, and ethics.

     5) Courage: The mental and physical ability to cope with a variety of difficult situations without worrying about the outcome.

     6) Health: A person's physical, mental, emotional, intellectual, and social state.

     7) Perseverance: To continue to work toward a goal despite challenges.

   b. Post the DECIDE Model in the classroom for easy reference when talking about making decisions.

   c. Use **Worksheet 7.6 Grades 6–8 Making Responsible Decisions** to model the decision-making process or to allow the children to read and parse the DECIDE steps on their own.

Sanchay is new to the middle school and wants to make friends. He is joining after-school clubs and sports teams to get to know other peers. Sanchay met Brady during soccer practice and the two became friends.

Brady invited Sanchay to his house Saturday night to watch a movie with some of the other boys. Finally, Sanchay is beginning to feel like he belongs! While watching the movie, Brady left and came back with a beer. He took a big gulp and passed it along. Sanchay doesn't drink alcohol and his family does not approve of teens drinking. (**I**) Plus, everyone was drinking out of the same can! No way. What can he do? (**D**) He doesn't want to look foolish in front of these new peers.

He could pretend to take a sip and pass it quickly (**E**). That way, no one will know, and he will act like everyone else (**C**). He could just pass the beer without taking any (**E**) and stay true to his beliefs but is afraid the other boys will make fun of him while he is trying to fit in (**C**). He could get up and grab a soda, so he already has a drink by the time the beer gets to him (**E**). That might be acceptable to the other boys but it still makes him feel uncomfortable and not true to himself (**C**).

Sanchay decided to pass the beer and see what happens (**D**). No one said anything. He went to the bathroom and texted his mom to pick him up. When his mother arrived, she beeped the horn. Sanchay's phone beeped and he told the boys he had to go. His mom was outside.

Sanchay told his mom what happened and that he has decided that he does not want to be friends with this group. (**E**)

   d. Use **Worksheet 7.7 Grades 6–8 Responsible Decision-Making Template** to play, "What would you do?"

     1) Adam is friends with Jerry. They have fun together but when they hang out with the whole group, Jerry changes. He makes fun of others, uses bad language, tells crude jokes, and other things Adam does not like. What would you do if you were Adam?

     2) During a sleepover, Leslie took a picture of Lisseth while she was sleeping. Her hair was a mess, her mouth was wide open, and she looked awful. The next day, Lisseth saw her picture posted online. She was hurt and angry. What would you do if you were Lisseth?

     3) Your friend, Allie, texts you all day. It is annoying. There is not anything important in the text, but "ping!" here comes another text! If you do not answer, Allie will think you are not a friend. What would you do if it happened to you? (Alex J. Packer, 2017)

4. Read the practice prompt. Students answer the reflection questions and discuss.

Practice Prompt: Scott

Scott likes to walk through the park on his way home from school. It is quiet and peaceful. While walking the other day, he saw Tanya and waved. He and Tanya worked on a health project last term and she was fun to be with.

Tanya was with a group of friends and called him over. She introduced Scott to her friends and invited him to stay. Scott knew a few of the people. He liked some of the friends but he doesn't like Bella because she talks/texts about her friends behind their backs. He does not want her to do that to him.

Bella and Trainer were behaving rather strangely. They were turning around, going into their back packs, then turning back. It looked like they were drinking something, but Scott couldn't see anything. After a while, they started to get silly.

Bella told everyone that her dad has a collection of nips. She described them as very small bottles of alcohol. She brought some with her today and asked if anyone wanted one. Trainer said, "I like the Schnapps. Try it! It tastes like root beer." A few of the group did take one of the little bottles and drank it. The little bottles were easy to hide if an adult came along.

Scott does not want to drink the alcohol. There is alcoholism in his family and drinking is too dangerous for him.

Tanya said, "Hey, Bella, what are you doing? You know you shouldn't have alcohol!" Bella just laughed. Tanya felt bad because she invited Scott into the group, and she knows he does not drink. Neither does she, and she does not want to stay any longer.

What should he do? He just got there and was having fun until Bella took out the nips. He looked at Tanya and after she called out Bella, she seemed just as uncomfortable as he was. Maybe the two of them could leave together? Tanya lives near Scott and he could offer to walk her home. He could tell everyone that he had to get going because his mom is waiting for him to babysit so she can go to work but he would be lying. He could stay and try the nip, but he knows alcohol is a problem in his family and he respects his parents' rule that he wait to drink until he is 21. He was curious and everyone looked like they were having fun. No one pressured him but he felt the pressure, anyway.

Scott looked at Tanya again and asked her if she wanted to leave. She said, "Yes," and they both got up, said "Goodbye," and walked away.

On the way home, Tanya apologized to Scott. She told him she had no idea that Bella brought alcohol to the park. Scott said it was OK and was glad she wanted to leave, too.

On the way home, Scott asked Tanya if she would like to hang out some time. With a lovely smile, she said, "Sure."

When Tanya went in the house, he was pleased with himself. He made a good decision and maybe a new friend!

5. Use the review questions in **Table 7.9** to help the students understand the effects of friends on responsible decision making.
6. End of class review. Instruct the students to put away their materials then ask review questions.

a. What is one benefit of having a positive friend when making a decision about alcohol? (1.8.7)
b. What is one barrier to having a negative friend when making a decision about alcohol? (1.8.7)

Table 7.9 Grades 6–8: Responsible Decision Making

Question	Answer
What were *three* benefits of making a decision about alcohol when positively influenced by peers and *three* barriers to making a decision about alcohol when negatively influenced by peers? (1.8.7)	*Three* benefits Scott experienced when making a decision about alcohol when positively influenced by Tanya. 1. Tanya confronted Bella about having alcohol. 2. Tanya didn't want to stay with the group because of the drinking. 3. Tanya agreed to leave the group with Scott. *Three* barriers Scott experienced when making a decision about alcohol when negatively influenced by peers. 1. A few members of the group did drink the alcohol and he felt the pressure to try it even though no one verbally pressured him. 2. The group was having fun and he was curious about the nips. 3. He did not want Bella to talk/text about him to other peers if he didn't try the nips.

How did Scott use the responsible decision-making model to make a good decision about drinking alcohol?	**D – Define the decision to be made.** The problem is Scott is feeling the pressure to drink alcohol. **E – Explore the options.** 1. Scott and Tanya could leave the group together. 2. Scott could tell everyone that he had to get going because his mom is waiting for him to babysit so she can go to work. 3. Scott could stay and try the nip. **C – Consider the consequences.** 1. Scott and Tanya could leave the group together. Both were uncomfortable being part of the group because of the alcohol. 2. Scott could tell everyone that he had to get going because his mom is waiting for him to babysit so she can go to work but that would be a lie and he does not lie. 3. Scott could stay and try the nip but that would be against his family's rules and he respects why his parents do not want him to drink. **I – Identify your values.** Scotts' values include integrity, family, honesty, and friendship. **D – Decide and act.** Scott asked Tanya if she would like to leave and she agreed. **E – Evaluate the results.** Scott made a good decision. On the way home, Tanya apologized to Scott and explained she had no idea that Bella brought alcohol to the park. Scott said it was OK and was glad she wanted to leave, too. On the way home, Scott asked Tanya if she would like to hang out some time. With a lovely smile, she said, "Sure." When Tanya went in the house, he was very pleased with himself. He made a good decision and maybe made a new friend!
SEL–Responsible Decision Making: Identifying the problem, analyzing the situation, solving the problem, evaluating the results, reflecting on the results, and demonstrating ethical responsibility.	Same as above.

c. Think of an example of a common decision made by teens and solve it through the responsible decision-making process.

7. Exit ticket (Relationship skills: Maintaining healthy and rewarding relationships)

Why is it important to base our decisions on positive values?

Grades 9–12: Responsible Decision Making

When teaching responsible decision making, explain the importance of taking time to think through a decision rather than acting impulsively. Also explain that the presence of peers increases risk taking among adolescents by heightening sensitivity to the peer potential approval of making risky decisions. (Jason Chein, 2011)

Lesson Overview: Distracted Driving

Students learn ways to prevent distracted driving and make a responsible decision about decreasing a distraction while driving.

Thirty-nine percent of high school students (38.4% girls and 39.6% boys) texted or e-mailed while driving a car or other vehicle on at least one day during the 30 days before the survey, among students who had driven a car or other vehicle during the 30 days before the survey. (Centers for Disease Control and Prevention, 2020)

More than 9% of the fatal crashes in the United States in the past seven years involved a distracted driver, according to the National Highway Traffic Safety Administration (NHTSA)

More than 2,800 people were killed as a result of distracted driving in 2018, including the use of cell phones while driving, resulting in injury and loss of life. (NHTSA)

An estimated 400,000 people were injured in crashes involving distracted drivers in 2018.

According to a National Occupant Protection Use Survey, handheld cell phone use continues to be highest among 16–24 year old drivers. (Federal Communications Commission, 2020)

Resources:

* Federal Communications Commission
* DMV.org

Materials needed:

* **Worksheet 7.8 Preventing Distracted Driving**
* **Worksheet 7.9 Grades 9–12 Making Responsible Decisions**
* **Worksheet 7.10 Grades 9–12 Responsible Decision-Making Template**

Table 7.10 provides an overview of the lesson objectives, assessment, and instruction for this lesson.

Step 3 Instruction

1. Define
   a. Identify: To recognize a particular person or an object.
   b. Analyze: To scrutinize something or someone in order to understand how it or they work(s).
   c. Solve: To find the solution to a problem or question. (Wordnet by Princeton University, Database: 3.0, 2020)
   d. Evaluate: To judge a person or thing after methodically examining the situation.
   e. Reflect: To think deeply about a subject. (Wordnet by Princeton University, Database: 3.0, 2020)
   f. Ethical responsibility: The obligation to behave according to the principles of right and wrong that are accepted by an individual or social group. Adapted from: (Wordnet by Princeton University, Database: 3.0, 2020)
2. 1.12.1 <u>Predict</u> how healthy behaviors, *such as not driving distracted*, affect health status.
   a. Use **Worksheet 7.8 Preventing Distracted Driving** to design a brochure that predicts 10 ways to prevent distracted driving.

Table 7.10 Lesson Objectives, Assessment, and Instruction

Step 1 – Lesson Objectives	Step 2 – Assessment
The verb of the *infused* performance indicator and the SEL competency generate the assessment and instruction.	Design the assessment based on the objectives. Ask yourself the question, "What can my students do to show me they have met the standard?"
1.12.1 Predict how healthy behaviors, *such as not driving distracted*, affect health status. (Joint Committee on National Health Education Standards, 2007, p. 25)	1.12.1 Students <u>predict</u> *five* ways not to be distracted when driving.
5.12.1–5.12.7 D – Define the decision to be made. E – Explore the options. C – Consider the consequences. I – Identify your values. D – Decide and act. E – Evaluate the results.	5.12.1–5.12.7 DECIDE Students <u>demonstrate</u> the responsible decision-making model when making a healthy decision about driving and being distracted.
SEL–Responsible Decision Making: Identifying the problem, analyzing the situation, solving the problem, evaluating the results, reflecting on the results, and demonstrating ethical responsibility.	Students <u>demonstrate</u> the responsible decision-making model when making a healthy decision about driving and being distracted.

Step 3 – Instruction
Design the instruction so that students learn the content, skill, and competency to be successful on the assessment. Ask yourself the question, "What do I need to teach so that the students will be successful when assessed?"

3. **DECIDE Model/Responsible Decision Making**
   a. To explore positive values as a foundation of decision making, place the following words and definitions on large post-its, and place around the classroom. Direct the students to walk from one to the other and comment on how that positive value helps teens make positive decisions about alcohol. Discuss
      1) Honesty: Being truthful; acting or speaking without deception.
      2) Compassion: A feeling of caring and wanting to help someone who is less fortunate.
      3) Sincerity: A quality of a person who is genuine, open, and not deceitful.
      4) Integrity: A code of positive principles including honesty, morality, and ethics.
      5) Courage: The mental and physical ability to cope with a variety of difficult situations without worrying about the outcome.
      6) Health: A person's physical, mental, emotional, intellectual, and social state.
      7) Perseverance: To continue to work toward a goal despite challenges.
   b. Place the DECIDE Model in the classroom for easy reference when speaking about making decisions.
   c. Use **Worksheet 7.9 Grades 9–12 Making Responsible Decisions** to model the decision-making process or to allow the students to read and parse the DECIDE steps on their own.

      Dellmar was excited! His dad is letting him take the family car to go to work. Usually, his dad drives him because Dellmar is a new driver but tonight is dad's night out with his friends and there is a friendly competition at the bowling lanes. Dellmar has his phone in case he is running late.

      During his break, he texted his friends that he drove himself to work and that it felt really good to be on his own and trusted by his parents. His friends know he will not answer a text or his phone while driving.

      On the way home, his phone started buzzing and beeping. Who is trying to reach him? What should he do **(D)**? It must be an emergency if people are trying to reach him when they know he is driving!

      Traffic is really slow. He could safely pick up his phone and see who is calling **(E)** but if he ever got in an accident, his parents would never trust him to drive alone again **(C)**. He could pull over and check things out **(E)**, which would be very safe **(C)** and consistent with family rules **(I)**. He could use his "hands off" dialing to call and text **(E)**, but he still will be distracted and knows it could be dangerous **(C)**.

      Dellmar decided to pull over and check his calls and texts **(D)**. His friends were getting together and they were trying to reach him so he could come over right from work instead of driving home first. Oh boy! He was glad it was not a family emergency but upset that his friends tried to reach him when they all agreed not to call or text when they knew one of them was driving **(I)**.

      Dellmar decided to go home **(D)**. He was tired and stressed. He told his parents that he pulled over to answer a call/texts because he thought it was an emergency. They were proud of him for making such a good and safe choice **(I)**. His dad told him, "Dellmar, you made a good decision and you can drive yourself to work from now on!" **(E)**

4. Use **Worksheet 7.10 Grades 9–12 Responsible Decision-Making Template** to play, "What would you do?"
   a. While at the mall with friends, Adrien sees something she really wants but doesn't have any money. The salesclerk is busy, and her friend says, "Quick, put it in your backpack. No one will ever know!" Adrien knows taking the item would be stealing, which is wrong, but she really wants it. If you were Adrien, what would you do?
   b. Jiel and Miguel are at the lake with Miguel's parents and there are no lifeguards. Jiel is a good but not great swimmer. Jiel knows the family rule, never swim where there are no lifeguards. Miguel says, "Let's see who can swim out to the middle the fastest!" If you were Jiel, what would you do? (Michigan Model for Health, 2016)
   c. Farlie's health project is due today. He does not have a good reason why it is not finished but knows if he gives the teacher a good reason, she will give him more time. Your friend says, "Tell the teacher the Internet

went down or the printer was out of ink and see if she accepts the excuse." Farlie knows lying is wrong but doesn't want a bad grade and needs more time. If you were Farlie, what would you do?

5. Read the practice prompt. Students answer the reflection questions and discuss.

Practice Prompt: Rafaela

Rafaela is a new driver and she is excited because her mom asked her to go pick up a pizza, fries, and rolls for supper. She was really hungry and eager to take the ride.

The ride was uneventful. There was little traffic and no wait at the take-out window. She put the take-out next to her, on the passenger side. All is going well!

The problems started on the way home. The pizza box moved around as she stopped and started. The smell was driving her crazy! She was really hungry and thought she could take a bite out of one of the pizza slices while at the red light. It seemed like every billboard showed a food ad and made her even more hungry. The fries were really close, and she knows she could take a few and eat them while driving.

What was she thinking!! Everything she learned about distracted driving was challenging her from the passenger's seat!

She started thinking about what she could do to get home safely. She could stop and put the package on the floor in the back. It wouldn't move around back there but she could still smell it and if she places it in the middle, she could still snag a few fries. It is not a good idea because she would still be distracted. She could stop and secure the takeout in the trunk. She wouldn't have to keep

moving the package when it shifts. If she doesn't see it, it will be easier to keep her mind on driving. She could also leave the package where it is and just concentrate on driving. She is almost home and she wouldn't have to stop in traffic.

She remembered what her mom used to tell her when she saw something she wanted, "Out of sight, out of mind, Rafaela!" That was it! She pulled into a parking lot and put the pizza, fries, and rolls in the trunk. She did take a few fries during the transfer and they were good! She got home safely and told her mother what she did.

Mom was pleased Rafaela made the good decision to put the food in the trunk. Rafaela didn't realize how distracted she would be just picking up takeout but now knows how to get food home safely, especially when hungry.

6. Use the review questions in **Table 7.11** to help the students predict ways of driving without distractions and to make a responsible decision about how to minimize distractions when driving.

7. End of class review. Instruct the students to put away their materials then ask review questions.
   a. What predictions can you make to minimize manual, cognitive, and visual distractions while driving? (1.12.8)
   b. What is another common teen problem and how can you demonstrate the responsible decision making to resolve it.

8. Exit ticket
   Why is it important to base our decisions on positive values?

Table 7.11 Benefits of Face-to-Face Communication Rather Than Texting

Question	Answer
What are three ways Rafaela could drive home with the takeout and not be distracted while driving? (1.12.1)	■ Rafaela could prevent a manual distraction by putting the takeout in the trunk so it doesn't move around and she would not have to keep repositioning it. ■ Rafaela could prevent a cognitive distraction by putting the takeout in the trunk, so she is not smelling it and being reminded of how hungry she is. ■ Rafaela could prevent a visual distraction by moving the takeout to the trunk, so she won't see it and not look at the billboards because they all seemed to be advertising food and that only made Rafaela more hungry.
How did Rafaela <u>demonstrate</u> how to use the responsible decision-making model when making a decision about not being distracted while driving?	**D – Define the decision to be made.** The problem is Rafaela is bringing home takeout and is very distracted by the package. Moving in the seat as she drives and her desire to snack on the takeout because she is very hungry.

E – Explore the options.

Rafaela could

1. Stop and put the package on the floor in the back.
2. Stop and secure the takeout in the trunk.
3. Leave the package where it is and just concentrate on driving.

C – Consider the consequences.

1. If Rafaela stops and puts the package on the floor in the back, it wouldn't move around but she could still smell it and if she places it in the middle, she could still snag a few fries. That is not a good idea because she would still be distracted.
2. If Rafaela stops and secures the takeout in the trunk, she will not have to keep moving the package when it shifts. If she does not see it, it will be easier to keep her mind on driving.
3. If Rafaela leaves the package where it is and just concentrates on driving, she is almost home, and she would not have to stop in traffic.

I – Identify your values.

Rafaela's values include honesty, trust, and family.

D – Decide and act.

Rafaela pulled into a parking lot and put the pizza, fries, and rolls in the trunk.

E – Evaluate the results.

1. Rafaela got home safely and told her mother what she did. Her mom was pleased Rafaela made the good decision to put the food in the trunk.
2. Rafaela didn't realize how distracted she would be just picking up takeout but now she knows how to get food home safely, especially if she is hungry.

SEL–Responsible Decision Making: Identifying the problem, analyzing the situation, solving the problem, evaluating the results, reflecting on the results, and demonstrating ethical responsibility.	See above.

Sample Lesson Plan for Responsible Decision Making

Unit: *State the unit of the lesson.*	Responsible Decision Making
Topic: *State the topic of the lesson.*	Distracted Driving
Grade level: *State the grade level of the lesson.*	Grades 9–12
Time allotment: *State the time allotted for the lesson.*	50 minutes
Lesson summary: *Provide a summary of the lesson.*	Students make a responsible decision about how to decrease driving distractions.
Risk behavior data: *Provide time rationale for this lesson by accessing the risk behavior the lesson reduces.*	39.2% of high school students (40.2% girls and 38.2% boys) texted or e-mailed while driving a car or other vehicle on at least one day during the 30 days before the survey, among students who had driven a car or other vehicle during the 30 days before the survey. (Centers for Disease Control and Prevention, 2020)

	More than 9% of the fatal crashes in the United States in the past seven years involved a distracted driver, according to the National Highway Traffic Safety Administration. (NHTSA)
	More than 2,800 people were killed as a result of distracted driving in 2018, including the use of cell phones while driving, resulting in injury and loss of life. (NHTSA)
	An estimated 400,000 people were injured in crashes involving distracted drivers in 2018.
	According to a National Occupant Protection Use Survey, handheld cell phone use continues to be highest among 16- to 24 year old drivers. (Federal Communications Commission, 2020)
Standards and SEL Competency to reduce the risk factor(s): *List the Standard 1 and skills standards and the SEL competency/ subcompetency.*	1.12.1 Predict how healthy behaviors affect health status. **DECIDE** Model/Responsible Decision Making D – Define the decision to be made. E – Explore the options. C – Consider the consequences. I – Identify your values. D – Decide and act. E – Evaluate the results. SEL–Responsible Decision Making
Objectives: *The objectives are the infused performance indicators and SEL competency.*	1.12.1 Predict how healthy behaviors, *such as not driving distracted*, affect health status. Use the DECIDE model to make a responsible decision about how to decrease distracted driving. **DECIDE** Model/Responsible Decision Making D – Define the decision to be made. E – Explore the options. C – Consider the consequences. I – Identify your values. D – Decide and act. E – Evaluate the results. SEL–Use the DECIDE model to make a responsible decision about how to decrease distracted driving.

Lesson assessment: *Design an assessment for each infused performance indicator and SEL competency.*	1.12.1 Students <u>predict</u> *five* ways not to be distracted when driving. Students <u>demonstrate</u> the responsible decision-making model when making a healthy decision about driving and being distracted. SEL–Students <u>demonstrate</u> the responsible decision-making model when making a healthy decision about driving and being distracted.

Lesson instruction: *Provide a detailed description of how content, skill, and SEL competency are taught, "bell to bell."*	Review/Preview
	    What is distracted driving?
	    What are the different ways a teen can be distracted while driving?
	    How dangerous is it to be distracted and driving? (refer to the data)
	    Review the lesson definitions, if needed.
	
	Lesson Objectives
	
	Students predict five ways not be distracted when driving and demonstrate how to use the DECIDE model to make a responsible decision about driving and being distracted.

Lesson

1. 1.12.1 <u>Predict</u> how healthy behaviors, *such as not driving distracted*, affect health status.
   a. Use **Worksheet 7.8 Preventing Distracted Driving** to design a brochure that predicts 10 ways to prevent distracted driving.

DECIDE
Model/Responsible Decision Making

D – Define the decision to be made.

E – Explore the options.

C – Consider the consequences.

I – Identify your values.

D – Decide and act.

E – Evaluate the results.

---

2. **DECIDE Model/Responsible Decision Making**
   a. To explore positive values as a foundation of decision making, place the following words and definitions on large post-its and place around the classroom. Direct the students to walk from one to the other and comment on how that positive value helps teens make positive decisions about alcohol. Discuss
      1) Honesty: Being truthful; acting or speaking without deception.
      2) Compassion: A feeling of caring and wanting to help someone who is less fortunate.
      3) Sincerity: A quality of a person who is genuine, open, and not deceitful.
      4) Integrity: A code of positive principles including honesty, morality, and ethics.
      5) Courage: The mental and physical ability to cope with a variety of difficult situations without worrying about the outcome.
      6) Health: A person's physical, mental, emotional, intellectual, and social state.
      7) Perseverance: To continue to work toward a goal despite challenges.
   b. Post the DECIDE Model in the classroom for easy reference when talking about making decisions.
   c. Use **Worksheet 7.9 Grades 9–12 Making Responsible Decisions** to model the decision-making process or to allow the children to read and parse the DECIDE steps on their own.

   Dellmar was excited! His dad is letting him take the family car to go to work. Usually, his dad drives him because Dellmar is a new driver but tonight is dad's night out with his friends and there is a friendly competition at the bowling lanes. Dellmar has his phone in case he is running late.

   During his break, he texted his friends that he drove himself to work and that it felt really good to be on his own and trusted by his parents. His friends know he will not answer a text or his phone while driving.

On the way home, his phone started buzzing and beeping. Who is trying to reach him? What should he do **(D)**? It must be an emergency if people are trying to reach him when they know he is driving!

Traffic is really slow. He could safely pick up his phone and see who is calling **(E)** but if he ever got in an accident, his parents would never trust him to drive alone again **(C)**. He could pull over and check things out **(E)**, which would be very safe **(C)** and consistent with family rules **(I)**. He could use his "hands off" dialing to call and text **(E)**, but he still will be distracted and knows it could be dangerous **(C)**.

Dellmar decided to pull over and check his calls and texts **(D)**. His friends were getting together and they were trying to reach him so he could come over right from work instead of driving home first. Oh boy! He was glad it was not a family emergency but upset that his friends tried to reach him when they all agreed not to call or text when they knew one of them was driving **(I)**.

Dellmar decided to go home **(D)**. He was tired and stressed. He told his parents that he pulled over to answer a call/texts because he thought it was an emergency. They were proud of him for making such a good and safe choice **(I)**. His dad told him, "Dellmar, you made a good decision and you can drive yourself to work from now on!" **(E)**

3. Use **Worksheet 7.10 Grades 9–12 Responsible Decision-Making Template** to play, "What would you do?"
   a. While at the mall with friends, Adrien sees something she really wants but doesn't have any money. The salesclerk is busy, and her friend says, "Quick, put it in your backpack. No one will ever know!" Adrien knows taking the item would be stealing, which is wrong, but she really wants it. If you were Adrien, what would you do?
   b. Jiel and Miguel are at the lake with Miguel's parents and there are no lifeguards. Jiel is a good but not great swimmer. Jiel knows the family rule: never swim where there are no lifeguards. Miguel says, "Let's see who can swim out to the middle the fastest!" If you were Jiel, what would you do? (Michigan Model for Health, 2016)
   c. Farlie's health project is due today. He does not have a good reason why it is not finished but knows if he gives the teacher a good reason, she will give him more time. Your friend says, "Tell the teacher the Internet went down or the printer was out of ink and see if she accepts the excuse." Farlie knows lying is wrong but doesn't want a bad grade and needs more time. If you were Farlie, what would you do?

4. Read the practice prompt then ask the students the re-enforcement questions.

Practice Prompt: Rafaela

Rafaela is a new driver and she is excited because her mom asked her to go pick up a pizza, fries, and rolls for supper. She was really hungry and eager to take the ride.

The ride was uneventful. There was little traffic and no wait at the takeout window. She put the takeout next to her, on the passenger side. All is going well!

The problems started on the way home. The pizza box moved around as she stopped and started. The smell was driving her crazy! She was really hungry and thought she could take a bite out of one of the pizza slices while at the red light. It seemed like every billboard showed a food ad and made her even more hungry. The fries were really close, and she knows she could take a few and eat them while driving.

What was she thinking! Everything she learned about distracted driving was challenging her from the passenger's seat!

She started thinking about what she could do to get home safely. She could stop and put the package on the floor in the back. It wouldn't move around back there but she could still smell it and if she places it in the middle, she could still snag a few fries. It is not a good idea because she would still be distracted. She could stop and secure the take out in the trunk. She wouldn't have to keep moving the package when it shifts. If she doesn't see it, it will be easier to keep her mind on driving. She could also leave the package where it is and just concentrate on driving. She is almost home and she wouldn't have to stop in traffic.

She remembered what her mom used to tell her when she saw something she wanted, "Out of sight, out of mind, Rafaela!" That was it! She pulled into a parking lot and put the pizza, fries, and rolls in the trunk. She did take a few fries during the transfer and they were good! She got home safely and told her mother what she did.

Mom was pleased Rafaela made the good decision to put the food in the trunk. Rafaela didn't realize how distracted she would be just picking up takeout but now knows how to get food home safely, especially when hungry.

What are three ways Rafaela could drive home with the takeout and not be distracted while driving? (1.12.1)	■ Rafaela could prevent a manual distraction by putting the takeout in the trunk so it doesn't move around and she would not have to keep repositioning it. ■ Rafaela could prevent a cognitive distraction by putting the takeout in the trunk, so she is not smelling it and being reminded of how hungry she is. ■ Rafaela could prevent a visual distraction by moving the takeout to the trunk, so she won't see it and not look at the billboards because they all seemed to be advertising food and that only made Rafaela more hungry.

How did Rafaela <u>demonstrate</u> how to use the responsible decision-making model when making a decision about not being distracted while driving?

D – Define the decision to be made.

The problem is Rafaela is bringing home takeout and is very distracted by the package moving in the seat as she drives and her desire to snack on the takeout because she is very hungry.

E – Explore the options.
■ Rafaela could stop and put the package on the floor in the back.
■ Rafaela could stop and secure the takeout in the trunk.
■ Rafaela could leave the package where it is and just concentrate on driving.

C – Consider the consequences.
■ If Rafaela stops and puts the package on the floor in the back, it wouldn't move around but she could still smell it and if she places it in the middle, she could still snag a few fries. That is not a good idea because she would still be distracted.
■ If Rafaela stops and secures the takeout in the trunk, she will not have to keep moving the package when it shifts. If she does not see it, it will be easier to keep her mind on driving.
■ If Rafaela leaves the package where it is and just concentrates on driving, she is almost home, and she would not have to stop in traffic.

		I – Identify your values. Rafaela's values include honesty, trust, and family. **D – Decide and act.** Rafaela pulled into a parking lot and put the pizza, fries, and rolls in the trunk. **E – Evaluate the results.** Rafaela got home safely and told her mother what she did. Her mom was pleased Rafaela made the good decision to put the food in the trunk. Rafaela didn't realize how distracted she would be just picking up takeout but now she knows how to get food home safely, especially if she is hungry.
	SEL–Responsible Decision Making: Identifying the problem, analyzing the situation, solving the problem, evaluating the results, reflecting on the results, and demonstrating ethical responsibility.	See above.

Materials: *List the materials used to plan and implement the lesson, including formative assessments.*	**Worksheet 7.8 Preventing Distracted Driving** **Worksheet 7.9 Grades 9–12 Making Responsible Decisions** **Worksheet 7.10 Grades 9–12 Responsible Decision-Making Template**
Resources: *What resources were used to plan and implement the lesson?*	■ Federal Communications Commission ■ DMV.org

Differentiated instruction: *What modifications are being made for students with disabilities and English learners?*	Students work in groups, specifically designed to support students with disabilities or English learners.
Sample student products: *Provide exemplars of how other students successfully complete this assignment.*	Show previously completed worksheets.
Collaboration: *Are the students completing the activity individually, in pairs, in groups, etc.?*	Students work in groups of four in order to pair up or work as a group.

Teacher reflection: *What can I do to improve this lesson next time it is taught?*	Will vary.

References

Bronson, B. M. (2007). *Teen Health, Course 2*. New York: McGraw-Hill.

CASEL. (2019, September 21). *What is SEL?* Retrieved from CASEL https://casel.org/what-is-sel/

Centers for Disease Control and Prevention. (2020). *2019 Middle School YRBS ever drank alcohol*. Retrieved from Centers for Disease Control and Prevention https://nccd.cdc.gov/youthonline/App/Results.aspx?TT=B&OUT=0&SID=MS&QID=M26&LID=LL&YID=RY&LID2=&YID2=&COL=&ROW1=&ROW2=&HT=&LCT=&FS=&FR=&FG=&FA=&FI=&FP=&FSL=&FRL=&FGL=&FAL=&FIL=&FPL=&PV=&TST=&C1=&C2=&QP=&DP=&VA=CI&CS=Y&SYID=&EYID=&SC=&SO=

Centers for Disease Control and Prevention. (2020). *2019 Middle School YRBS Middle school students report drinking before age 11*. Retrieved from Centers for Disease Control and Prevention: https://nccd.cdc.gov/youthonline/App/Results.aspx?TT=B&OUT=0&SID=MS&QID=M27&LID=LL&YID=RY&LID2=&YID2=&COL=&ROW1=&ROW2=&HT=&LCT=&FS=&FR=&FG=&FA=&FI=&FP=&FSL=&FRL=&FGL=&FAL=&FIL=&FPL=&PV=&TST=&C1=&C2=&QP=&DP=&VA=CI&CS=Y&SYID=&EYID=&SC=&SO=

Centers for Disease Control and Prevention. (2020). *High School YRBS 2019 Results High school students who texted while driving*. Retrieved from Centers for Disease Control and Prevention https://nccd.cdc.gov/youthonline/App/Results.aspx?TT=B&OUT=0&SID=HS&QID=H11&LID=LL&YID=RY&LID2=&YID2=&COL=&ROW1=&ROW2=&HT=&LCT=&FS=&FR=&FG=&FA=&FI=&FP=&FSL=&FRL=&FGL=&FAL=&FIL=&FPL=&PV=&TST=&C1=&C2=&QP=&DP=&VA=CI&CS=Y&SYID=&EYID=&SC=&SO=

Chein, J., Albert, D., O'Brien, L., Uckert, K., & Steinberg, L. (2011). Peers increase adolescent risk taking by enhancing activity in the brain's reward circuitry. *Developmental Science, 14*(2), F1–F10.

Childcare. (2019). *Ways Child Care Providers Can Teach Young Children to Resolve Conflicts*. Retrieved from eXtension Alliance for Better Child Care https://childcare.extension.org/ways-child-care-providers-can-teach-young-children-to-resolve-conflicts/

Cohn-Vargas, B. (2020). *Helping Students Through a Period of Grief*. Retrieved from George Lucas Educational Foundation, Edutopia: https://www.edutopia.org/article/helping-students-through-period-grief

Collaborative for Academic and Social Emotional Learning. (2020). *CASEL Competencies*. Retrieved from CASEL https://casel.org/wp-content/uploads/2019/12/CASEL-Competencies.pdf

Collaborative for Academic Social Emotional Learning. (2020). *www.casel.org/.../08/Sample-Teaching-Activities-to-Support-Core-Competencies-8-20-17.pdf*. Retrieved from CASEL.org https://casel.org/wp-content/uploads/2017/08/Sample-Teaching-Activities-to-Support-Core-Competencies-8-20-17.pdf

Connolly, M. (2020). *Skills-Based Health Education, Second Edition*. Burlington, MA: Jones and Bartlett.

Federal Communications Commission. (2020). *The Dangers of Distracted Driving*. Retrieved from Federal Communications Commission https://www.fcc.gov/consumers/guides/dangers-texting-while-driving

Frey, N., Fisher, D., & Smith, D. (2019). *All learning is social and emotional: Helping students develop essential skills for the classroom and beyond*. Alexandria: ASCD.

Hanway, S. M. (2017). *Injuries and Investigated Deaths Associated with Playground Equipment, 2009-2014*. Bethesda, M.D.: U.S. Consumer Product Safety Commission. Retrieved from https://www.cpsc.gov/s3fs-public/Injuries%20and%20Investigated%20Deaths%20Associated%20with%20Playground%20Equipment%202009%20to%202014_1.pdf?29GwYlhQ6fUwXskAQxLoGaHaE8aHZSsY

Hurley, K. (2018). *5 Strategies to Help Kids Resolve Conflict*. Retrieved from PBS for Parents https://www.pbs.org/parents/thrive/5-strategies-to-help-kids-resolve-conflict

John W. Gardner Center. (2007). *Youth Engaged in Leadership and Learning YELL: A Handbook for Program, Staff, Teachers, and Community Leaders*. California: John W. Gardner Center for Youth and Their Communities. Retrieved from file:///C:/Users/Mary's%20Surface%20Pro%206/OneDrive/Desktop/YELL%20Handbook.pdf

Joint Committee on National Health Education Standards. (2007). *National Health Education Standards, Second Edition*. American Cancer Society.

Kay, J. (2020). *The D.E.C.I.D.E. Model, A Tool For Teaching Students How To Make Healthy Decisions*. Retrieved from Project School Wellness https://www.projectschoolwellness.com/the-d-e-c-i-d-e-model-a-tool-for-teaching-students-how-to-making-healthy-decisions/

KidsHealth from Nemours. (2020). *Playground Safety*. Retrieved from KidsHealth from Nemours: https://kidshealth.org/en/parents/playground.html?ref=search

KidsMatter, Learning to Resolve Conflict. (2011). *How Children Learn to Resolve Conflict*. Retrieved from KidsMatter www.kidsmatter.edu.au/resources/information-resources

Krueger, K. R., Wilson, R. S., Kamenetsky, J. M., Barnes, L. L., Bienias, J. L., & Bennett, D. A. (2009). Social engagement and cognitive function in old age. *Experimental Aging Research, 35*(1), 45–60.

Lynch, A. E. (2012). *Choosing Health*. San Francisco: Pearson Education.

Meeks, L. H. (2020). *Comprehensive School Health Education, Ninth Edition*. New York: McGraw Hill.

Mendler, D. A. (2013). *Teaching Your Students How to Have a Conversation*. Retrieved from George Lucas Educational Foundation, Edutopia https://www.edutopia.org/blog/teaching-your-students-conversation-allen-mendler

Michigan Model for Health. (2013). *Michigan Model for Health, High School Edition, Skills for Health and Life*. Mt. Pleasant, Michigan: Michigan Model for Health Clearninghouse.

Michigan Model for Health. (2016). Lesson 9 Finding Ways to Resolve Conflict. *Michigan Model for Health, Grade 6 Curriculum*. Holt, Michigan, United States: Michigan Model for Health Clearinghouse.

Michigan Model for Health. (2016). *Michigan Model for Health, Alcohol, Tobacco, and Other Drugs, Grade 1, Lesson 1*. Holt, Michigan: Michigan Model for Health Clearinghouse.

Michigan Model for Health. (2016). *Michigan Model for Health, Grade 5*. Holt, Michigan: Michigan Model for Health Clearinghouse.

Michigan Model for Health. (2016). *Michigan Model for Health, Grade 6*. Holt, Michigan: Michigan Model for Health Clearinghouse.

Michigan Model for Health. (2016). *Safe and Sound for Life, Middle School*. Michigan Model for Health Clearinghouse.

Michigan Model for Health. (2016). *Stay Drug Free for a Successful Tomorrow, Lesson 7*. Michigan Model for Health Clearinghouse.

Michigan Model for Health. (2019). *Michigan Model for Health, Grade 2*. Holt, MI: Michigan Model for Health Clearinghouse.

Michigan Model for Health. (2019). *Michigan Model for Health, Kindergarten*. Holt, MI: Michigan Model for Health Clearinghouse.

Michigan Model for Health Clearinghouse. (2016). Lesson 9, Finding Ways to Resolve Conflicts. *Michigan Model for Health, Grade 6 Curriculum*. Michigan, United States: Michigan Model for Health Clearinghouse.

Michigan Model for Health Clearinghouse. (2016). *Michigan Model for Health, Grade 1, Lesson 7*. Holt, Michigan: Michigan Model for Health Clearinghouse.

Minnesota Department of Education. (2019). *SEL Implementation Guidance, Responsible Decision Making*. Retrieved from Minnesota Department of Education: https://education.mn .gov/mdeprod/groups/communications/documents/hidden content/bwrl/mdcz/~edisp/mde073493.pdf

National Institute on Drug Abuse. (2019). *Vaping of marijuana on the rise among teens*. Retrieved from National Institute of Drug Abuse https://www.drugabuse.gov/news-events/news releases/2019/12/vaping-of-marijuana-on-the-rise-among -teens

National Institute of Drug Abuse. (2020). *Marijuana*. Retrieved from NIDA for Teens: https://teens.drugabuse.gov/drug-facts /marijuana#:~:text=Marijuana%20use%20has%20been %20linked%20with%20depression%20and,people%20 with%20a%20genetic%20risk%20for%20developing%20 schizophrenia

National Safety Council. (2020). *How Many Teen Passengers Can Safely Ride with New Drivers?* Retrieved from National Safety Council https://www.nsc.org/driveithome/teen-driver-risks /passengers

National Safety Council. (2020). *Inexperience is the Leading Cause of Teen Crashes*. Retrieved from National Safety Council https:// www.nsc.org/driveithome/teen-driver-risks/inexperience

NIDA, National Institutes of Health. (2013). *Marijuana Facts for Teens*. U.S. Department of Health and Human Services. Retrieved from file:///C:/Users/Mary's%20Surface%20Pro %206/OneDrive/Jones%20and%20Bartlett-Teaching %20SEL/Chapter%206-Teaching%20Relationship%20Skills /NIDA%20teens_brochure_2013.pdf

Office on Women's Health, Office of the Assistant Secretary for Health, Human Services. (2015). *Healthy Relationships*. Retrieved from Girls Health: https://www.girlshealth.gov /relationships/healthy/index.html

Packer, A. J. (2017). *Oh, the Drama! 11 Scenarios to Help Teens Work Through Sticky Social Situations*. Retrieved from Free Spirit Publishing Blog https://freespiritpublishingblog.com /2017/04/25/oh-the-drama-11-scenarios-to-help-teens-work -through-sticky-social-situations/#:~:text=Oh%2C%20 the%20Drama%21%2011%20Scenarios%20to%20 Help%20Teens,you%20drooling%20in%20your%20sleep .%20More%20items...%20

Page, Page, T. S. (2015). *Promoting Health and Emotional Well-Being in Your Classroom*. Burlington, MA: Jones and Bartlett.

Ponta, E. (2020). *The Positive Side of Peer Pressure*. Retrieved from Center for Parent & Teen Communication https:// parentandteen.com/positive-peer-pressure/

Robert Wood Johnson Foundation. (2015). *New Research: Children With Strong Social Skills in Kindergarten More Likely to Thrive as Adults*. Retrieved from Robert Wood Johnson Foundation https://www.rwjf.org/en/library/articles-and-news/2015/07 /new-research--children-with-strong-social-skills-in -kindergarten.html

Schneiderman, K. (2013). *The trouble with texting*. Retrieved from *Psychology Today* https://www.psychologytoday.com/us/blog /the-novel-perspective/201301/the-trouble-texting

Scholastic. (2015). *The Science of Decision Making and Peer Pressure*. Retrieved from Scholastic http://headsup.scholastic .com/teachers/lesson-the-science-of-decision-making-and -peer-pressure#:~:text=%22The%20Science%20of%20 Decision%20Making%20and%20Peer%20Pressure%22 ,%20%20%20%20%20%20

Scholastic. (2020). *Peer Pressure: Its Influence on Teens and Decision Making*. Retrieved from Scholastic http://headsup.scholastic .com/students/peer-pressure-its-influence-on-teens-and -decision-making

Scholastic and the Scientists of the National Institute of Drug Abuse. (2020). *Teens and Decision Making: What Brain Science Reveals*. Retrieved from Heads Up, Real News About Drugs and Your Body: http://headsup.scholastic.com /students/teens-and-decision-making-what-brain-science -reveals

Suler, J. (2010). Interpersonal guidelines for texting. *International Journal of Applied Psychoanalytic Studies, 7*(4), 358–361.

Telljohann, S. K. (2009). *Health Education, Elementary and Middle School Applications*. New York: McGraw-Hill.

The Nemours Foundation/KidsHealth. (2016). *Grades 3 to 5 • Personal Health Series, Conflict Resolution*. Retrieved from KidsHealth in the Classroom: https://kidshealth.org /classroom/3to5/personal/growing/conflict_resolution.pdf

Transforming Education. (2020). *Introduction to Social Awareness*. Retrieved from Transforming Education https://www .transformingeducation.org/wp-content/uploads/2019/04 /Introduction-to-Social-Awareness.pdf

Victoria Rideout, M. M. (2018). *Social Media, Social Life: Teens Reveal Their Experiences*. Retrieved from www.commonsense .org: https://www.commonsensemedia.org/sites/default/files /uploads/research/2018_cs_socialmediasociallife_executive summary-final-release_3_lowres.pdf

Wilson, D. C. (2017). *4 Proven Strategies for Teaching Empathy*. Retrieved from George Lucas Educational Foundation, Edutopia https://www.edutopia.org/article/4-proven-strategies -teaching-empathy-donna-wilson-marcus-conyers

Wordnet by Princeton University, Database: 3.0. (2020). *Ethics*. Retrieved from English Dictionary http://Wordnet.princeton .edu

Wordnet by Princeton University, Database:3.0. (2020). *Reflect*. Retrieved from Wordnet.princeton.edu: http://Wordnet .princeton.edu

Wordnet by Princeton University, Database: 3.0. (2020). *Solve*. Retrieved from Wordnet.princeton.edu: http://Wordnet .princeton.edu

Youth.gov. (2020). *Characteristics of Healthy and Unhealthy Relationships*. Retrieved from Youth.gov: https://youth.gov /youth-topics/teen-dating-violence/characteristics

Chapter 7—Appendix A

Responsible Decision Making: Scope, Sequence, Content, SEL Competency/Subcompetencies

<u>Note:</u> This page is organized by grade span, Standard 1, skill standards, the HECAT content areas, and SEL Competency/Subcompetencies.

The HECAT content areas include: AOD – Alcohol and Other Drugs; HE – Healthy Eating; MEH – Mental/Emotional Health; PHW – Personal Health and Wellness; PA – Physical Activity; S – Safety; SH – Sexual Health; T – Tobacco; V – Violence Prevention

Making Constructive Choices

Grade span	Standard 1	Skill	HECAT Content Areas and Specific Content	SEL Competency and Subcompetencies
PreK–2	1.2.1 <u>Recognize</u> that healthy behaviors, *such as taking medicine safely*, affect personal health.	**D – Define the decision to be made;** (5.2.1 Identify situations when a health-related decision is needed—NHES; identify the problem—CASEL) **E – Explore the Options;** (5.2.2 Differentiate between situations when a health-related decision can be made individually or when assistance is needed—NHES; Analyze the situation—CASEL) **C – Consider the consequences** **I – Identify your values;** (ethical responsibility—CASEL) **D – Decide and act;** (solving the problem—CASEL) **E – Evaluate the results;** (Evaluate, Reflect—CASEL)	Safety: Taking medicine safely.	Responsible Decision Making ■ Identifying problems ■ Analyzing situations ■ Solving problems ■ Evaluating ■ Reflecting ■ Ethical responsibility
3–5	1.5.2 Identify examples of emotional, intellectual, physical, and social health *when making a responsible decision about getting together with friends.*	**D – Define the decision to be made;** (5.2.1 Identify situations when a health-related decision is needed—NHES; identify the problem—CASEL)	Mental/Emotional Health – Making responsible decisions about getting together with friends.	Responsible Decision Making ■ Identifying problems ■ Analyzing situations ■ Solving problems ■ Evaluating ■ Reflecting ■ Ethical Responsibility

(continues)

Making Constructive Choices (continued)

Grade span	Standard 1	Skill	HECAT Content Areas and Specific Content	SEL Competency and Subcompetencies
		E – Explore the Options; (5.2.2 Differentiate between situations when a health-related decision can be made individually or when assistance is needed—NHES; Analyze the situation—CASEL)		
		C – Consider the consequences		
		I – Identify your values; (ethical responsibility—CASEL)		
		D – Decide and act; (solving the problem—CASEL		
		E – Evaluate the results; (evaluate, reflect—CASEL)		
6 8	1.8.7 Describe the benefits of and barriers to practicing healthy behaviors such as *making a healthy decision about alcohol when influenced by peers.*	**D – Define the decision to be made;** (5.2.1 Identify situations when a health-related decision is needed—NHES; identify the problem—CASEL)	Alcohol and Other Drugs–Alcohol	Responsible Decision Making ■ Identifying problems ■ Analyzing situations ■ Solving problems ■ Evaluating ■ Reflecting ■ Ethical Responsibility
		E – Explore the Options; (5.2.2 Differentiate between situations when a health-related decision can be made individually or when assistance is needed—NHES; Analyze the situation—CASEL)		
		C – Consider the consequences		
		I – Identify your values; (Ethical responsibility—CASEL)		
		D – Decide and act; (solving the problem—CASEL		
		E – Evaluate the results; (evaluate, reflect—CASEL)		

9–12	1.12.1 Predict how healthy behaviors, *such as not driving distracted*, affect health status.	**D – Define the decision to be made;** (5.2.1 Identify situations when a health-related decision is needed—NHES; identify the problem—CASEL)	Safety - Distracted driving	Responsible Decision Making
		E – Explore the Options; (5.2.2 Differentiate between situations when a health-related decision can be made individually or when assistance is needed—NHES; Analyze the situation—CASEL)		■ Identifying problems ■ Analyzing situations ■ Solving problems ■ Evaluating ■ Reflecting ■ Ethical Responsibility
		C – Consider the consequences		
		I – Identify your values; (ethical responsibility—CASEL)		
		D – Decide and act; (solving the problem—CASEL		
		E – Evaluate the results; (evaluate, reflect—CASEL)		

Glossary

A

appreciating diversity The positive acknowledgement of the attributes of people from different races and cultures and how valuable their contributions to society are.

authentic assessment Occurs when students demonstrate their proficiency of the content, skill, and SEL competency. (Connolly, 2018, p. 99)

B

backwards design A planning strategy that begins with data assessment, a selection of performance indicators and SEL competency to reduce the risk factor, selection of assessment, and planning of instruction. (Connolly, 2018, p. 48)

C

communication Sharing ideas, thoughts, and opinions in writing, through speaking, or using some other nonverbal communication method.

E

emotions Human feelings, including love, happiness, anger, and fear, which also often involves a physical reaction.

empathy Imagining the feelings experienced by another even when not personally experienced.

ethical responsibility The obligation to behave according to the principles of right and wrong that are accepted by an individual or social group.

ethical standards Principles of right and wrong that are accepted by an individual or social group. (Wordnet by Princeton University, Database: 3.0, 2020)

Every Student Succeeds Act A federal law that is the reauthorization of the Elementary and Secondary Education Act. In 2012, states developed rigorous and comprehensive plans to close achievement gaps, increase equity, improve the quality of instruction, and increase student outcomes. (US Department of Education, 2019)

F

fixed mindset A mindset in which a person believes their basic qualities, including intelligence and talent, are (fixed) unchanging and unchangeable. They are full of doubt and do not believe effort has a role in learning something new. (Frey, Fisher, & Smith, 2019, pp. 30–31)

G

goal setting Aspiring to achieve a goal and then creating milestones to accomplish the goal(s) including a timeline.

growth mindset A mindset in which a person believes their innate abilities are improved with effort, hard work, and dedication. They see failure as something to overcome, not a reflection of their innate ability. (Frey, Fisher, & Smith, 2019, pp. 30–31)

I

impulse control The ability to resist a strong, sudden urge.

infused performance indicators NHES performance indicators that have content added that generates assessment and instruction.

N

neuroplasticity (neuroplastic response) The ability of the brain's synapses, neuron, dendrites, and myelin-coated axons to change their properties in response to usage. (McTighe & Judy Willis, 2019, p. 166)

neuroscience The scientific discipline that encompasses nervous tissue, anatomy, biochemistry (molecular biology of nerves), physiology. Neuroscience specifically embraces the scientific disciplines and their connection to learning and human behavior.

O

organizational skills The capability to use knowledge, skills, and procedures to complete a project.

P

pedagogy The educational approach that includes teaching and learning of science, art, and culture.

performance task An authentic assessment that consists of prompts, the rubric, and back-up materials and resources the students need to be successful on the summative assessment. (Connolly, 2018, p. 99)

personal strengths A talent or positive quality of a person.

perspective-taking A person's capability of seeing a situation from several different points of view.

R

relationship building The development of a healthy relationship based on honesty, trust, respect, communication, personal freedom, enjoyment of common interests and activities, kindness, and mutual affection. (Lynch, 2012, p. 198)

respect for others Holding others in high esteem and treating them in a sensitive manner.

S

self-awareness The ability to accurately recognize one's own emotions, thoughts, and values and how they influence behavior. The ability to accurately assess one's strengths and limitations, with a well-grounded sense of confidence, optimism, and a "growth mindset." (CASEL, 2019)

self-confidence The ability to depend on one's own strength, talent, and ability.

self-discipline A person's capacity to control his/her behavior.

self-efficacy The ability to take action, complete a task, and attain goals. (Frey, Fisher, & Smith, 2019)

self-motivation The ability to encourage one's self to accomplish a task.

self-perception The complete understanding that a person has of who they are as a whole (physically, emotionally, mentally, and psychologically).

social awareness The ability to take the perspective of another person and empathize including those from diverse backgrounds and cultures. The ability to understand social and ethical norms for behavior and to recognize family, school, and community resources and supports. (CASEL, 2019)

social emotional learning (SEL) The process through which children and adults understand and manage emotions, set and achieve positive goals, feel and show empathy for others, establish and maintain positive relationships, and make responsible decisions. (CASEL, 2019)

social engagement The maintenance of social connections and participation in social activities. (Krueger, 2009)

stress management A person's ability to identify stress and use healthy coping strategies to reduce it.

T

teamwork More than one person working together to achieve the same collective goal.

W

Whole School, Whole Community, Whole Child (WSCC) Model A framework, designed by the Centers for Disease Control and Prevention (CDC) and the Association for Supervision and Curriculum Development (ASCD) for addressing health in schools. The 10 components (health education, physical education/physical activity, nutrition environment and services, social and emotional school climate, physical environment, health services, counseling, psychological and social services, employee wellness, community involvement, and family engagement) along with school policy, procedures, and practice and community support, all work together to enhance the health of students. (Centers for Disease Control and Prevention, CDC Healthy Schools, 2020)

References

Centers for Disease Control and Prevention. (2020). *CDC Healthy Schools*. Retrieved from https://www.cdc.gov/healthyschools/index.htm

Collaborative for Academic, Social and Emotional Learning. (2020). *What is SEL?* Retrieved from CASEL.org: https://casel.org/what-is-sel/CASEL, 2019

Connolly, M. (2018). *Skills-based health education* (2nd ed.) Burlington: Jones and Bartlett.

Frey, N., Fisher, D., & Smith, D. (2019). *All learning is social and emotional; helping students develop essential skills for the classroom and beyond*. Alexandria: ASCD.

Krueger, K. R., Wilson, R. S., Kanenetsky, J. M., Barnes, L. L., Bienias, J. L., & Bennett, D. A. (2009). Social engagement and cognitive function in old age. *Experimental Aging Research*, 35(1), 45–60.

Lynch, A. E. (2012). *Choosing Health*. San Francisco: Pearson Education.

McTighe, J., & Judy Willis, M. (2019). *Upgrade your teaching, understanding by design meets neuroscience*. Alexandria: ASCD.

Understood. (2020). *The 3 types of self-control*. Retrieved from Understood https://www.understood.org/en/friends-feelings/common-challenges/self-control/the-3-types-of-self-control?_ul=1*q4cwmp*domain_userid*YW1wLUdnNFdocGNScm9xUmlvQ1dXNmVRRVE

Wordnet by Princeton University, Database 3:0. (2020). *Analyze*. Retrieved from http://Wordnet.princeton.edu

Your Dictionary. (2020). Retrieved from Your Dictionary https://www.yourdictionary.com/goal-setting

Index

Note: Page numbers followed by *f* or *t* represent figures or tables respectively.

A

Academic performance, 2
Accurate self-perception/recognizing
 strengths
  bicycle safety, 55–58, 55*t*–57*t*
  interests and strengths, 60–62,
   60*t*–62*t*
  sexually transmitted infections (STIs),
   62–64, 62*t*–64*t*
  sun safety, 58–60, 58*t*, 59*f*
Active listening skills, 211*f*
Alcohol, 267–271, 267*t*–268*t*, 270*t*–271*t*
Appreciating diversity, 166
Art/creative project, 32
ASCD. *See* Association for Supervision
 and Curriculum Development
 (ASCD)
Association for Supervision and
 Curriculum Development
 (ASCD), 13
Authentic assessment, 21, 22*t*

B

Backwards design, 23, 27, 27*f*
 assessment, 28
 data analysis, 27–28
 example of, 29–31
 instruction, 28–29
 standards/SEL selection, 28
 youth risk behavior data, 29*t*
Bicycle safety, 55–58, 55*t*–57*t*
Body mass index, 51*t*
Bullying, effects of, 45–48, 45*t*–46*t*, 49*t*

C

CASEL. *See* Collaborative for Academic,
 Social, and Emotional Learning
 (CASEL)
CASEL competencies, 2, 7*f*, 8*t*–10*t*
CASEL framework, 36*f*
CDC. *See* Centers for Disease Control
 and Prevention (CDC)

Centers for Disease Control and
 Prevention (CDC), 13, 27
Cognitive empathy, 167
Cognitive regulation, 11
Cognitive regulation skill development,
 17
Collaborative for Academic, Social, and
 Emotional Learning (CASEL), 2
Communication, 204
Conversation skills, 213–216, 214*t*, 216*t*
Cultural diversity, 183
Cycle of life, 211*f*

D

DECIDE Model, 255*t*–258*t*, 260, 264,
 273
Demonstrate respect, 188*t*
Dental health, 77–78, 77*t*, 79*t*
Dimensions of health, 168–169, 168*f*
Discrimination
 effects on components of health, 192,
  193*t*
 types of, 192*t*
Distracted driving, 271–275, 272*t*

E

Emotional intelligence, 3
Emotional processes, 11–12
Emotions, 35
Empathy, 164, 166–167
 coping with bullying, 169–173,
  170*t*–173*t*
 for friend and accessing community
  resources, 167–169, 167*t*–170*t*
 for LGBTQ middle school students,
  173–176, 173*t*–176*t*
 physical activity, 176–179, 177*t*, 179*t*
ESSA. *See* Every Student Succeeds Act
 (ESSA)
Ethical responsibility, 254, 255
Ethical standards, 255
Ethics, definition of, 254
Every Student Succeeds Act (ESSA), 1–2

Expressing appreciation and respect-
 friendship, 207–209, 207*t*, 210*t*

F

Face-to-face communication
 benefits of, 274*t*–275*t*
Family influences emotions, 39–41, 40*t*,
 41*f*, 42*t*–43*t*
Fixed mindset, 19, 35, 86
 vs. growth mindset, 92*f*
Formative assessment, 22–23, 23*t*–26*t*
 tools, 23, 23*t*–26*t*

G

Gay Straight Alliance (GSA), 175
Goal setting, 111
 eat breakfast, 148–152, 149*t*, 151*t*
 eat healthy and increase physical
  activity, 142–145, 142*t*–143*t*,
  143*f*, 144*t*–145*t*
 steps of, 143*f*
 use myplate to eat healthy, 145–148,
  145*t*–146*t*, 146*f*, 147*t*, 148*t*
Growth mindset, 13, 35, 86
 feedback in helping students, 87–88
 vs. fixed mindset, 92*f*
 making friends, 91–93, 92*f*, 92*t*, 97*t*
 mindset, 97–100, 97*t*–100*t*
 pedagogical strategies to, 88–89
 to quit marijuana, 93–97, 94*t*–96*t*
 self-confidence and self-efficacy, 88–89
 and self-efficacy, 55
 working in group, 89–91, 89*t*, 91*t*
GSA. *See* Gay Straight Alliance (GSA)

H

Healthy dating relationship,
 characteristics of, 229
Healthy weight maintenance, 52*t*, 54*t*
HEAR method of effective listening, 167*f*

I

Impulse control, 111
    controlling/not controlling impulses,
        118*t*
    effect of, 113–117, 113*t*–114*t*,
        116*t*–117*t*
    self-discipline, and self-motivation,
        117–119, 117*t*–118*t*, 120*t*
    in sexual relationships, 123–125,
        123*t*–124*t*, 124*f*, 126*t*
    and texting, 119–123, 120*t*–123*t*
Infused performance indicators, 19

L

LGBTQ (Lesbian, gay, bisexual,
    transsexual, and queer/
    questioning) middle school
    students, 173–176, 173*t*–176*t*

M

Mastery experiences, 76
Medicine safety rules, 260

N

National Health Education Standards
    (NHES), 2, 3*t*–10*t*, 21, 39,
    255*t*–257*t*
National Highway Traffic Safety
    Administration (NHTSA), 272
Neuro-friendly teaching practices, 20
Neuroplasticity, 20
Neuroplastic response, 19–20
Neuroscience, 19–21, 21*t*
NHES. *See* National Health Education
    Standards (NHES)
NHTSA. *See* National Highway Traffic
    Safety Administration (NHTSA)

O

Organizational skills, 109

P

Pedagogical practices, 19–21, 21*t*
    assessment, 21
        authentic, 21, 22*t*
        formative, 22–23, 23*t*–26*t*
        performance task, 21
        summative, 23, 26–27

backwards design, 27, 27*f*
    assessment, 28
    data analysis, 27–28
    example of, 29–31
    instruction, 28–29
    standards/SEL selection, 28
    youth risk behavior data, 29*t*
developmental considerations, 17–19,
    18*f*, 18*t*–19*t*
skills-based health/social emotional
    learning, 19–21, 21*t*
    delivery of, 30–33
    effective teaching strategies, 31–33
    and neuroscience, 19–21, 21*t*
    student brain learn by, 21*t*
Pedagogy, 20
Performance task, 21
Personal strengths, 69
Perspective-taking, 166–167
    coping with bullying, 169–173,
        170*t*–173*t*
    for friend and accessing community
        resources, 167–169, 167*t*–170*t*
    for LGBTQ middle school students,
        173–176, 173*t*–176*t*
    physical activity, 176–179, 177*t*, 179*t*
Plutchik's Wheel of Emotion, 37, 37*f*
Positive emotional state, 77
Practicing yoga
    belly (balloon) breathing, 127*f*
    cat pose, 131*f*
    child's pose, 132*f*
    cow pose, 131*f*
    downward-facing dog, 128*f*
    easy pose, 132*f*
    four square breathing, 135*f*
    hero pose, 132*f*
    horse stance, 128*f*
    table pose, 128*f*
PreK-2 Responsible Decision Making,
    262*t*

Q

Quit marijuana. growth mindset to,
    93–97, 94*t*–96*t*

R

Recognizing/identifying emotions, 39–54
    body image, 48, 50–54, 50*t*–52*t*, 51*f*,
        54*t*
    bullying, effects of, 45–48, 45*t*–46*t*,
        49*t*
    family influences emotions, 39–41,
        40*t*, 41*f*, 42*t*–43*t*
    reducing screen time, 41, 43–45,
        43*t*–45*t*

Refusal skills, 232, 233
    to avoid risks of driving with newly
        licensed driver, 240–243,
        241*t*–243*t*
    to avoid risks of, pressured to smoke
        marijuana, 238–240, 238*t*, 240*t*
    to reject being pressured to be bully,
        235–237, 235*t*, 237*t*
Relationship building, 205
Relationship skills, 203
    alignment of, 204, 205*t*
    competency on, 204
    establishing and maintaining healthy
        and rewarding relationships/
        communication
        conversation skills, 213–216, 214*t*,
            216*t*
        coping with grief, 209–212, 210*t*,
            211*f*, 213*t*
        expressing appreciation and respect-
            friendship, 207–209, 207*t*, 210*t*
        value of face-to-face conversation
            with friend rather than texting,
            217–219, 217*t*, 219*t*
    negotiating conflict constructively/
        seeking and offering help,
        219–220
        dating relationship, resolving
            conflict in, 228–231, 229*t*, 231*t*
        resolving conflict, 220–228, 220*t*,
            222*t*, 223*t*, 225*t*–228*t*
    organization, 206
    resisting inappropriate social pressure/
        seeking and offering help when
        needed, 231–232
        preventing injuries on playground,
            232–235, 232*t*, 234*t*
        refusal skills to avoid risks of driving
            with newly licensed driver,
            240–243, 241*t*–243*t*
        refusal skills to avoid risks of,
            pressured to smoke marijuana,
            238–240, 238*t*, 240*t*
        refusal skills to reject being
            pressured to be bully, 235–237,
            235*t*, 237*t*
    skills-based lesson infrastructure,
        205–206
    skills-based lesson plan, 204–205
    strategies to, develop healthy
        relationships, 206–207
    by subcompetency, 206*t*
    unit plan, 204
Respect for others, 165
Responsible decision-making skills, 254*f*
    benefits of and barriers to, 254*f*
    DECIDE, 255*t*–258*t*
    making constructive choices, 259
        alcohol, 267–271, 267*t*–268*t*,
            270*t*–271*t*
        distracted driving, 271–275, 272*t*

making responsible decisions about getting together with friends, 263–267, 263t, 265t–267t
taking medicine safely, 259–262, 259t–260t, 261f, 262t–263t
NHES, 255t–257t
organization, 258–259
skills-based lesson infrastructure, 258
skills-based lesson plan, 258
by subcompetencies, 259t
unit plan, 258
RULER model, 13

S

SAFE plan (Sequenced, Active forms of learning, Focused time for skill development, and has Explicit learning goals), 18t–19t
School Connectedness, 193f
Self-awareness, 35
  accurate self-perception/recognizing strengths
    bicycle safety, 55–58, 55t–57t
    interests and strengths, 60–62, 60t–62t
    sexually transmitted infections (STIs), 62–64, 62t–64t
    sun safety, 58–60, 58t, 59f
  analyzing influences, sample lesson plan for, 101–104
  CASEL framework, 36f
  growth mindset, 86
    feedback in helping students, 87–88
    making friends, 91–93, 92f, 92t, 97t
    mindset, 97–100, 97t–100t
    pedagogical strategies to, 88–89
    to quit marijuana, 93–97, 94t–96t
    self-confidence and self-efficacy, 88–89
    working in group, 89–91, 89t, 91t
  organization, 39
  Plutchik's Wheel of Emotion, 37, 37f
  recognizing/identifying emotions, 39–54
    body image, 48, 50–54, 50t–52t, 51f, 54t
    bullying, effects of, 45–48, 45t–46t, 49t
    family influences emotions, 39–41, 40t, 41f, 42t–43t
    reducing screen time, 41, 43–45, 43t–45t
  self-confidence/recognizing strengths, 65
    body image, 72–76, 73t–76t
    reducing screen time, with friends, 71–72, 71t, 73t

responding to emergency, 69–71, 69t, 70t
    spread of communicable disease, prevention of, 65–69, 66t–68t
  self-efficacy, 76–77
    CPR, 84–86, 84t–85t, 87t
    dental health, 77–78, 77t, 79t
    and growth mindset, 55
    influence of advertising on vaping, 80–84, 82t–84t
    mastery experiences, 76
    positive emotional state, 77
    transition to middle school, 78–80, 79t, 81t
    verbal persuasion, 77
    vicarious experiences, 76–77
  skills-based lesson infrastructure, 39
  skills-based lesson plan, 39
  Standard 2 of the National Health Education Standards, 38t
  by subcompetency, 39t
  unit plan, 38
Self-check, 65
Self-confidence, 35, 65, 88–89
  body image, 72–76, 73t–76t
  reducing screen time, with friends, 71–72, 71t, 73t
  responding to emergency, 69–71, 69t, 70t
  spread of communicable disease, prevention of, 65–69, 66t–68t
Self-discipline, 111, 117–119, 117t–118t, 120t
Self-efficacy, 35, 76–77, 88–89
  CPR, 84–86, 84t–85t, 87t
  dental health, 77–78, 77t, 79t
  and growth mindset, 55
  influence of advertising on vaping, 80–84, 82t–84t
  mastery experiences, 76
  positive emotional state, 77
  transition to middle school, 78–80, 79t, 81t
  verbal persuasion, 77
  vicarious experiences, 76–77
Self-esteem, 76
Self-management, 112
  alignment of, 112t
  competency on, 110f, 113t
  development of, 110t–111t
  goal setting
    eat breakfast, 148–152, 149t, 151t
    eat healthy and increase physical activity, 142–145, 142t–145t, 143f
    steps of, 143f
    use myplate to eat healthy, 145–148, 145t–148t, 146f
  impulse control, 111
    controlling/not controlling impulses, 118t

effect of, 113–117, 113t–114t, 116t–117t
  self-discipline, and self-motivation, 117–119, 117t–118t, 120t
  in sexual relationships, 123–125, 123t–124t, 124f, 126t
  and texting, 119–123, 120t–123t
  organization, 113
  skills-based lesson, 112–113
  skills-based unit, 112
  SMARTHR goal setting, 152–158, 152t, 154t
  stress management
    effects of anxiety, 133–137, 134t–137t, 135f
    mindful eating exercise, 137–141, 138t, 141t–142t
    practicing yoga, 125–129, 126t–127t, 127f–128f, 129t
    using stress reduction, 129–133, 129t–130t, 131f–132f, 133t
Self-motivation, 113, 117–119, 117t–118t, 120t
Self-perception, 35
Sequenced, Active forms of learning, Focused time for skill development, and has Explicit learning goals (SAFE), 18t–19t
Sexually transmitted infections (STIs), 62–64, 62t–64t
Skill practice, 31
Skills-based health education, 17, 18
Skills-based health/social emotional learning (SBH/SEL), 19–21, 21t
  delivery of, 30–33
  effective teaching strategies, 31–33
    art/creative project, 32
    book/story, 31
    discussions in, 31
    drawing, 32
    games, 33
    role play, 31
    skill practice, 31
    songs, 32–33
    teaching skills, 31–32, 31f
    tools and handouts, 32
    video, 32
    visual display, 32, 32f
    vocabulary, 32
    writing, 32
  implementation, 18t–19t
  summative assessment for, 23, 26–27
Social and interpersonal skills, 12, 12t
Social awareness, 163, 180, 203
  accepting differences, 183–191, 183t–184t, 186t–191t, 189f
  alignment of, 164, 165t
  appreciating diversity, 191–196, 191t–193t, 193f, 195t–196t
  competency on, 164f
  organization, 166

Social awareness (*cont.*)
  perspective-taking, empathy, and
    community resources, 166–167
  coping with bullying, 169–173,
    170*t*–173*t*
  for friend and accessing
    community resources, 167–169,
    167*t*–170*t*
  for LGBTQ middle school students,
    173–176, 173*t*–176*t*
  physical activity, 176–179, 177*t*,
    179*t*
  respecting differences, 180–183,
    180*t*–183*t*
  skills-based lesson infrastructure, 166
  skills-based lesson plan, 165
  by subcompetency, 166*t*
  unit plan, 165
Social emotional learning (SEL), 17, 18
  and academic performance, 2
  CASEL competencies, 2, 7*f*, 8*t*–10*t*
  curriculum, 2
  and Every Student Succeeds Act
    (ESSA), 1–2
  evolution of, 3
    collaborative for academic and,
      9–10
    Wallace Foundation, 10–13, 11*f*
    Yale Center for Emotional
      Intelligence, 13
  National Health Education Standards,
    2, 3*t*–7*t*

selection, 28
  Whole School, Whole Community,
    Whole Child Model, 13–15,
    14*t*, 15*f*
Social engagement, 205
SPAT method, 174, 175*t*
Spread of communicable disease,
    prevention of, 65–69, 66*t*–68*t*
STIs. *See* Sexually transmitted infections
    (STIs)
Stress management, 28
  effects of anxiety, 133–137, 134*t*–137*t*,
    135*f*
  mindful eating exercise, 137–141,
    138*t*, 141*t*–142*t*
  practicing yoga, 125–129, 126*t*–127*t*,
    127*f*–128*f*, 129*t*
  using stress reduction, 129–133,
    129*t*–130*t*, 131*f*–132*f*, 133*t*
Student Assistance Program (SAP), 240
Summative assessment, performance
    task, 26–27
Sun safety, 58–60, 58*t*, 59*f*

Taking medicine safely, 259–262,
    259*t*–260*t*, 261*f*, 262*t*–263*t*
Teaching skills, 31–32, 31*f*
Teamwork, 205

Value of face-to-face conversation
    with friend rather than texting,
    217–219, 217*t*, 219*t*
Verbal persuasion, 77
Vicarious experiences, 76–77
Virus *vs.* bacteria, 67*t*, 68*t*
Visual display, 32, 32*f*
Vocabulary, 32

W

Wallace Foundation, 10–13, 11*f*
  character, 13
  cognitive regulation, 11
  emotional processes, 11–12
  mindset, 13
  social and interpersonal skills, 12, 12*t*
Whole School, Whole Community,
    Whole Child Model, 13–15, 14*t*,
    15*f*
Word respect, meaning of, 188*t*

Y

Yale Center for Emotional Intelligence,
    13
Youth risk behavior data, 29*t*